T0314045

More than 230 videos are available for viewing on MediaCenter.Thieme.com!

Simply visit MediaCenter.thieme.com and, when prompted during the registration process, enter the code below to get started today.

5W65-6Q83-QJJ2-89PQ

	WINDOWS & MAC	**TABLET**
Recommended Browser(s)	Recent browser versions on all major platforms and any mobile operating system that supports HTML5 video playback. *All browsers should have JavaScript enabled.*	
Flash Player Plug-in	Flash Player 9 or higher. *For Mac users, ATI Rage 128 GPU doesn't support full-screen mode with hardware scaling.*	Tablet PCs with Android OS support Flash 10.1.
Recommended for optimal usage experience	Monitor resolutions: • Normal (4:3) 1024×768 or higher • Widescreen (16:9) 1280×720 or higher • Widescreen (16:10) 1440×900 or higher A high-speed internet connection (minimum 384 Kps) is suggested.	WiFi or cellular data connection is required.

Connect with us on social media

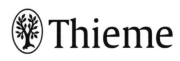

Clinical Breast Tomosynthesis

A Case-Based Approach to Screening and Diagnosis

Lonie R. Salkowski, MD, MS
Professor
Section of Breast Imaging
Department of Radiology
University of Wisconsin School of Medicine and Public Health
Madison, Wisconsin

Tanya W. Moseley, MD
Professor
Breast Imaging Section
Division of Diagnostic Imaging
The University of Texas M.D. Anderson Cancer Center
Houston, Texas

1,193 illustrations

Thieme
New York • Stuttgart • Delhi • Rio de Janeiro

Executive Editor: William Lamsback
Managing Editor: J. Owen Zurhellen IV
Director, Editorial Services: Mary Jo Casey
Editorial Assistant: Keith Palumbo
Production Editor: Sean Woznicki
International Production Director: Andreas Schabert
International Marketing Director: Fiona Henderson
International Sales Director: Louisa Turrell
Director of Sales, North America: Mike Roseman
Senior Vice President and Chief Operating Officer: Sarah Vanderbilt
President: Brian D. Scanlan

Library of Congress Cataloging-in-Publication Data

Names: Salkowski, Lonie, author. | Moseley, Tanya W., author.
Title: Clinical breast tomosynthesis : a case-based approach / Lonie R.
    Salkowski, Tanya W. Moseley.
Description: First edition. | New York : Thieme, [2017] | Includes
    bibliographical references and index.
Identifiers: LCCN 2016018936 (print) | LCCN 2016019459 (ebook) |
    ISBN 9781626232082 | ISBN 9781626232099 (eISBN) |
    ISBN 9781626232099
Subjects: | MESH: Mammography—methods | Breast
    Neoplasms—radiography | Tomography, X-Ray—methods |
    Imaging, Three-Dimensional—methods | Image
    Processing, Computer-Assisted—methods | Radiographic Image
    Enhancement—methods | Case Reports
Classification: LCC RG493.5.R33 (print) | LCC RG493.5.R33 (ebook) |
    NLM WP 815 | DDC 618.1/907572—dc23
LC record available at https://lccn.loc.gov/2016018936

© 2017 Thieme Medical Publishers, Inc.
Thieme Publishers New York
333 Seventh Avenue, New York, NY 10001 USA
+1 800 782 3488, customerservice@thieme.com

Thieme Publishers Stuttgart
Rüdigerstrasse 14, 70469 Stuttgart, Germany
+49 [0]711 8931 421, customerservice@thieme.de

Thieme Publishers Delhi
A-12, Second Floor, Sector-2, Noida-201301
Uttar Pradesh, India
+91 120 45 566 00, customerservice@thieme.in

Thieme Publishers Rio de Janeiro, Thieme Publicações Ltda.
Rua do Matoso 170
Tijuca, RJ CEP 20270-135
Rio de Janeiro
Brazil
+55 21 2563-9700

Cover design: Thieme Publishing Group
Typesetting by Thomson Digital, India

Printed in India by Replika Press Pvt. Ltd.   5 4 3 2 1

ISBN 978-1-62623-208-2

Also available as an e-book:
eISBN978-1-62623-209-9

Important note: Medicine is an ever-changing science undergoing continual development. Research and clinical experience are continually expanding our knowledge, in particular our knowledge of proper treatment and drug therapy. Insofar as this book mentions any dosage or application, readers may rest assured that the authors, editors, and publishers have made every effort to ensure that such references are in accordance with **the state of knowledge at the time of production of the book**.

Nevertheless, this does not involve, imply, or express any guarantee or responsibility on the part of the publishers in respect to any dosage instructions and forms of applications stated in the book. **Every user is requested to examine carefully** the manufacturers' leaflets accompanying each drug and to check, if necessary in consultation with a physician or specialist, whether the dosage schedules mentioned therein or the contraindications stated by the manufacturers differ from the statements made in the present book. Such examination is particularly important with drugs that are either rarely used or have been newly released on the market. Every dosage schedule or every form of application used is entirely at the user's own risk and responsibility. The authors and publishers request every user to report to the publishers any discrepancies or inaccuracies noticed. If errors in this work are found after publication, errata will be posted at www.thieme.com on the product description page.

Some of the product names, patents, and registered designs referred to in this book are in fact registered trademarks or proprietary names even though specific reference to this fact is not always made in the text. Therefore, the appearance of a name without designation as proprietary is not to be construed as a representation by the publisher that it is in the public domain.

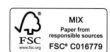

This book, including all parts thereof, is legally protected by copyright. Any use, exploitation, or commercialization outside the narrow limits set by copyright legislation, without the publisher's consent, is illegal and liable to prosecution. This applies in particular to photostat reproduction, copying, mimeographing, preparation of microfilms, and electronic data processing and storage.

Dedicated to my patients, past, present, and future, for the privilege to care for you and learn from you; to my students, who compel me to be a better teacher and person; and to my family and friends, who have stood beside me and supported me.

—*LRS*

This book is lovingly dedicated to all my teachers and all my students. Mom, you were my first teacher and gave me the love of teaching and learning. Dad, who believes I can do anything and everything. My brother, Daryl, who was my first student. My husband, Riasell, who is teaching me about myself.

—*TWM*

Contents

Contents

Contents

Part VII: Cases with Known Cancer Diagnosis Needing Additional Evaluation

Part VIII: Intervention: Biopsy Using Tomosynthesis or Stereotactic Guidance

Menu of Accompanying Videos

Key
Dxm = diagnostic
LCC = left craniocaudal view
LCCID = left craniocaudal implant-displaced view
LLM = left lateromedial view
LML = left mediolateral view
LMLO = left mediolateral oblique view
LMLOID = left mediolateral oblique implant-displaced view
LSCC = left craniocaudal spot-compression view
LSLM = left lateromedial spot-compression view
LSML = left mediolateral spot-compression view
LXCCL = left craniocaudal exaggerated lateral view
RCC = right craniocaudal view
RCCID = right craniocaudal implant-displaced view
RLM = right lateromedial view
RML = right mediolateral view
RMLO = right mediolateral oblique view
RMLOID = right mediolateral oblique implant-displaced view
RSCC = right craniocaudal spot-compression view
RSLM = right lateromedial spot-compression view
RSMLO = right mediolateral oblique spot-compression view
Scm = screening

1. Chapter 003 RCC
2. Chapter 003 RMLO
3. Chapter 004 LCC tomo
4. Chapter 004 LMLO tomo
5. Chapter 004 RCC tomo
6. Chapter 004 RMLO tomo
7. Chapter 005 RCC tomo
8. Chapter 005 RLM tomo
9. Chapter 006 RCC
10. Chapter 006 RMLO
11. Chapter 007 LCC tomo
12. Chapter 007 LMLO tomo
13. Chapter 007 RCC tomo
14. Chapter 007 RMLO tomo
15. Chapter 008 LCC
16. Chapter 008 LMLO
17. Chapter 009 LCC
18. Chapter 009 LMLO
19. Chapter 009 RCC
20. Chapter 009 RMLO
21. Chapter 010 LCC
22. Chapter 010 LMLO
23. Chapter 011 LCC tomo
24. Chapter 011 LMLO tomo
25. Chapter 011 RCC tomo
26. Chapter 011 RMLO tomo
27. Chapter 012 RCC
28. Chapter 012 RMLO
29. Chapter 013 RCC tomo
30. Chapter 013 RMLO tomo
31. Chapter 014 RCC
32. Chapter 014 RMLO
33. Chapter 015 LCC tomo
34. Chapter 015 LMLO tomo
35. Chapter 016 LCC tomo
36. Chapter 016 LMLO tomo
37. Chapter 017 RCC
38. Chapter 017 RMLO
39. Chapter 018 LCCID tomo
40. Chapter 018 LMLOID tomo
41. Chapter 018 RCCID tomo
42. Chapter 018 RMLOID tomo
43. Chapter 019 RCC
44. Chapter 019 RMLO
45. Chapter 020 LCC tomo
46. Chapter 020 LMLO tomo
47. Chapter 021 RCC
48. Chapter 021 RMLO
49. Chapter 022 2014 LCC
50. Chapter 022 2014 LMLO
51. Chapter 022 2014 RCC
52. Chapter 022 2014 RMLO
53. Chapter 022 2015 LCC
54. Chapter 022 2015 LMLO
55. Chapter 022 2015 RCC
56. Chapter 022 2015 RMLO
57. Chapter 023 RCC tomo
58. Chapter 023 RMLO tomo
59. Chapter 024 LCC tomo current
60. Chapter 024 LCC tomo prior
61. Chapter 024 LLM tomo current
62. Chapter 024 LLM tomo prior
63. Chapter 024 RCC tomo current
64. Chapter 024 RCC tomo prior
65. Chapter 024 RLM tomo current
66. Chapter 024 RLM tomo prior
67. Chapter 025 RCC
68. Chapter 025 RMLO
69. Chapter 026 LCC
70. Chapter 026 LMLO
71. Chapter 027 LCC
72. Chapter 027 LMLO

Preface

The cases presented in this book represent a compilation of common cases seen while using digital breast tomosynthesis (DBT). This book is not meant to be an all-inclusive tome of all breast pathologies. Many patients will have had a bilateral mammogram evaluation and the appropriate diagnostic imaging. The cases presented will not include all images in the patient's work-up however will demonstrate the images that were integral in the diagnostic process. If there were imaging findings only present in one breast, often only the pertinent imaging of the one breast is presented. The contralateral breast is omitted to optimize space for the presentation of imaging examples.

Within each case a captured image corresponding to the key DBT image for the case is presented. A few cases will not include a captured DBT image either because the abnormality was not seen on DBT or the abnormality covered multiple images such that one DBT would not optimally display its essence. The on-line component of this text contains the DBT movies for review.

Image presentation for the cases includes a FFDM and/or synthetic 2D mammogram. The synthetic images will be clearly designated. We felt it was important to include both FFDM and synthetic mammograms as it covers the cases as will be seen in any DBT breast-imaging program.

The format chosen for this textbook is as follows. The first section is dedicated to the basis physics principles of DBT including reconstruction methods, acquisition parameters and considerations to patient dose and data size. The next two sections will be case-based presentation of DBT in clinical practice. These will be divided into screening DBT and diagnostic DBT. Some screening exams will be taken through to their diagnostic evaluation as deemed necessary. All the cases in the diagnostic DBT section presented initially as a diagnostic use of DBT. Some of these cases may have started as a conventional screening mammogram and the diagnostic evaluation incorporated DBT or cases were diagnostic DBT from presentation.

Contributors

Tanya W. Moseley, MD
Professor
Breast Imaging Section
Division of Diagnostic Imaging
The University of Texas M.D. Anderson Cancer Center
Houston, Texas

Walter W. Peppler, PhD
Professor of Medical Physics and Radiology
Wisconsin Institutes for Medical Research (WIMR)
University of Wisconsin
Madison, Wisconsin

Lonie R. Salkowski, MD, MS
Professor
Section of Breast Imaging
Department of Radiology
University of Wisconsin School of Medicine and
    Public Health
Madison, Wisconsin

Part I

**Introduction to Clinical Breast
Tomosynthesis**

I

1 The Physics of Digital Breast Tomosynthesis

Walter W. Peppler

1.1 Introduction

Digital breast tomosynthesis (DBT) is a technology that produces three-dimensional slice images of the breast. The technology is related to conventional film tomography, which was widely used in radiography until the advent of computed tomography (CT). DBT has a lot in common with digital mammography as well. The spatial resolution in the individual reconstructed plane images is similar to that in a digital mammogram. The limited acquisition angle used in DBT is similar to that used for conventional tomography. On the other hand, CT generally has lower spatial resolution and utilizes data collected from all 360 degrees around the patient. The acquisition of data from 360 degrees means that the detector and source need to rotate around the object of interest, in this case, the breast. There are systems under development that place the patient prone on a table with the breast suspended in a hole in the table. The detector and X-ray source are then rotated around the pendulous breast. Such systems show some promise, but none are currently approved for clinical use. Although in many ways DBT of the breast seems very different from CT of the breast, DBT can really be considered to be a limited-angle CT device. Because DBT uses a digital mammography detector, it has very high resolution within the reconstructed plane. But, because of the limited acquisition angles, it has much poorer resolution in the direction perpendicular to the reconstructed plane.

1.2 History

Tomosynthesis was originally proposed in the 1930s by Ziedes des Plantes and was first implemented as conventional tomography. Tomosynthesis, the formation of a series of slices through an object from a series of projection images, was not practical until recently. In the late 1990s, high-quality full-field digital detectors became available. This added technology was required to successfully implement breast tomosynthesis. Flat-panel digital detectors, which are now commonly used in digital mammography, exhibit the necessary properties for a DBT detector; they are highly dose efficient, have low noise, and have high data-acquisition rates.

The first full-field digital mammography (FFDM) system (GE Senographe 2000D, GE Healthcare, Waukesha, Wisconsin) was approved for use in January 2000. Several other full-field digital detector systems were developed and approved for use over the next decade. Tomosynthesis imaging was first demonstrated by Niklason in 1997 but was not commercially available until 2011. In February 2011, the first digital breast tomosynthesis (DBT) system (Hologic Selenia Dimensions) was introduced. Two other systems have been approved since then, GE SenoClaire (August 2014) and Siemens MAMMOMAT Inspiration (April 2015). Early DBT studies were viewed on dedicated workstations due to the large data sets involved and due to the proprietary compression algorithms that were originally employed. The digital imaging and communication (DICOM) standard now supports DBT, allowing viewing and reading of DBT studies on conventional picture archiving and communication systems (PACS) workstations. The workstations need to conform to the mammographic quality standards act (MQSA) with 5-megapixel (MP) monitors and regular physics testing. ▶ Table 1.1 provides key definitions of terms in the field of FFDM and DBT.

1.3 Principles of Tomosynthesis: How Does Tomosynthesis Work?

The basic principles of DBT can be understood with a simple example. As seen in ▶ Fig. 1.1, there is a digital detector, an object with two features (a star and a pentagon), and an X-ray tube that can be moved from position A to position B. If we make an exposure with the X-ray tube at position A, we get an image A, as shown on the top right side of ▶ Fig. 1.1. We then move the X-ray tube to position B and make another exposure and obtain the image labeled B. Notice that the positions of the features (the star and the pentagon) are at different locations in the two images. As one can see by the blue lines in ▶ Fig. 1.1, the position of the star moves by a greater amount between exposure A and exposure B than the position of the pentagon. So if we shift the two images relative to each other by an amount *x* that corresponds to the change in position of the pentagon and add the two images, we get the image labeled A + B. Both the images of the pentagon are superimposed and the signal intensities add together.

However, the images of the star do not superimpose and their intensities do not add together. So the intensity of the two stars will be half that of the pentagon. You can imagine that if we took more images at positions between A and B and properly shifted each image and added them all together, then we could get all the pentagon images to superimpose and the intensity of the pentagon would continue to increase, while the intensity of the star would remain the same. Alternatively, we could adjust the image so that the intensity of the pentagon remained the same, in which case the intensity of the star images would decrease by a factor equal to the number of X-ray exposures. If we took enough exposures close together, the individual images of the star would begin to overlap each other. The result would be a low-intensity, blurry image of the star.

Table 1.1 Digital mammography and tomosynthesis definitions

- **FFDM:** Full-field digital mammography

- **Projection image:** For regular mammography, a projection image is simply the mammography image. For DBT, this is one of a set of images that are taken as the tube rotates in an arc across the breast.

- **Reconstructed slice:** The reconstructed slice is produced from a set of projection images and depicts a slice through the breast, parallel to the detector. Multiple reconstructed slices can be produced from a set of projection images.

- **Synthesized view:** A synthesized view is a single two-dimensional (2D) image of the breast that is formed from either the projection images or the reconstructed slices. The synthesized view may serve as a surrogate for a conventional 2D mammogram.

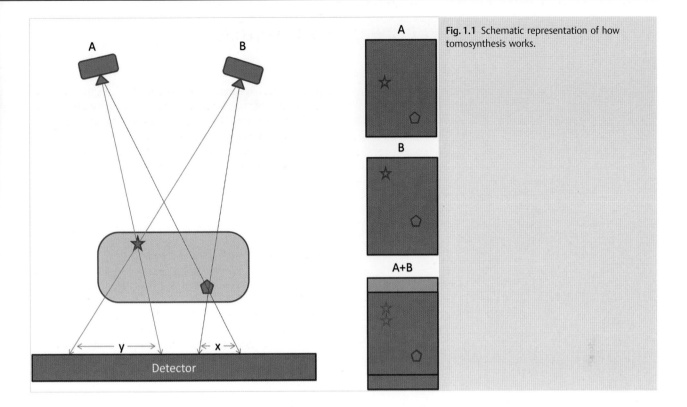

Fig. 1.1 Schematic representation of how tomosynthesis works.

The sharp, full-intensity characteristics of the pentagon would also be true for any other structure that was in the same horizontal plane as the pentagon. So the appropriately shifted and added images from all the exposures would produce a final image that showed all the structures in the plane of the pentagon in sharp focus and any structure that was not in that plane, such as the star, would be of lower intensity and would be blurred. Structures in planes slightly above or below the pentagon would be only slightly blurred, while structures in planes further from the plane of the pentagon would be significantly blurred. Since the detector is a digital detector, we can save all the individual images. If we shift the images by a different amount (for example, y) and then add them together, we can obtain an image where the plane of the star is in sharp focus and the plane of the pentagon is blurred. In general, we can shift and add the individual images with a range of shift amounts and can therefore produce a series of planes through the object.

In conventional tomography, the addition was performed by accumulating the exposures on a single film, and the shifting was accomplished by moving the film during the exposure. In that way, the shifting and adding was accomplished on a single film. Generally the exposure was a single continuous exposure as the tube was moved from A to B. A downside of conventional tomography was that only a single plane could be imaged at a time, and additional exposures were required to obtain images of other planes.

1.3.1 Reconstruction Methods

Shift and Add

The synthesis of the tomographic plane described in the previous section is accomplished by shifting and adding the individual images. Not surprisingly the first algorithm for reconstructing tomographic slices was called the *shift and add (SAA) method*. It is the original method that was developed and is still commonly used to reconstruct DBT images. The SAA method does not perfectly reconstruct the plane of interest. Information from structures in other planes is also superimposed on the information from the plane of interest. The reduced-intensity, blurry structures from other planes may be more or less of a problem depending on the contrast of the structure and the distance of the structure from the plane of interest. High-contrast structures and structures from planes that are close to the plane of interest produce greater artifacts. In ▶ Fig. 1.2 a conventional mammographic right caudocranial (RCC) view (left) is placed side-by-side with a tomosynthesis slice (right). In the tomosynthesis image on the right, you can observe significant residual artifacts from the high-contrast objects seen in the RCC image on the left.

Alternative reconstruction algorithms are attempts to reduce the effects of structures from other planes.

Filtered Back-Projection

The SAA method is a straightforward algorithm that is relatively easy to understand and to implement. Essentially it represents the method of reconstruction that is used when a conventional tomogram is produced. However, it is true that DBT can also be considered to be limited-angle computed tomography. "Limited-angle" means that data was not acquired from all the angles surrounding the breast. DBT utilizes at most 60 degrees of acquisition whereas complete CT utilizes at least 180 degrees and generally acquires and uses all 360 degrees. Since it is a limited-angle CT, it is not surprising that a common reconstruction

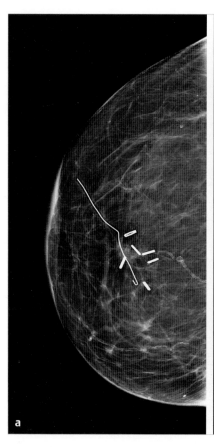
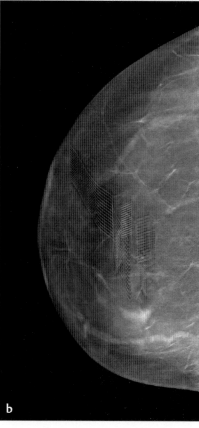

Fig. 1.2 Right craniocaudal (RCC) views demonstrating the artifact effect of high-contrast objects placed either on or within the breast. (a) Full-field digital mammographic (FFDM) view demonstrating the wire placed on the skin overlying the surgical scar and the surgical clips at the surgical bed. (b) A tomosynthesis slice demonstrating the artifact created by these high-contrast objects.

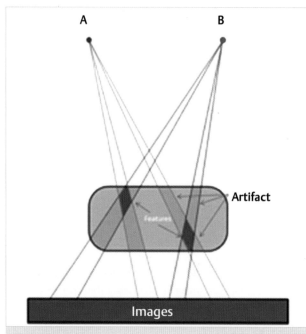

Fig. 1.3 Filtered back-projection.

method used for CT, filtered back-projection (FBP), is also used for DBT. FBP takes the transmitted information and, after applying a filter to the data, back-projects it through the object (▶ Fig. 1.3).

Every voxel (volume pixel) that is along a ray between a pixel in the image and the focal spot of the X-ray tube is given the value of the data in the pixel. This is repeated for all the pixels in the projection image and for all the projection images (for all the angles of acquisition). The blue lines in ▶ Fig. 1.3 correspond to the back projection of the data from the image taken with the X-ray tube at position A and the red lines correspond to the back projection of the data from the image taken with the X-ray tube at position B. The reconstructed volume is not very accurate when only two projection images are acquired. As the number of acquisitions and number of angles of acquisition increase, the accuracy of the reconstruction improves; the features are more accurately displayed and the artifacts are reduced. The filter in "filtered back-projection" is a modification of the projection data that is used to help correct the accuracy of the reconstruction.

The acquisition over a limited angle leads to residual artifacts, and there are various methods used to reduce the effects of those artifacts. All commercially available DBT systems use either FBP or an iterative reconstruction method.

Iterative Reconstruction Algorithms

One class of reconstruction algorithm is based on iterative reconstruction. The basic premise of this class of algorithms is that a first estimate of the reconstructed slices is produced. The algorithm assumes the reconstructed slices represent what is actually in all the planes and simulates what the projection images would look like if an X-ray were directed through those planes. The simulation is done mathematically on a computer, not with real imaging. The resulting simulated image does not look exactly like the actual projection image that was taken. The algorithm then adjusts the reconstructed slices to correct for the differences. Then it again simulates what the projection image would look like for the current reconstructed slices. The details of how the reconstructed slices are adjusted are beyond the scope of this text. The iteration continues until the corrections to the reconstructed slices become smaller than some predetermined threshold. The main advantage of iterative algorithms is that they produce more accurate reconstructions. The main disadvantages are that the iterative process can be time consuming and may introduce image noise.

All commercially available DBT systems use either FBP or an iterative reconstruction method.

1.3.2 Acquisition Parameters

The details of how the projection images are obtained can vary significantly from one system to another and can have a significant impact on image quality, speed of the exam, and patient comfort. Some of the considerations are how many projection images to take and over how great of an angle. The greater the angle over which the images are obtained the more sharply you can define the plane of interest. But larger angles generally require a longer acquisition time. The range of angles employed in commercial systems range from 15 to 50 degrees.

A greater number of images also improves the ability to reconstruct the plane of interest. But if the total X-ray dose is to be held constant, the greater the number of images then the less dose per individual projection image. While digital detectors are very dose efficient, it is possible to reduce the signal strength (dose per image) to a point where the detector characteristics degrade the quality of the image.

Another consideration is whether to acquire images with the tube in motion or whether to stop it for each exposure. If the tube is in motion, the resolution in the direction of motion is decreased due to an effective increase in the focal spot size in that direction. This effect can be minimized by taking short exposures, but tube loading limits how short the exposure can be while still producing adequate X-ray intensity. Stopping the tube before each exposure eliminates that issue, but it results in a longer acquisition time. It takes time to start and stop the tube and while waiting for the tube to stop vibrating from the sudden stop. With longer acquisition times comes the increased possibility of patient motion and increased patient discomfort. Commercially available systems take between 9 and 25 projection images with overall acquisition times between 3.7 and 20 seconds per acquisition.

Another consideration is how many planes to reconstruct. This is primarily limited by the data acquisition because the number of reconstructed planes is dictated by the resolution in the direction perpendicular to the image planes. Typically between-plane resolution is ~ 1 mm and consequently most systems reconstruct planes with 1-mm spacing. For a 5-cm compressed breast that would yield 50 images. Most imaging

software allows you to recombine individual slices into thicker slabs.

1.3.3 Anti-Scatter Grid

The use of a grid in DBT can be problematic. First, it can be difficult to use a grid because the tube is moving and, to avoid grid cutoff, the grid would need to move in synchrony with the tube. Secondly, the advantage of the grid is that it reduces scatter radiation, but it also reduces the primary signal. For DBT projection images, the dose per image is quite low, at least a factor of ten less than that for a conventional 2D digital mammographic image. This is so that the total dose of all the projection images is comparable to the dose of a single 2D digital image. The problem is that detector dose efficiency, commonly measured as detective quantum efficiency (DQE), and electronic noise can be a problem for very low exposures. So the detector itself may cause a degradation of the image quality if care is not taken. Most manufacturers have opted not to use a grid for DBT. However, one vendor does use a grid (GE SenoClaire).

1.3.4 Radiation Dose Considerations

It was generally accepted that the DBT data acquisition should require a patient radiation dose no more than that of a conventional 2D digital mammogram under the assumption that a single DBT acquisition would be adequate to provide comparable diagnostic information to that of a conventional two-view mammography study. Studies have not borne that out. The data suggests that two DBT acquisitions per breast perform better than one. The data also suggests that conventional 2-view 2D mammography acquisitions combined with DBT provide more accuracy than either alone. However, this results in roughly double the patient radiation dose. The manufacturers have developed synthesized 2D images (Hologic C-view) that are created from the DBT data. The hope is that the synthesized 2D images (synthetic mammograms) combined with the DBT reconstructed slices will provide the diagnostic information needed without requiring the conventional 2D mammography and the additional radiation dose.

Other alternatives for keeping the patient radiation dose as low as possible while obtaining the most accurate diagnostic information include producing DBT projection images that do not all have the same exposure. One proposal is to deliver half of the total dose to a central projection image with the remaining half distributed to all the remaining projection images, approximately the dose that they received before. The dose for this arrangement would be higher than DBT (or 2D mammography) alone but would only require one acquisition per view (two per breast). Other distributions of dose might also produce a more optimal image quality for a given dose since not all the projection angles provide the same amount of image information. An increased dose generally provides improved image quality. While we have optimized the image quality of conventional digital mammography using the accepted patient dose, it is not clear that the same dose would necessarily be the optimal dose for a technology such as DBT that provides at least different (if not better) diagnostic information. The essential question is, "What extra dose would be justified if we can produce a study with improved diagnostic accuracy?"

1.3.5 Data Size

DBT projection images have pixel sizes of between 85 and 100 μm (microns). For a 24×30 cm detector with 2 bytes per pixel that corresponds to between 14.4 and 20 megabytes (MB) per image. Manufacturers may recombine pixels for tomosynthesis projection images and/or for the reconstructed slices in order to reduce noise (by averaging pixels) and also to reduce data requirements. A set of projection images is between 9 and 25 images yielding a total size of up 500 MB per set. Generally lossless compression can reduce that to ~ 150 MB. The reconstructed slices are of a similar size. Therefore a four-view (two per breast) DBT study can be ~ 600 MB. These numbers can be important when designing the amount of memory per workstation, the storage capacity of the archive, and network capacity.

1.4 Conclusion

This brief overview provides the fundamental physics underlying the DBT technology. Understanding the basics will assist you when making the many decisions involved in implementing a DBT program within a breast imaging program. Beyond choosing a DBT vendor and the supporting infrastructure, some additional decisions regarding clinical imaging need to be considered. These decisions may include whether DBT will be offered for screening or for diagnosis, or for both. Will exams involve combination imaging, with FFDM and DBT or with synthetic 2D mammogram and DBT? Additionally, will DBT imaging be collected in two views or one view? The answers to these questions will ultimately impact your infrastructure and data storage.

References

[1] Chawla AS, Lo JY, Baker JA, Samei E. Optimized image acquisition for breast tomosynthesis in projection and reconstruction space. Med Phys. 2009; 36 (11):4859–4869

[2] Dobbins JT, III, Godfrey DJ. Digital x-ray tomosynthesis: current state of the art and clinical potential. Phys Med Biol. 2003; 48(19):R65–R106

[3] Dobbins JT, III. Tomosynthesis imaging: at a translational crossroads. Med Phys. 2009; 36(6):1956–1967

[4] Niklason LT, Christian BT, Niklason LE, et al. Digital tomosynthesis in breast imaging. Radiology. 1997; 205(2):399–406

[5] Reiser I, Sechopoulos I. A Review of Digital Breast Tomosynthesis. Medical Physics International Journal. 2014; 2(1):57–66

[6] Sechopoulos I. A review of breast tomosynthesis. Part I. The image acquisition process. Med Phys. 2013; 40(1):014301

[7] Sechopoulos I, Ghetti C. Optimization of the acquisition geometry in digital tomosynthesis of the breast. Med Phys. 2009; 36(4):1199–1207

[8] Sechopoulos I. A review of breast tomosynthesis. Part II. Image reconstruction, processing and analysis, and advanced applications. Med Phys. 2013; 40(1):014302

[9] Suryanarayanan S, Karellas A, Vedantham S. Physical characteristics of a full-field digital mammography system. NIM B. 2004; 533(11):560–570

[10] Van de Sompel D, Brady SM, Boone J. Task-based performance analysis of FBP, SART and ML for digital breast tomosynthesis using signal CNR and Channelised Hotelling Observers. Med Image Anal. 2011; 15(1):53–70

[11] Ziedes des Plantes BG. Eine neue methode zur differenzierung in der roentgenographie (planigraphie). Acta Radiol. 1932; 13:182–192

2 BI-RADS Nomenclature for Mammography and Ultrasound

Lonie R. Salkowski and Tanya W. Moseley

2.1 Introduction

The American College of Radiologists (ACR) Breast Imaging Reporting and Data System (BI-RADS) has become an integral component of breast imaging reporting. BI-RADS has served as a universal language beginning in the late 1980s, with the first edition of BI-RADS put into practice in 1993. Through the use of the BI-RADS lexicon, standardization and uniformity has been brought to breast imaging reporting. The lexicon takes into consideration the overall features of a mammogram that may interfere with image interpretation such as the breast density pattern. It provides an effective means of communication to

Table 2.1 Terminology for mammography based on ACR BI-RADS, 5th edition

Breast composition	The breasts are almost entirely fatty	
	There are scattered areas of fibroglandular density	
	The breasts are heterogeneously dense, which may obscure small masses	
	The breasts are extremely dense, which lowers the sensitivity of mammography	
Masses	Shape	Oval
		Round
		Irregular
	Margin	Circumscribed
		Obscured
		Microlobulated
		Indistinct
		Spiculated
	Density	High density
		Equal density
		Low density
		Fat-containing
Calcifications	Typically benign	Skin
		Vascular
		Coarse or "popcorn"
		Large rodlike
		Round
		Rim
		Dystrophic
		Milk of calcium
		Suture
	Suspicious morphology	Amorphous
		Coarse heterogeneous
		Fine pleomorphic
		Fine linear or fine-linear branching
	Distribution	Diffuse
		Regional
		Grouped
		Linear
		Segmental
Architectural distortion		
Asymmetries	Asymmetry	
	Global asymmetry	
	Focal asymmetry	
	Developing asymmetry	

Source: Adapted from ACR BI-RADS Mammography, p 171-175.

Table 2.2 Terminology for ultrasound based on ACR BI-RADS, 5th edition

Masses	Shape	Oval
		Round
		Irregular
	Orientation	Parallel
		Not parallel
	Margin	Circumscribed
		Not circumscribed
		• Indistinct
		• Angular
		• Microlobulated
		• Spiculated
	Echo pattern	Anechoic
		Hyperechoic
		Complex cystic and solid
		Hypoechoic
		Isoechoic
		Heterogeneous
	Posterior features	No posterior features
		Enhancement
		Shadowing
		Combined pattern
Calcifications	Calcifications in a mass	
	Calcifications outside of a mass	
	Intraductal calcifications	

Source: Adapted from ACR BI-RADS Ultrasound, p149-152.

Table 2.3 Lesion location terminology based on ACR BI-RADS, 5th edition

Laterality
Quadrant and clock face
Depth
Distance from the nipple

Source: Adapted from ACR BI-RADS Mammography, p 119.

Table 2.4 BI-RADS classification

Category 0: Mammography: Incomplete – need additional imaging evaluation and/or prior mammograms for comparison Ultrasound & MRI: Incomplete – need additional imaging evaluation
Category 1: Negative
Category 2: Benign
Category 3: Probably benign
Category 4: Suspicious mammography & ultrasound:
• Category 4A: Low suspicion for malignancy
• Category 4B: Moderate suspicion for malignancy
• Category 4C: High suspicion for malignancy
Category 5: Highly suggestive of malignancy
Category 6: Known biopsy-proven malignancy

Source: Adapted from ACR BI-RADS Mammography, p135-138.

discriminate between benign and malignant features through terminology and structured reporting of lesions seen on mammography, ultrasound, and magnetic resonance imaging (MRI). Finally, it aids in imparting an overall assessment of the level of concern for malignancy and the appropriate action that should be taken for patient management. The cases in this text use the terminology of the ACR BI-RADS® Atlas, 5th edition,[1] as they apply to the imaging findings of mammography (which also apply to digital breast tomosynthesis [DBT]) and for corresponding ultrasound imaging when it further aids the findings of DBT. Therefore, to assist in using this text, we have provided the following abbreviated terminology and classification tables

(▶ Table 2.1, ▶ Table 2.2, ▶ Table 2.3, and ▶ Table 2.4) adapted from ACR BI-RADS® Atlas, 5th edition, for these imaging modalities. These tables are not intended to be comprehensive. For more complete details, the reader should refer to the ACR BI-RADS® Atlas, 5th edition.

References

[1] D Orsi CJ, Sickles EA, Mendelson EB, Morris EA, et al. ACR BI-RADS® Atlas, Breast Imaging Reporting and Data System. Reston, VA, American College of Radiology; 2013.

Part II

**Cases with Screening
Tomosynthesis Evaluation Needing
No Further Evaluation**

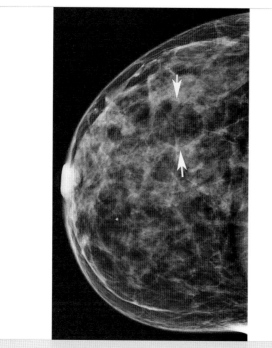

Fig. 3.5 Right craniocaudal (RCC) mammogram with label.

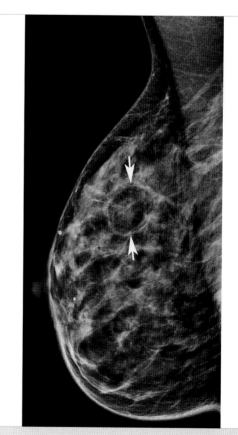

Fig. 3.6 Right mediolateral oblique (RMLO) mammogram with label.

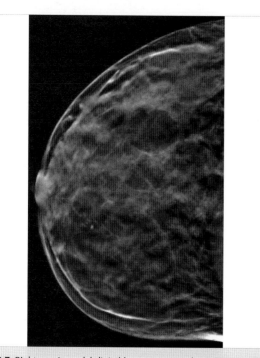

Fig. 3.7 Right craniocaudal digital breast tomosynthesis (RCC DBT), slice 16 of 40.

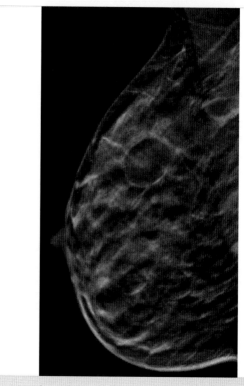

Fig. 3.8 Right mediolateral oblique (RMLO DBT), slice 8 of 43.

4 Radiolucent Lesions with Calcifications

Tanya W. Moseley

4.1 Presentation and Presenting Images

(▶ Fig. 4.1, ▶ Fig. 4.2, ▶ Fig. 4.3, ▶ Fig. 4.4, ▶ Fig. 4.5, ▶ Fig. 4.6, ▶ Fig. 4.7, ▶ Fig. 4.8)

A 72-year-old female with a history of invasive ductal carcinoma of the right breast treated with segmentectomy followed by oncoplastic tissue rearrangement and left breast mastopexy presents for asymptomatic screening mammography.

4.2 Key Images

(▶ Fig. 4.9, ▶ Fig. 4.10, ▶ Fig. 4.11, ▶ Fig. 4.12, ▶ Fig. 4.13)

4.2.1 Breast Tissue Density

The breasts are heterogeneously dense, which may obscure small masses.

4.2.2 Imaging Findings

The imaging of the right breast demonstrates a postsurgical scar with architectural distortion and postsurgical clips (*arrows* in ▶ Fig. 4.9, ▶ Fig. 4.10, and ▶ Fig. 4.11) in the central aspect of the right breast middle and posterior depths. The imaging of both breasts demonstrates postsurgical changes consistent with mastopexy. In the right subareolar region there are radiolucent lesions with linear and curvilinear calcifications (*circles*).

The right craniocaudal (CC) tomosynthesis movie demonstrates the radiolucent lesions and calcifications on slices 17 to 52 of 90. A representative slice is shown (slice 24 of 90 in ▶ Fig. 4.12). Similarly, the area is seen on the right mediolateral oblique (MLO) tomosynthesis movie on slices 20 to 52 of 92. A representative slice is shown (slice 41 of 92 in ▶ Fig. 4.13).

4.3 BI-RADS Classification and Action

Category 2: Benign

4.4 Differential Diagnosis

1. **Fat necrosis**: The radiolucent lesions (fat) associated with linear and curvilinear calcifications are pathognomonic of fat necrosis.

2. *Ductal carcinoma in situ (DCIS)*: While linear calcifications may be a presentation of DCIS, curvilinear calcifications are not.

3. *Fibrocystic changes*: Fibrocystic changes usually present as amorphous calcifications, not linear or curvilinear calcifications.

4.5 Essential Facts

- The postsurgical history is important in this case. The patient has had right segmentectomy followed by right oncoplastic tissue rearrangement and left breast mastopexy. The right breast surgeries removed the breast malignancy and reestablished cosmesis. The left breast surgery established cosmesis. This history explains the appearance of both breasts.
- There are many ways that fat necrosis may present mammographically, including lipid cysts, calcifications, focal asymmetries, or spiculated masses. If minimal fibrosis occurs, as in this case, then the mass appears radiolucent or as an oil cyst.
- Oil cysts have a predictable evolution with linear and curvilinear calcifications developing and central calcifications developing later.

4.6 Management and Digital Breast Tomosynthesis Principles

- Tomosynthesis, by removing overlapping tissue, easily delineates the radiolucent oil cysts and clearly demonstrates the associated calcifications along the edge of the oil cysts.
- Even when unrecognized on conventional mammography, fat is commonly seen in both benign and malignant masses on tomosynthesis.
- With tomosynthesis, the radiologist can confidently classify encapsulated fat-containing masses as benign.
- Alternatively, radiologists must be careful not to misclassify all fat-containing lesions as benign or probably benign. Due to the growth of cancer, it can encapsulate fat and on tomosynthesis appear to contain fat. Fat-containing lesions should be carefully assessed for margins and other morphological features that could suggest a more suspicious lesion.

4.7 Further Reading

[1] Freer PE, Wang JL, Rafferty EA. Digital breast tomosynthesis in the analysis of fat-containing lesions. Radiographics. 2014; 34(2):343–358

[2] Taboada JL, Stephens TW, Krishnamurthy S, Brandt KR, Whitman GJ. The many faces of fat necrosis in the breast. AJR Am J Roentgenol. 2009; 192(3): 815–825

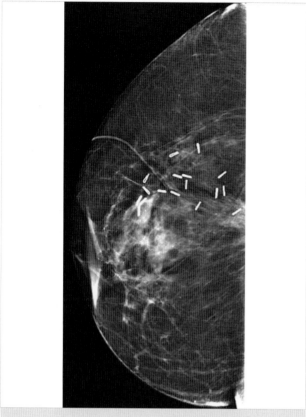

Fig. 4.1 Right craniocaudal (RCC) mammogram.

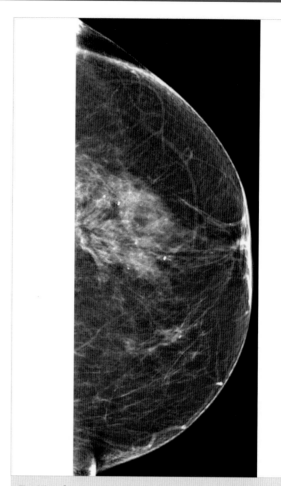

Fig. 4.2 Left craniocaudal (LCC) mammogram.

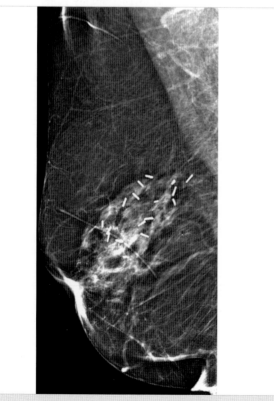

Fig. 4.3 Right mediolateral oblique (RMLO) mammogram.

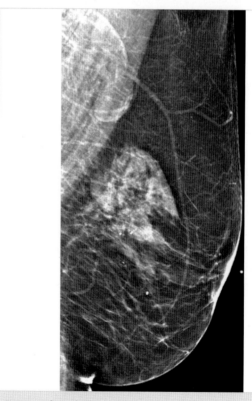

Fig. 4.4 Left mediolateral oblique (LMLO) mammogram.

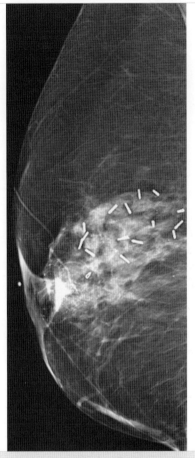

Fig. 4.5 Right lateromedial (RLM) mammogram.

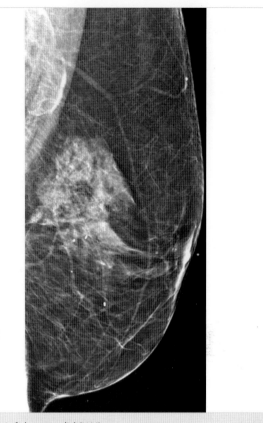

Fig. 4.6 Left lateromedial (LLM) mammogram.

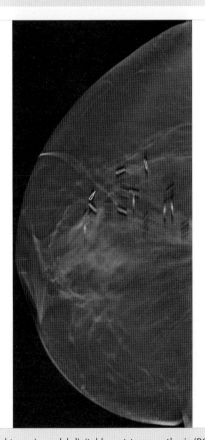

Fig. 4.7 Right craniocaudal digital breast tomosynthesis (RCC DBT), slice 24 of 90.

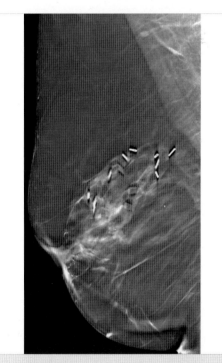

Fig. 4.8 Right mediolateral oblique digital breast tomosynthesis (RMLO DBT), slice 41 of 92.

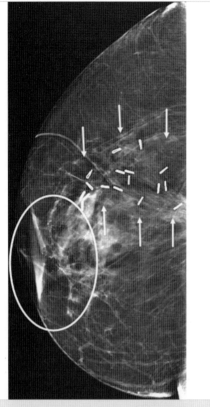

Fig. 4.9 Right craniocaudal (RCC) mammogram with label.

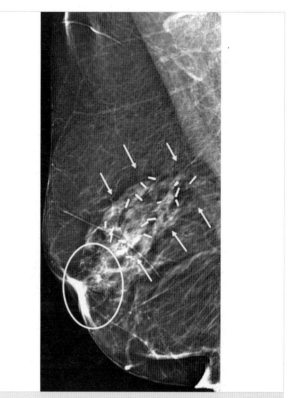

Fig. 4.10 Right mediolateral oblique (RMLO) mammogram with label.

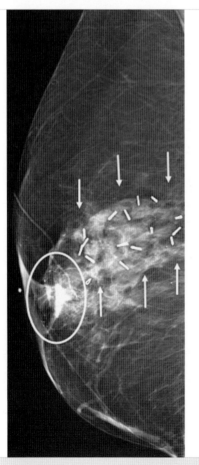

Fig. 4.11 Right lateromedial (RLM) mammogram with label.

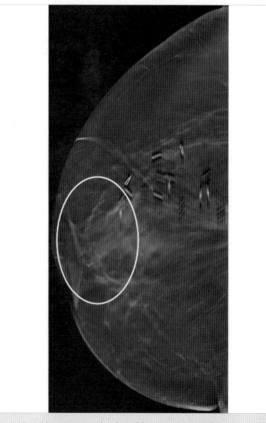

Fig. 4.12 Right craniocaudal digital breast tomosynthesis (RCC DBT), slice 24 of 90 with label.

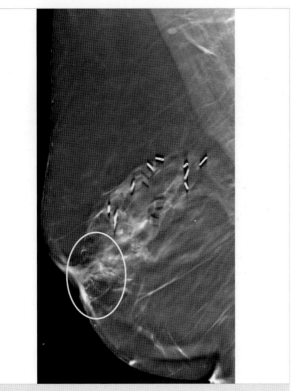

Fig. 4.13 Right mediolateral oblique digital breast tomosynthesis (RMLO DBT), slice 41 of 92 with label.

5 Architectural Distortion

Tanya W. Moseley

5.1 Presentation and Presenting Images

(▶ Fig. 5.1, ▶ Fig. 5.2, ▶ Fig. 5.3, ▶ Fig. 5.4, ▶ Fig. 5.5, ▶ Fig. 5.6)

A 62-year-old female with a history of left mastectomy for invasive ductal carcinoma and right reduction mammoplasty presents for routine mammography.

5.2 Key Images

(▶ Fig. 5.7, ▶ Fig. 5.8, ▶ Fig. 5.9, ▶ Fig. 5.10, ▶ Fig. 5.11)

5.2.1 Breast Tissue Density

The breasts are heterogeneously dense, which may obscure small masses.

5.2.2 Imaging Findings

There is no imaging of the left breast as the patient had a mastectomy. The right breast demonstrates architectural distortion centrally (*circle* in ▶ Fig. 5.7, ▶ Fig. 5.8, ▶ Fig. 5.10, and ▶ Fig. 5.11) and elevation of the nipple (*arrow* in ▶ Fig. 5.8 and ▶ Fig. 5.9).

5.3 BI-RADS Classification and Action

Category 2: Benign

5.4 Differential Diagnosis

1. **Postsurgical changes**: There is central architectural distortion and elevation of the nipple. These imaging findings correlate with the surgical changes of reduction mammoplasty.
2. *Radial scar*: Although a radial scar may present as architectural distortion, the clinical history is less appropriate for this diagnosis.
3. *Breast cancer*: Patients with a prior history of breast cancer are at increased risk for developing another cancer, but the findings in this case are most consistent with postsurgical changes.

5.5 Essential Facts

- According to Danikas and colleagues (2001), the most common mammographic findings seen after reduction mammoplasty were parenchymal redistribution and elevation of the nipple. These authors felt that mammographic findings after reduction mammoplasty are predictable; therefore knowledge of these findings will prevent unnecessary biopsies and make the diagnosis of lesions unrelated to the procedure easier.
- All patients over 35 years of age having reduction mammoplasty surgery should have a preoperative and a postoperative mammogram for future reference.
- Postsurgical changes following reduction mammoplasty do not significantly hinder evaluation of screening mammograms and the detection of breast cancers.

5.6 Management and Digital Breast Tomosynthesis Principles

- Obtaining the two-dimensional (2D) mammogram along with tomosynthesis allowed direct comparison between the 2D mammogram and tomosynthesis. Comparing the two studies in this example, the breast is smaller, the nipple position is higher, and there is central architectural distortion.
- Tomosynthesis is helpful in identifying lesions unrelated to the reduction mammoplasty procedure and the postsurgical changes.
- The process of reviewing the images acquired with tomosynthesis takes longer, but early studies suggest that the number of callbacks are reduced.

5.7 Further Reading

[1] Danikas D, Theodorou SJ, Kokkalis G, Vasiou K, Kyriakopoulou K. Mammographic findings following reduction mammoplasty. Aesthetic Plast Surg. 2001; 25(4):283–285

[2] Muir TM, Tresham J, Fritschi L, Wylie E. Screening for breast cancer post reduction mammoplasty. Clin Radiol. 2010; 65(3):198–205

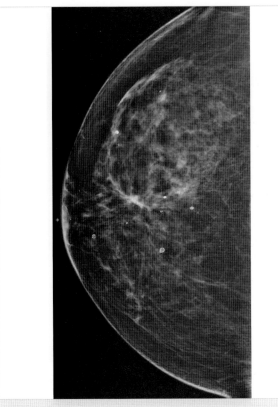

Fig. 5.1 Right craniocaudal (RCC) mammogram.

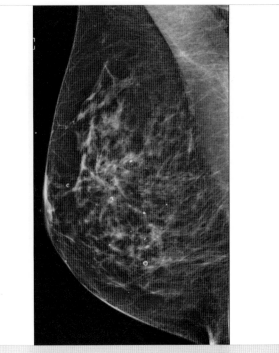

Fig. 5.2 Right mediolateral oblique (RMLO) mammogram.

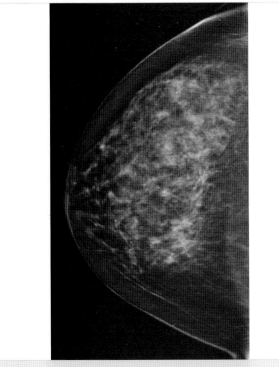

Fig. 5.3 Right craniocaudal (RCC) mammogram comparison.

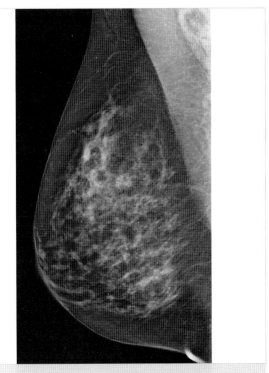

Fig. 5.4 Right mediolateral oblique (RMLO) mammogram comparison.

6 Architectural Distortion on a Full-Field Digital Mammogram

Lonie R. Salkowski

6.1 Presentation and Presenting Images

(▶ Fig. 6.1, ▶ Fig. 6.2, ▶ Fig. 6.3, ▶ Fig. 6.4)
A 54-year-old female presents for screening mammography.

6.2 Key Images

(▶ Fig. 6.5, ▶ Fig. 6.6)

6.2.1 Breast Tissue Density

There are scattered areas of fibroglandular density.

6.2.2 Imaging Findings

In the anterior depth of the right breast at the 11 o'clock location on the two-dimensional (2D) digital mammogram, there is an area of possible architectural distortion (▶ Fig. 6.6). This area appears more convincing on the craniocaudal (CC) view (▶ Fig. 6.5). The corresponding digital breast tomosynthesis (DBT) images (*not shown*) confirm that this is normal overlapping tissue.

6.2.3 BI-RADS Classification and Action

Category 1: Negative

6.3 Differential Diagnosis

1. **Normal breast tissue (superimposition of breast tissue)**: Superimposition of tissue is a common occurrence in breast imaging and is a source of many recalled mammograms.
2. *Surgical scar*: Surgical scars are a source of architectural distortion on mammograms; however, this patient did not have any history of a surgical procedure. If in doubt, it is important to check the medical record.
3. *Breast cancer*: Breast cancer can present as architectural distortion; however, it is not very common. When architectural distortion is suspected to be breast cancer, it has a high positive predictive value. But in this case, the distortion was due to overlapping tissue.

6.4 Essential Facts

- Summation artifacts, or superimposition of breast tissue, accounts for a substantial portion of the recalls (5%–25%) in a mammographic screening program.
- A summation artifact occurs when normal breast tissue from different planes superimpose upon each other mimicking a lesion (also called a "pseudomass").
- Tomosynthesis technique, which limits the effects of overlapping structures, enhances lesion detection and can aid in determining if no lesion is present.
- The decreased recall rate of digital breast tomosynthesis (DBT) increases the specificity of screening mammography.

6.5 Management and Digital Breast Tomosynthesis Principles

- Tomosynthesis can decrease the number of benign recalls (false-positives) at screening mammography. Reports suggest DBT reduces the recall rate by 15 to17%.
- There are significant added costs for unnecessary mammographic recalls – that of the diagnostic mammogram, the added patient time and anxiety, and the added radiation exposure.
- Controversy exists as to whether DBT needs to be performed in both the craniocaudal (CC) and the mediolateral (MLO) projections. In a study by Rafferty and colleagues (2007), they found that in 35% of cases, the lesion was better visualized in one projection over the other. Most investigators have recommended performing DBT in both imaging planes to optimize lesion visualization.
- Performing a combination 2D digital mammogram and DBT examination involves increased breast irradiation.
- The appearance of radial scars stand out on DBT and thus are a source of false-positive findings.

6.6 Further Reading

[1] Kopans DB. Digital breast tomosynthesis from concept to clinical care. AJR Am J Roentgenol. 2014; 202(2):299–308
[2] Rafferty EA. Digital mammography: novel applications. Radiol Clin North Am. 2007; 45(5):831–843, vii

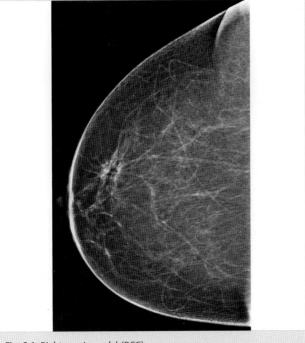

Fig. 6.1 Right craniocaudal (RCC) mammogram.

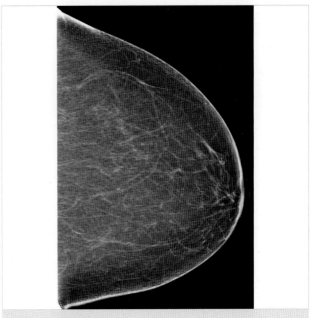

Fig. 6.2 Left craniocaudal (LCC) mammogram.

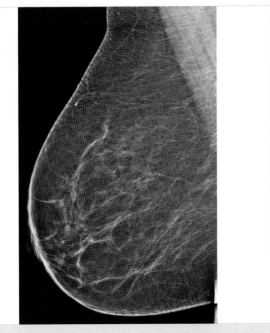

Fig. 6.3 Right mediolateral oblique (RMLO) mammogram.

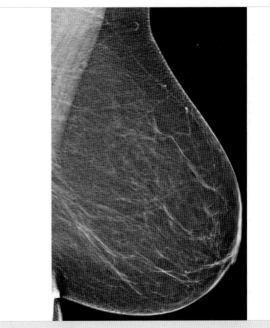

Fig. 6.4 Left mediolateral oblique (LMLO) mammogram.

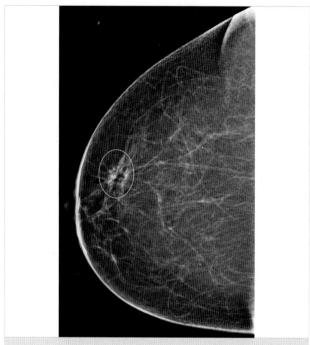

Fig. 6.5 Right craniocaudal (RCC) mammogram with label.

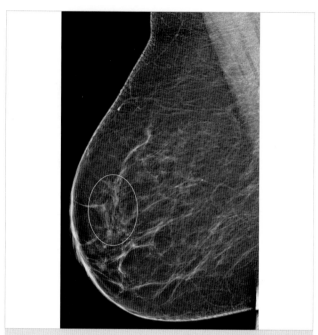

Fig. 6.6 Right mediolateral oblique (RMLO) mammogram with label.

7 No Skin Edge

Tanya W. Moseley

7.1 Presentation and Presenting Images

(▶ Fig. 7.1, ▶ Fig. 7.2, ▶ Fig. 7.3, ▶ Fig. 7.4, ▶ Fig. 7.5, ▶ Fig. 7.6, ▶ Fig. 7.7, ▶ Fig. 7.8, ▶ Fig. 7.9)

A 43-year-old female presents for routine screening mammography.

7.2 Key Images

(▶ Fig. 7.10, ▶ Fig. 7.11, ▶ Fig. 7.12, ▶ Fig. 7.13)

7.2.1 Breast Tissue Density

There are scattered areas of fibroglandular density.

7.2.2 Imaging Findings

Conventional mammography (▶ Fig. 7.1, ▶ Fig. 7.2, ▶ Fig. 7.3, and ▶ Fig. 7.4), synthetic mammography (▶ Fig. 7.5, ▶ Fig. 7.6, ▶ Fig. 7.7, and ▶ Fig. 7.8), and tomosynthesis imaging (*not shown*) demonstrate no suspicious calcifications, asymmetries, masses, or architectural distortions in either breast.

The inferior aspect of the right breast on the mediolateral oblique (MLO) view is incompletely imaged (▶ Fig. 7.3). A repeat right MLO view is shown in ▶ Fig. 7.9.

The skin line is absent from both the synthetic mammograms (*arrow* in ▶ Fig. 7.10 and ▶ Fig. 7.12) and tomosynthesis imaging (*not shown*). The skin line is clearly seen on the conventional mammograms (*arrow* in ▶ Fig. 7.11 and ▶ Fig. 7.13).

7.3 BI-RADS Classification and Action

Category 1: Negative

7.4 Differential Diagnosis

1. ***Technical artifact***: There was a detector failure on the tomosynthesis movie, which resulted in nonvisualization of the skin edge on both the digital breast tomosynthesis (DBT) movies and the synthetic mammogram. This did not affect the conventional digital mammogram.
2. *Negative/benign study*: There are no suspicious findings in either breast; however, this case is not "completely negative" due to positioning.
3. *Missed finding*: Sometimes mammograms are interpreted as negative or benign when there is an abnormality. There is not a missed finding on this mammogram.

7.5 Essential Facts

- The imaging from this case was reviewed by imaging physicists and the loss of the skin line was believed secondary to undercompression of the breast tissue during the examination. The compression thickness for the current study was 80 mm compared to 60 mm on the prior study.
- Artifacts can be subtle and escape detection. Tomosynthesis is a relatively new modality, and, with each new modality, there is a learning curve for both technologists and radiologists.
- Each view in this case for the conventional mammography, synthetic mammography and tomosynthesis studies was performed without repositioning the patient. This is why the right MLO view is poorly positioned on each of the three studies. A conventional right MLO view was repeated later.
- Positioning and obtaining adequate compression are important for both conventional mammography and tomosynthesis.

7.6 Management and Digital Breast Tomosynthesis Principles

- High-quality mammograms should be performed at the lowest radiation dose possible.
- Mammographic compression is important because it immobilizes the breast, reducing motion and geometric blur, and it prevents overpenetration by the radiation beam by decreasing the thickness of the breast.
- The Monte Carlo study of mass and microcalcification conspicuity in tomosynthesis[1] showed that reduced compression will have a minimal effect on the radiologist's performance interpreting tomosynthesis studies.
- Less compression will increase women's comfort with DBT; however, adequate compression must be applied to prevent artifacts.
- Technologists and radiologists must be aware of artifacts associated with DBT. As we gain more experience, we will easily detect and correct the artifacts.

7.7 Further Reading

[1] Saunders RS, Jr, Samei E, Lo JY, Baker JA. Can compression be reduced for breast tomosynthesis? Monte Carlo study on mass and microcalcification conspicuity in tomosynthesis. Radiology. 2009; 251(3):673–682

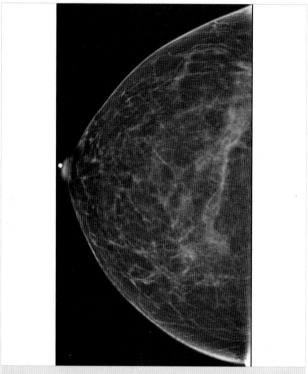

Fig. 7.1 Right craniocaudal (RCC) mammogram.

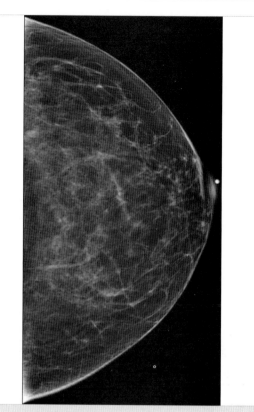

Fig. 7.2 Left craniocaudal (LCC) mammogram.

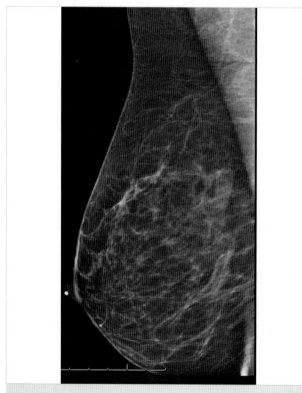

Fig. 7.3 Right mediolateral oblique (RMLO) mammogram.

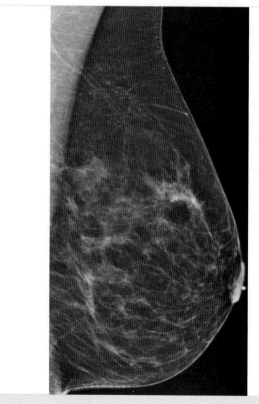

Fig. 7.4 Left mediolateral oblique (LMLO) mammogram.

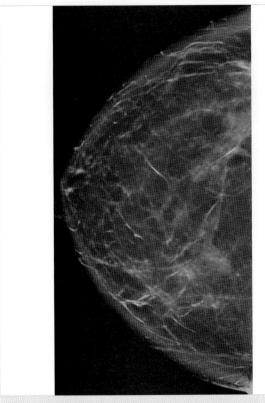

Fig. 7.5 Right craniocaudal (RCC) synthetic mammogram.

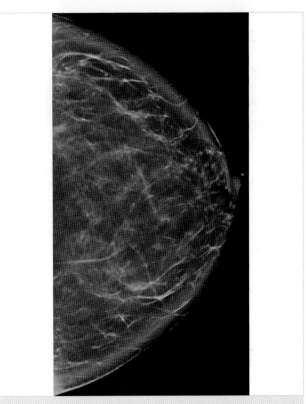

Fig. 7.6 Left craniocaudal (LCC) synthetic mammogram.

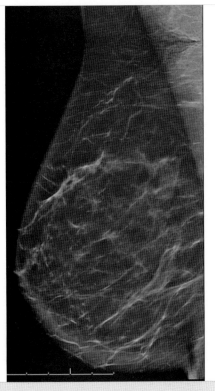

Fig. 7.7 Right mediolateral oblique (RMLO) synthetic mammogram.

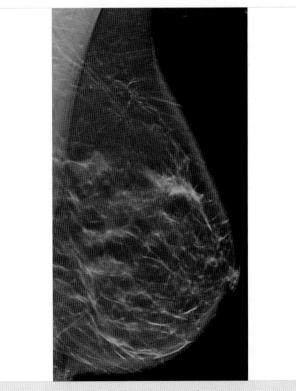

Fig. 7.8 Left mediolateral oblique (LMLO) synthetic mammogram.

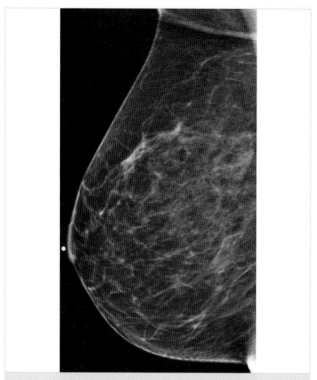

Fig. 7.9 Repeat right mediolateral oblique (RMLO) mammogram.

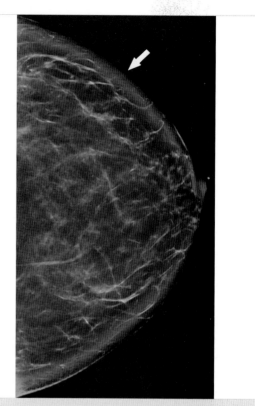

Fig. 7.10 Left craniocaudal (LCC) synthetic mammogram with label.

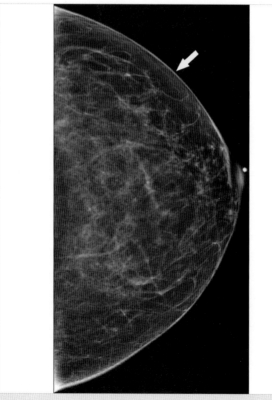

Fig. 7.11 Left craniocaudal (LCC) mammogram with label.

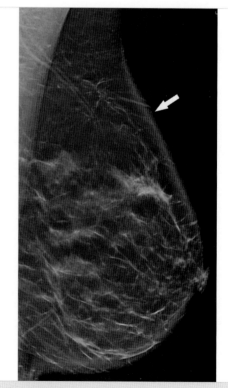

Fig. 7.12 Left mediolateral oblique (LMLO) synthetic mammogram with label.

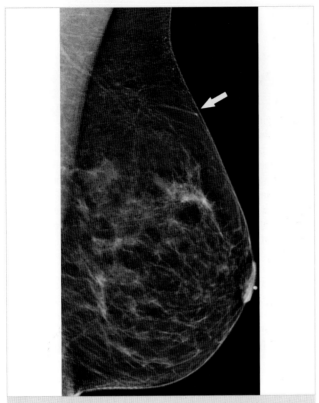

Fig. 7.13 Left mediolateral oblique (LMLO) mammogram with label.

8 Grouped Calcifications

Lonie R. Salkowski

8.1 Presentation and Presenting Images

(▶ Fig. 8.1, ▶ Fig. 8.2, ▶ Fig. 8.3, ▶ Fig. 8.4)
   A 55-year-old female presents for screening mammography.

8.2 Key Images

(▶ Fig. 8.5, ▶ Fig. 8.6, ▶ Fig. 8.7)

8.2.1 Breast Tissue Density

The breasts are heterogeneously dense, which may obscure small masses.

8.2.2 Imaging Findings

In the upper outer quadrant of the left breast at the 1 o'clock location in the posterior depth, there are grouped amorphous and round calcifications (▶ Fig. 8.5 and ▶ Fig. 8.6). The close-up of the calcifications on the mediolateral (MLO) view demonstrates their amorphous and loosely grouped appearance (▶ Fig. 8.7). They are difficult to localize to one digital breast tomosynthesis (DBT) slice in either imaging plane as they are loosely grouped. Comparison to earlier mammograms shows that these calcifications have been stable more than 5 years. The exam from 5 years ago was an analog mammogram and so not as easily reproduced. Therefore, the comparatives from 3 years ago are presented here as representative of the earlier mammograms showing the calcifications.

8.3 BI-RADS Classification and Action

Category 2: Benign

8.4 Differential Diagnosis

1. **Benign calcifications**: The punctate and amorphous calcifications are very loosely grouped and have been stable for more than 5 years. There are several areas of calcifications in the same breast that appear similarly.
2. *Calcifications needing further evaluation*: The stability of the calcifications suggest that they are benign and require no further evaluation.
3. *Suspicious calcifications*: Amorphous calcifications are part of the suspicious BI-RADS lexicon; however, some amorphous calcifications can be due to benign pathology. The stability of these calcifications suggests a benign etiology.

8.5 Essential Facts

- DBT is not as good for identifying calcifications as it is for identifying masses and architectural distortion.
- Only a few calcifications of a group of small and dispersed calcifications may show on a single reconstructed DBT slice.
- Large calcifications can cause significant artifacts with repeating ghostlike objects bordered by dark shadows in the direction of the X-ray tube motion.
- Spangler and colleagues (2011) noted that full-field digital mammography (FFDM) was significantly better for calcification detection than DBT (84% vs. 75%). In addition, FFDM had a higher specificity for calcifications over BDT (71% vs. 64%).
- Kopans and colleagues (2011) noted that calcifications can be seen equally well if not with superior clarity on DBT compared to conventional mammography (this study used both analog and digital mammograms for comparisons).
- Further research is needed to evaluate calcification detection on DBT.

8.6 Management and Digital Breast Tomosynthesis Principles

- DBT slices are generally reconstructed as 1-mm slices; however, increasing the slice thickness may help the three-dimensional perception of calcifications. The trade-off is that the spatial resolution of the individual calcifications is decreased with the increased slice reconstruction thickness.
- DBT slices are generally reconstructed as 1-mm slices. The thinness of the slices can cause calcifications in a group or a linear distribution to appear over several slices, thus not allowing the distribution of the individual calcifications to be observed in a single slice. The corresponding two-dimensional, conventional or synthetic mammogram may better provide this overview of calcifications. A synthesized view is a single two-dimensional (2D) image of the breast that is formed from either the projection images or the reconstructed slices. The synthesized view may serve as a surrogate for a conventional 2D mammogram.

8.7 Further Reading

[1] Conant EF. Clinical implementation of digital breast tomosynthesis. Radiol Clin North Am. 2014; 52(3):499–518

[2] Kopans D, Gavenonis S, Halpern E, Moore R. Calcifications in the breast and digital breast tomosynthesis. Breast J. 2011; 17(6):638–644

[3] Spangler ML, Zuley ML, Sumkin JH, et al. Detection and classification of calcifications on digital breast tomosynthesis and 2D digital mammography: a comparison. AJR Am J Roentgenol. 2011; 196(2):320–324

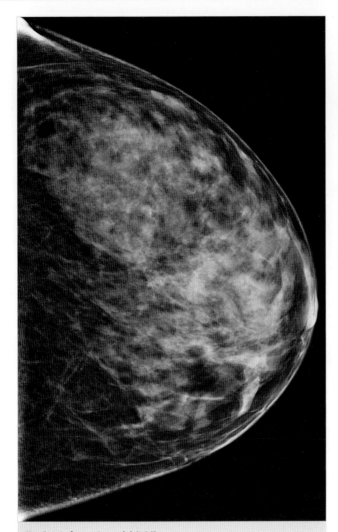

Fig. 8.1 Left craniocaudal (LCC) mammogram.

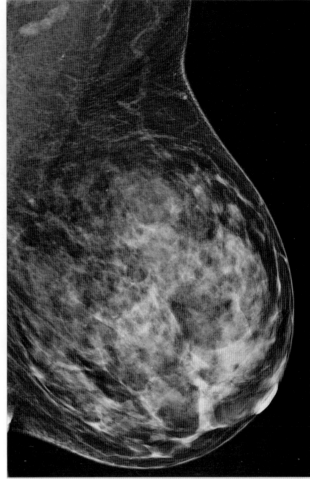

Fig. 8.2 Left mediolateral oblique (LMLO) mammogram.

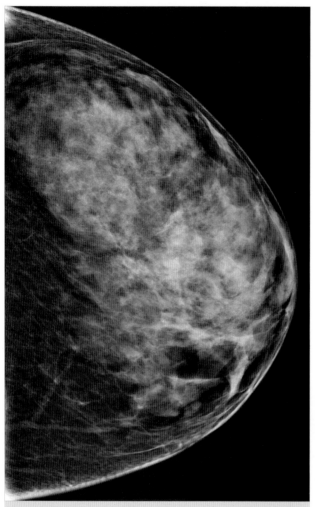

Fig. 8.3 Left craniocaudal (LCC) mammogram from 3 years ago.

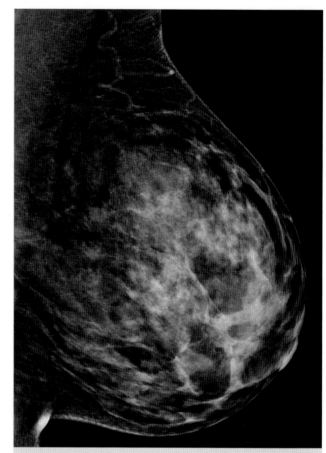

Fig. 8.4 Left mediolateral oblique (LMLO) mammogram from 3 years ago.

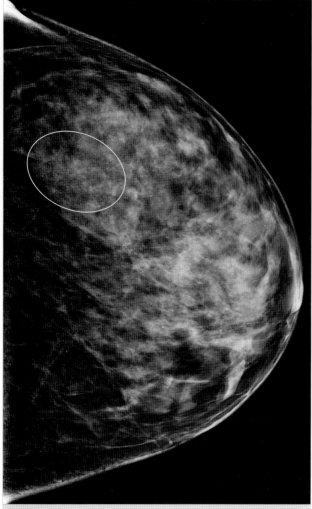

Fig. 8.5 Left craniocaudal (LCC) mammogram with label.

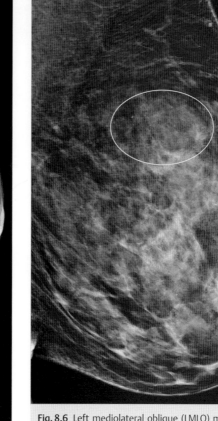

Fig. 8.6 Left mediolateral oblique (LMLO) mammogram with label.

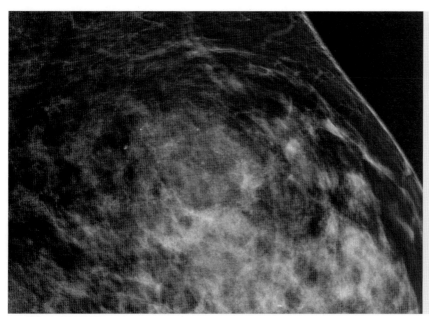

Fig. 8.7 Left mediolateral oblique (LMLO) mammogram, close-up [view.]

9 Scattered Masses

Lonie R. Salkowski

9.1 Presentation and Presenting Images

(► Fig. 9.1, ► Fig. 9.2, ► Fig. 9.3, ► Fig. 9.4)

A 42-year-old female whose mother had postmenopausal breast cancer presents for screening mammography.

9.2 Key Images

(► Fig. 9.5, ► Fig. 9.6, ► Fig. 9.7, ► Fig. 9.8, ► Fig. 9.9, ► Fig. 9.10, ► Fig. 9.11)

9.2.1 Breast Tissue Density

The breasts are heterogeneously dense, which may obscure small masses.

9.2.2 Imaging Findings

Scattered throughout both breasts, there are multiple masses of variable size. On the digital breast tomosynthesis (DBT) images at least two-thirds of the margins of the masses are circumscribed and the remaining margins are obscured (► Fig. 9.5, ► Fig. 9.6, ► Fig. 9.7, and ► Fig. 9.8). The patient had an ultrasound last year (► Fig. 9.9, ► Fig. 9.10, and ► Fig. 9.11) that demonstrated multiple simple cysts (anechoic masses with circumscribed margins and posterior acoustic enhancement).

9.3 BI-RADS Classification and Action

Category 2: Benign

9.4 Differential Diagnosis

1. **Multiple bilateral masses, benign**: All of the masses have similar features with at least 75% of the margins circumscribed and the remaining margins obscured by adjacent fibroglandular tissue.
2. *Fibroadenomas*: Patients can have multiple bilateral masses that are fibroadenomas. These would be benign as long as they fit the criteria of bilateral benign-appearing masses. In this case, the prior ultrasound of this patient revealed that these masses are cysts.
3. *Metastases*: Metastases can occur to the breast and occasionally can be the presenting sign of an unknown cancer. However, this is much less common than a benign etiology. This patient has no history of a confirmed cancer.

9.5 Essential Facts

- The BI-RADS classification of masses used for mammography should be similarly applied to DBT.
- Multiple bilateral masses is defined as having at least three masses, with at least one in each breast. The masses are at least partially circumscribed, with at least 75% of the margins circumscribed and the remaining margins obscured by adjacent fibroglandular tissue.

9.6 Management and Digital Breast Tomosynthesis Principles

- It is possible that DBT could greatly increase the cases that can be defined as multiple bilateral masses, because of DBTs ability to unmask the obscuring tissues and better define the underlying circumscribed masses.
- Thus, DBT may increase the number of masses that can be assigned a BI-RADS 2 assessment.
- A limitation of DBT can also be associated with an advantage of DBT. DBT decreases the effect of overlapping tissue, thus benign lesions that were previously concealed will be detected. Additional further evaluation may be prompted by this unmasking.

9.7 Further Reading

[1] Leung JW, Sickles EA. Multiple bilateral masses detected on screening mammography: assessment of need for recall imaging. AJR Am J Roentgenol. 2000; 175(1):23–29

[2] Roth RG, Maidment AD, Weinstein SP, Roth SO, Conant EF. Digital breast tomosynthesis: lessons learned from early clinical implementation. Radiographics. 2014; 34(4):E89–E102

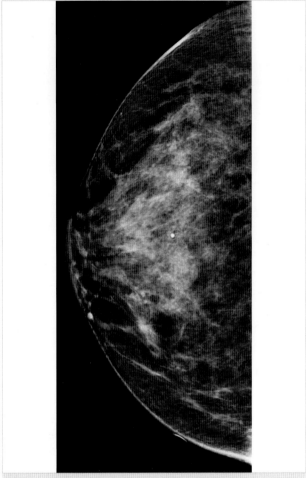

Fig. 9.1 Right craniocaudal (RCC) mammogram.

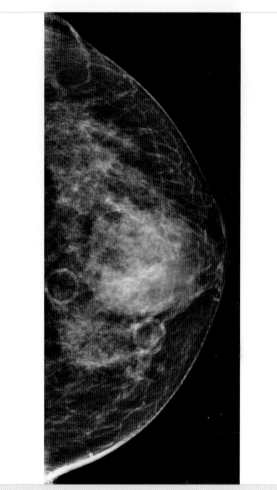

Fig. 9.2 Left craniocaudal (LCC) mammogram.

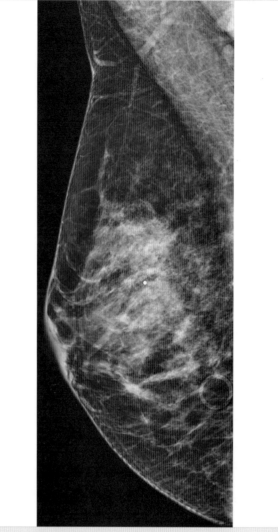

Fig. 9.3 Right mediolateral oblique (RMLO) mammogram.

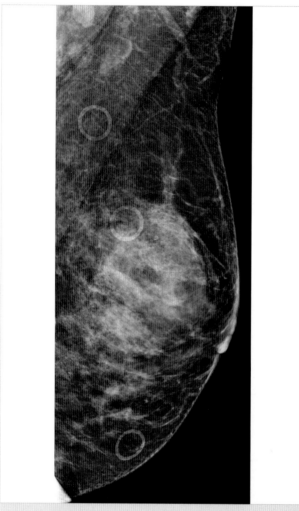

Fig. 9.4 Left mediolateral oblique (LMLO) mammogram.

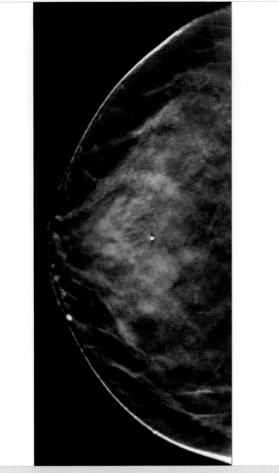

Fig. 9.5 Right craniocaudal digital breast tomosynthesis (RCC DBT), slice 37 of 73.

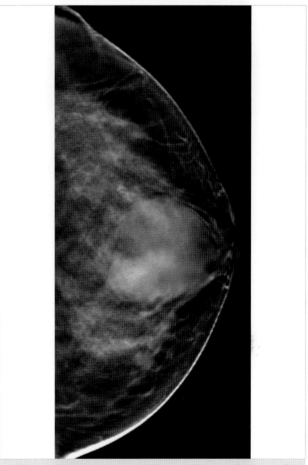

Fig. 9.6 Left craniocaudal digital breast tomosynthesis (LCC DBT), slice 37 of 75.

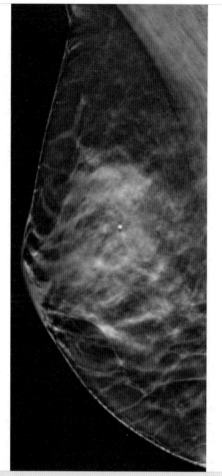

Fig. 9.7 Right mediolateral oblique digital breast tomosynthesis (RMLO DBT), slice 36 of 66.

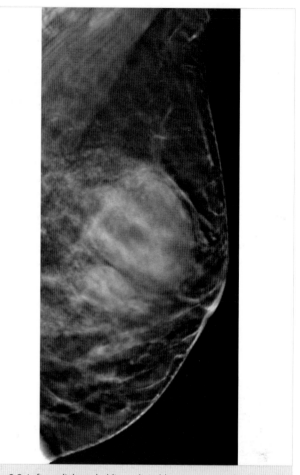

Fig. 9.8 Left mediolateral oblique digital breast tomosynthesis (LMLO DBT), slice 37 of 70.

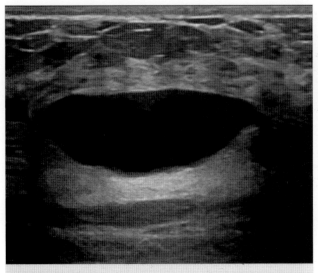

Fig. 9.9 Left breast ultrasound image from the 12 o'clock location from 1 year ago.

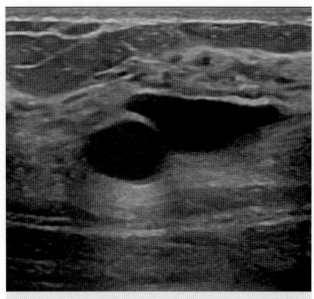

Fig. 9.10 Left breast ultrasound, transverse image from the subareolar region from 1 year ago.

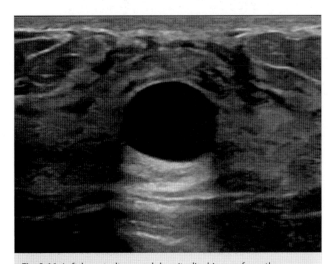

Fig. 9.11 Left breast ultrasound, longitudinal image from the subareolar region from 1 year ago.

10 Treated Breast Cancer

Lonie R. Salkowski

10.1 Presentation and Presenting Images

(▶ Fig. 10.1, ▶ Fig. 10.2, ▶ Fig. 10.3, ▶ Fig. 10.4)

A 73-year-old female with a history of left breast cancer treated with lumpectomy and radiation therapy more than 10 years ago presents for screening mammography.

10.2 Key Images

(▶ Fig. 10.5, ▶ Fig. 10.6)

10.2.1 Breast Tissue Density

There are scattered areas of fibroglandular density.

10.2.2 Imaging Findings

In the upper outer quadrant of the left breast in the middle depth at the 2 o'clock location, there is architectural distortion (▶ Fig. 10.5 and ▶ Fig. 10.6). It is located inferior and posterior to the radiopaque line marker placed on the skin over the surgical scar.

10.3 BI-RADS Classification and Action

Category 2: Benign

10.4 Differential Diagnosis

1. **Lumpectomy surgical scar**: Scars from surgery can have a variable appearance from person to person and within a person over time. The proximity of the architectural distortion to the skin marker and also the clinical history strongly favor that that this architectural distortion is due to surgery.
2. *Recurrent cancer*: The changes are stable from prior mammograms (*not shown*). There does not appear to be a new mass, increased density, or calcifications, which would suggest recurrence.
3. *Skin-fold changes*: The changes appear to be internal to the breast. Skin folds and skin lesions can simulate breast lesions; however, the digital breast tomosynthesis (DBT) images would localize the findings to the skin.

10.5 Essential Facts

- Skin markers on surgical scars can greatly assist in determining if an architectural distortion is due to surgery or represents a finding needing further evaluation.
- Similar to conventional mammography, postsurgical changes seen on DBT should have similar appearances and conventions (and intervals) for following to ascertain stability and change.
- Typical breast-conserving–treatment (BCT) changes are skin thickening, increased parenchymal markings, a stellate or masslike density at the surgical site, and dystrophic calcifications. These changes will vary over time.
- The lumpectomy site appears as a spiculated, poorly defined soft-tissue density with interspersed radiolucent areas of trapped fat.

10.6 Management and Digital Breast Tomosynthesis Principles

- Architectural distortion seen on DBT that is not attributed to a surgical scar and not seen on mammography or sonography should be considered suspicious. Biopsy would be warranted. DBT needle localization or DBT-guided core needle biopsy are options for tissue sampling.
- Patients treated with BCT have a long-term risk of recurrence estimated at 1 to 2.5% per year.
- Recurrence at a lumpectomy site is suggested by the lack of central radiolucent areas, a central mass, fine straight spiculations, and an increase in size or nodularity of the scar. On DBT, a partial central lucent area may be seen due to the unmasking of the summation effects of conventional mammography.

10.7 Further Reading

[1] Dershaw DD. Breast imaging and the conservative treatment of breast cancer. Radiol Clin North Am. 2002; 40(3):501–516
[2] Freer PE, Niell B, Rafferty EA. Preoperative Tomosynthesis-guided Needle Localization of Mammographically and Sonographically Occult Breast Lesions. Radiology. 2015; 275(2):377–383

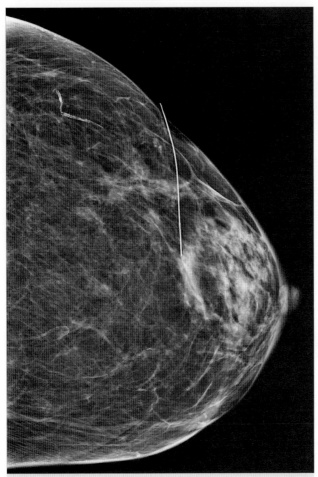

Fig. 10.1 Left craniocaudal (LCC) mammogram.

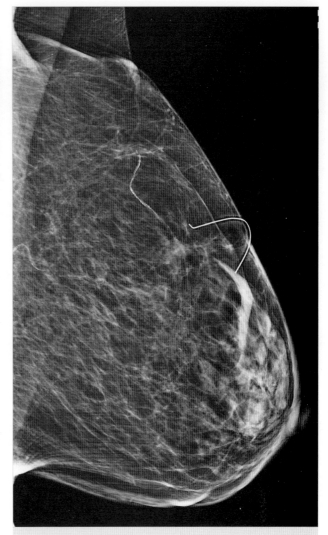

Fig. 10.2 Left mediolateral oblique (LMLO) mammogram.

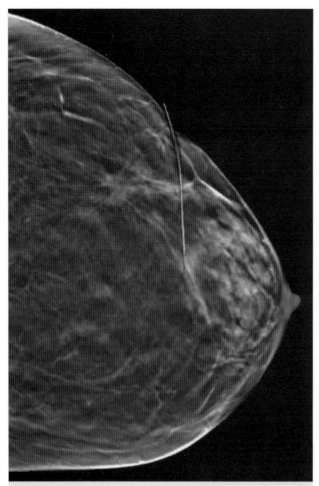

Fig. 10.3 Left craniocaudal digital breast tomosynthesis (LCC DBT), slice 20 of 49.

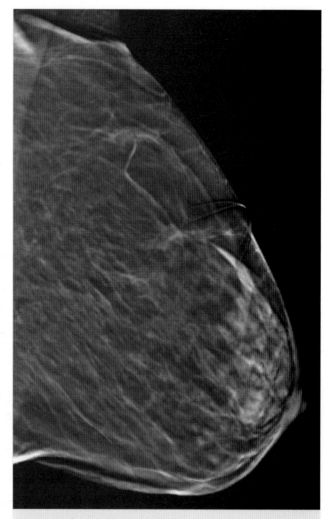

Fig. 10.4 Left mediolateral oblique digital breast tomosynthesis (LMLO DBT), slice 19 of 56.

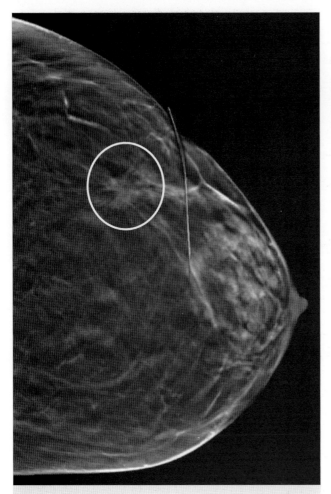

Fig. 10.5 Left craniocaudal digital breast tomosynthesis (LCC DBT), slice 20 of 49 with label.

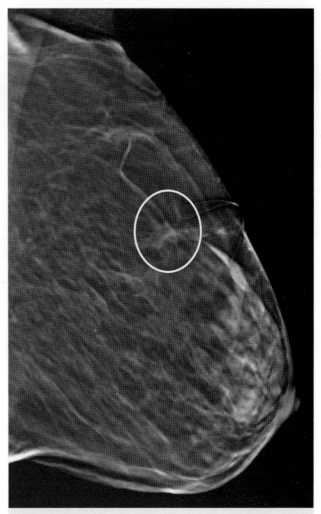

Fig. 10.6 Left mediolateral oblique digital breast tomosynthesis (LMLO DBT), slice 19 of 56 with label.

11 "Hairy" Skin Edge

Tanya W. Moseley

11.1 Presentation and Presenting Images

(▶ Fig. 11.1, ▶ Fig. 11.2, ▶ Fig. 11.3, ▶ Fig. 11.4, ▶ Fig. 11.5, ▶ Fig. 11.6, ▶ Fig. 11.7, ▶ Fig. 11.8)

A 67-year-old female presents for routine screening mammography.

11.2 Key Images

(▶ Fig. 11.9, ▶ Fig. 11.10, ▶ Fig. 11.11, ▶ Fig. 11.12, ▶ Fig. 11.13, ▶ Fig. 11.14, ▶ Fig. 11.15, ▶ Fig. 11.16, ▶ Fig. 11.17, ▶ Fig. 11.18)

11.2.1 Breast Tissue Density

There are scattered areas of fibroglandular density.

11.2.2 Imaging Findings

Postbiopsy clips (*arrows* in ▶ Fig. 11.12) are noted in the middle depth of the upper outer quadrant of each breast. The conventional mammograms and the synthetic mammograms demonstrate no suspicious calcifications, asymmetries, masses, or architectural distortions. Unread lines with the appearance of 'hair on end' (*box*) are seen on the synthetic mammograms (▶ Fig. 11.9, ▶ Fig. 11.10, ▶ Fig. 11.11, and ▶ Fig. 11.12) and on the first and last slices of both of the craniocaudal (CC) tomosynthesis movies (▶ Fig. 11.13, ▶ Fig. 11.14, ▶ Fig. 11.15, and ▶ Fig. 11.16) and on the last slices of both of the mediolateral oblique (MLO) tomosynthesis movies (▶ Fig. 11.17 and ▶ Fig. 11.18).

11.3 BI-RADS Classification and Action

None: Technical recall

11.4 Differential Diagnosis

1. **Technical artifact**: There is detector failure occurring causing the line artifacts on the synthetic mammograms and the tomosynthesis movies. Note that these lines are in the direction of the acquisition of the tomosynthesis images.

2. *Negative/benign study*: There are no suspicious findings in either breast; however, this case is not"completely negative" due to technical factors. It should be recalled to resolve the issues.

3. *Missed finding*: Sometimes mammograms are interpreted as negative or benign when there is an abnormality. There is not a missed finding on this mammogram.

11.5 Essential Facts

- As detectors become damaged the result is the failure of a line reading out during the reading of the detector. If noticed immediately by the technologist, the image can be repeated. The system may correct itself on repeat exposure.
- Artifacts can obscure findings that warrant attention and can create pseudolesions.
- Artifacts in digital mammography can involve the imaging detector, the equipment, the patient, and the processing and storage of the images.
- Detector-based artifacts are dead pixels, dead or unread lines, non-uniformities, and ghosting.

11.6 Management and Digital Breast Tomosynthesis Principles

- Imaging artifacts can occur in conventional digital mammography and during tomosynthesis. It is important to recognize these promptly. Some artifacts occur due to individual patient factors (hair, clothing, motion) and others are due to technical equipment issues. It is important to recognize equipment and processing-related artifacts so they can be promptly addressed and not compromise patient care.
- There is an increased radiation dose with combined conventional and tomosynthesis mammography. Having to repeat a study further increases the radiation exposure.

11.7 Further Reading

[1] Geiser W, Whitman G, Haygood T, et al. Artifacts in digital mammography. http://www.aapm.org/meetings/amos2/pdf/41–10046–70873–266.pdf

[2] Sechopoulos I. A review of breast tomosynthesis. Part II. Image reconstruction, processing and analysis, and advanced applications. Med Phys. 2013; 40(1):014302

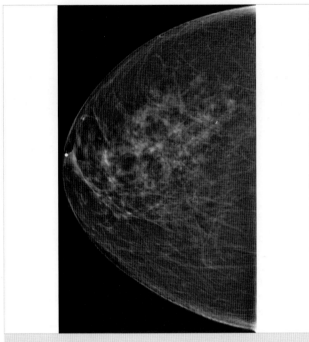

Fig. 11.1 Right craniocaudal (RCC) mammogram.

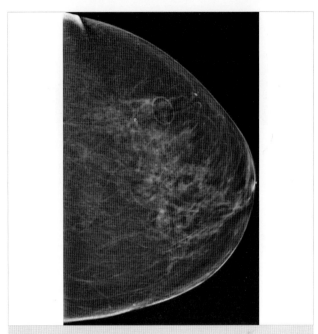

Fig. 11.2 Left craniocaudal (LCC) mammogram.

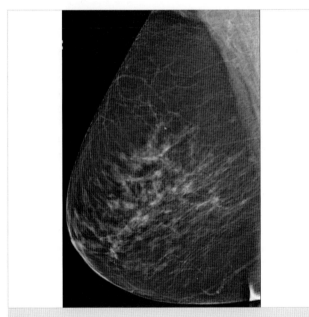

Fig. 11.3 Right mediolateral oblique (RMLO) mammogram.

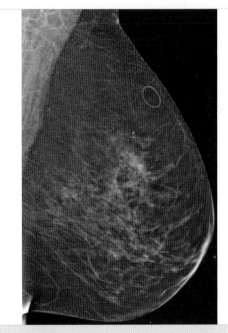

Fig. 11.4 Left mediolateral oblique (LMLO) mammogram.

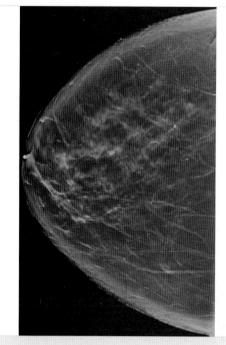

Fig. 11.5 Right craniocaudal (RCC) synthetic mammogram.

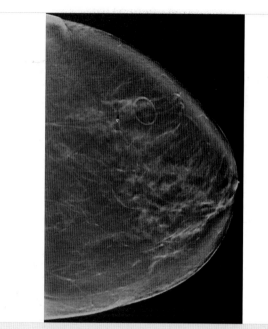

Fig. 11.6 Left craniocaudal (LCC) synthetic mammogram.

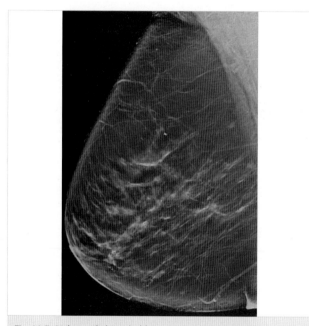

Fig. 11.7 Right mediolateral oblique (RMLO) synthetic mammogram.

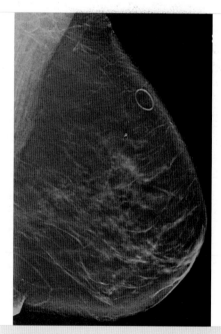

Fig. 11.8 Left mediolateral oblique (LMLO) synthetic mammogram.

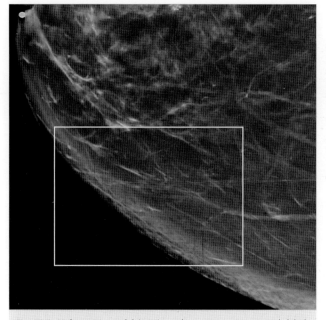

Fig. 11.9 Right craniocaudal (RCC) synthetic mammogram with label.

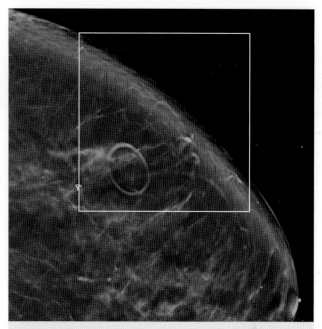

Fig. 11.10 Left craniocaudal (LCC) synthetic mammogram with label.

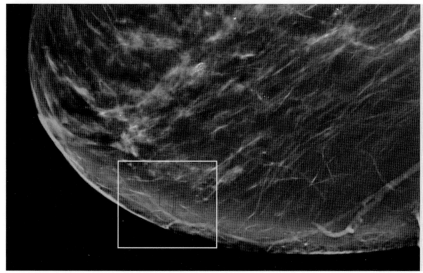

Fig. 11.11 Right mediolateral oblique (RMLO) synthetic mammogram with label.

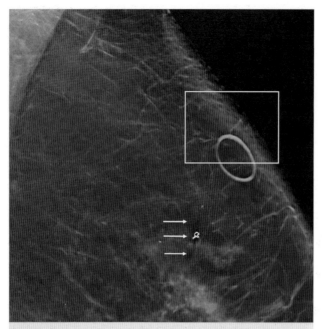

Fig. 11.12 Left mediolateral oblique (LMLO) synthetic mammogram with label.

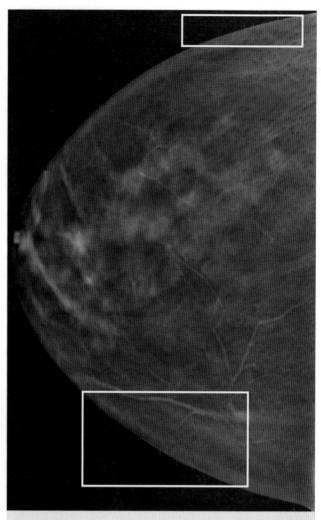

Fig. 11.13 Right craniocaudal digital breast tomosynthesis (RCC DBT), slice 1 of 101.

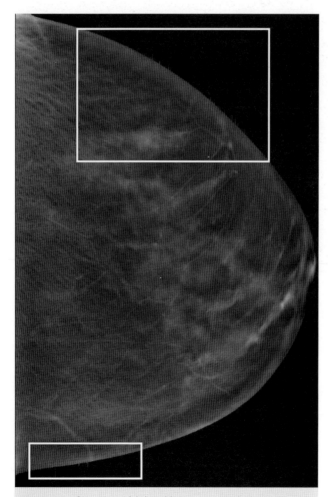

Fig. 11.14 Left craniocaudal digital breast tomosynthesis (LCC DBT), slice 1 of 107.

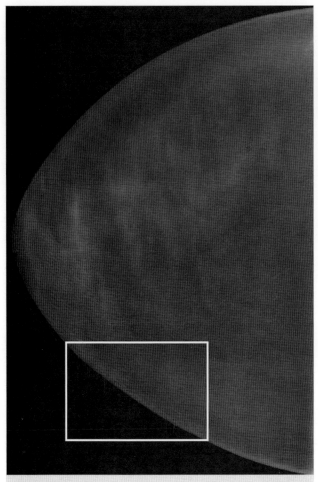

Fig. 11.15 Right craniocaudal digital breast tomosynthesis (RCC DBT), slice 101 of 101.

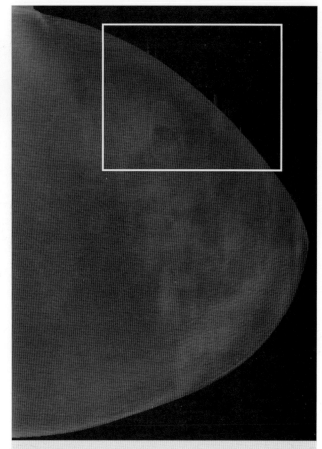

Fig. 11.16 Left craniocaudal digital breast tomosynthesis (LCC DBT), slice 107 of 107.

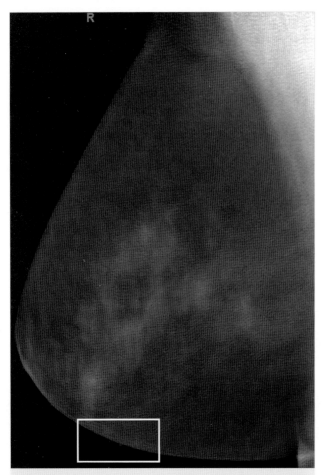

Fig. 11.17 Right mediolateral oblique digital breast tomosynthesis (RMLO DBT), slice 95 of 95.

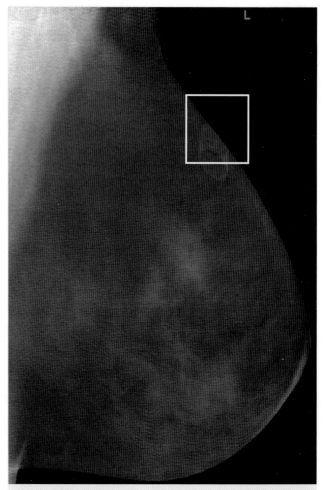

Fig. 11.18 Left mediolateral oblique digital breast tomosynthesis (LMLO DBT), slice 96 of 96.

12 Linear Calcifications

Lonie R. Salkowski

12.1 Presentation and Presenting Images

(▶ Fig. 12.1, ▶ Fig. 12.2, ▶ Fig. 12.3, ▶ Fig. 12.4)

A 60-year-old female with history of right breast cancer treated with lumpectomy and radiation therapy presents for a screening mammogram.

12.2 Key images

(▶ Fig. 12.5, ▶ Fig. 12.6)

12.2.1 Breast Tissue Density

There are scattered areas of fibroglandular density.

12.2.2 Imaging Findings

In the upper outer and the lower inner quadrants of the right breast, there are large linear rodlike calcifications. The calcifications in the lower inner quadrant are well seen in a ductal distribution on the DBT images (▶ Fig. 12.5 and ▶ Fig. 12.6).

12.3 BI-RADS Classification and Action

Category 2: Benign

12.4 Differential Diagnosis

1. *Secretory calcifications*: These calcifications are thick and rodlike in a ductal pattern radiating from the nipple.
2. *Ductal carcinoma in situ (DCIS)*: DCIS and secretory calcifications can have the same distribution as they both involve the ducts. The calcifications in DCIS are often finer, irregular, and not smooth like those seen in secretory calcifications.
3. *Vascular calcifications*: In the early phase of vessel-wall calcification, the hallmark parallel "tram-track" appearance

may not be present. The calcifications are less dense and can appear as "dot-dash" and linear. These calcifications do not have this appearance.

12.5 Essential Facts

- Secretory calcifications are often described as large rodlike. They are greater than or equal to 1 mm in diameter and can be 3 to 10 mm in length.
- Secretory calcifications require no treatment or intervention, except for routine follow-up.
- The large size of secretory calcifications makes them clearly delineated on DBT.
- The orientation of the secretory calcifications in this case allow for large regions of the ductal distribution to be identified in both the craniocaudal (CC) and mediolateral oblique digital breast tomosynthesis (MLO DBT) image sets.

12.6 Management and Digital Breast Tomosynthesis Principles

- Most secretory calcifications are detected on routine screening.
- Secretory calcifications can increase over time.
- DBT likely does not contribute much to making the diagnosis of secretory calcifications compared to full-field digital mammography (FFDM). It is important to be aware of the different patterns of benign calcifications on DBT.
- When secretory calcifications are extensive, it can be difficult to identify suspicious calcifications in their midst.
- The early phase of secretory calcifications can mimic DCIS.

12.7 Further Reading

[1] Baker JA, Lo JY. Breast tomosynthesis: state-of-the-art and review of the literature. Acad Radiol. 2011; 18(10):1298–1310
[2] Spangler ML, Zuley ML, Sumkin JH, et al. Detection and classification of calcifications on digital breast tomosynthesis and 2D digital mammography: a comparison. AJR Am J Roentgenol. 2011; 196(2):320–324

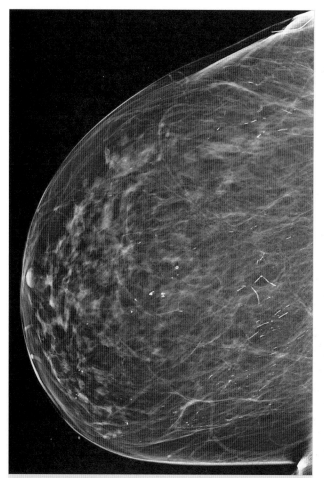

Fig. 12.1 Right craniocaudal (RCC) mammogram.

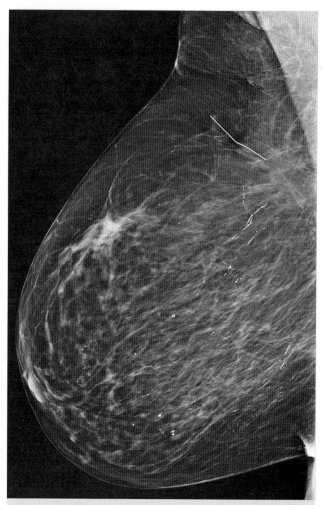

Fig. 12.2 Right mediolateral oblique (RMLO) mammogram.

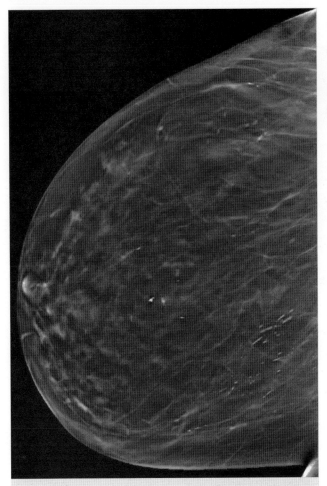

Fig. 12.3 Right craniocaudal digital breast tomosynthesis (RCC DBT), slice 17 of 80.

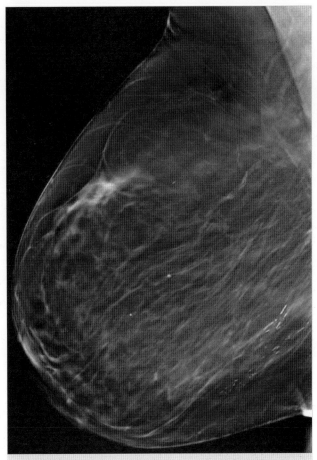

Fig. 12.4 Right mediolateral oblique digital breast tomosynthesis (RMLO DBT), slice 44 of 89.

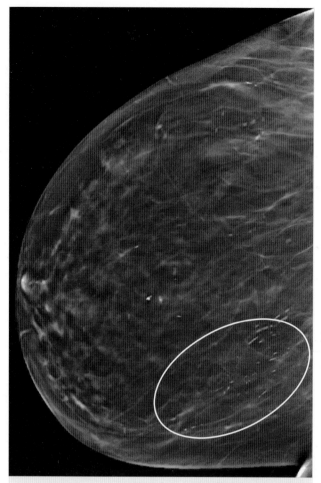

Fig. 12.5 Right craniocaudal digital breast tomosynthesis (RCC DBT), slice 17 of 80 with label.

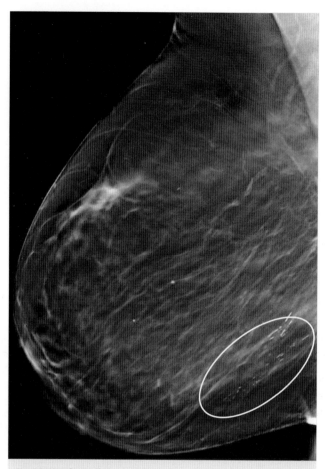

Fig. 12.6 Right mediolateral oblique digital breast tomosynthesis (RMLO DBT), slice 44 of 89 with label.

13 Multiple Masses

Tanya W. Moseley

13.1 Presentation and Presenting Images

(▶ Fig. 13.1, ▶ Fig. 13.2, ▶ Fig. 13.3, ▶ Fig. 13.4, ▶ Fig. 13.5, ▶ Fig. 13.6)

A 58-year-old female with a history of Crohn's disease presents for routine screening mammography.

13.2 Key images

(▶ Fig. 13.7, ▶ Fig. 13.8, ▶ Fig. 13.9, ▶ Fig. 13.10)

13.2.1 Breast Tissue Density

The breasts are heterogeneously dense, which may obscure small masses.

13.2.2 Imaging Findings

The imaging of the left breast is normal (*not shown*). The right breast demonstrates multiple obscured masses with a dominant mass (*circle*) at the 5 to 6 o'clock location. This mass is well-circumscribed on both conventional mammographic (▶ Fig. 13.7, ▶ Fig. 13.8) and tomosynthesis imaging (▶ Fig. 13.9, ▶ Fig. 13.10). The tomosynthesis images further define the margins of the smaller lesions (best seen on the tomosynthesis movie). The dominant mass is stable compared to prior mammographic evaluations (▶ Fig. 13.5, ▶ Fig. 13.6) and its borders are well-circumscribed on conventional mammographic imaging.

13.3 BI-RADS Classification and Action

Category 2: Benign

13.4 Differential Diagnosis

1. *Cyst*: Cysts are often multiple, usually bilateral, and may be painful and fluctuate in size. They are most common in 30- to 50-year-old patients. Cysts can appear as well-circumscribed masses.
2. *Fibroadenoma*: Fibroadenomas are the most common benign masses in young women. They may be multiple in 10 to 15% of patients. Fibroadenomas can appear as well-circumscribed masses.
3. *Breast cancer*: Breast cancer may present as a well-circumscribed mass; however, it is much less common. Careful evaluation of imaging characteristics is necessary, and, if there is doubt, then additional diagnostic imaging should be performed including an ultrasound.

13.5 Essential Facts

- By definition, the term multiple bilateral masses refers to at least three masses total with at least one mass in each breast.
- Multiple obscured or partially obscured masses have margins hidden by overlying breast tissue. Tomosynthesis and ultrasound are helpful to define the margins of these masses.
- Leung and Sickles (2000) found that the frequency of cancer development and the stage of cancer diagnosis in patients not recalled for multiple bilateral breast masses are similar to those seen in the general screening population. The authors concluded that recall for multiple masses did not appear to be justified.
- To be considered partially circumscribed, at least 75% of the margins should be circumscribed and the remaining 25% should be obscured. No portion of the margins should be considered indistinct.

13.6 Management and Digital Breast Tomosynthesis Principles

- In the study by Rafferty and colleagues (2013), it was discovered that care must be taken to avoid misclassification of malignant lesions. Some cancers seen on tomosynthesis as circumscribed lobular masses were being dismissed by some readers. This is because radiologists most often associate circumscribed masses with benign or probably benign lesions.
- In this case each mass could be evaluated individually.
- The slices on tomosynthesis reduce or eliminate breast tissue overlap and structural noise seen in single slice conventional mammographic imaging. Only findings on the imaged section appear sharp, whereas those above or below appear out of focus. This allows each lesion to be carefully assessed independent from the other lesions or distractions in the breast tissue.
- Tomosynthesis reduces callbacks for benign findings but increases interpretation time.

13.7 Further Reading

[1] Leung JW, Sickles EA. Multiple bilateral masses detected on screening mammography: assessment of need for recall imaging. AJR Am J Roentgenol. 2000; 175(1):23–29

[2] Rafferty EA, Park JM, Philpotts LE, et al. Assessing radiologist performance using combined digital mammography and breast tomosynthesis compared with digital mammography alone: results of a multicenter, multireader trial. Radiology. 2013; 266(1):104–113

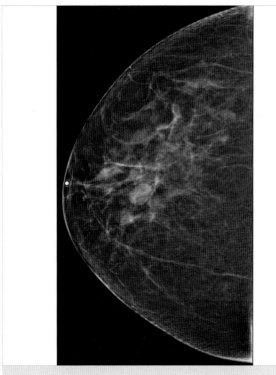

Fig. 13.1 Right craniocaudal (RCC) mammogram.

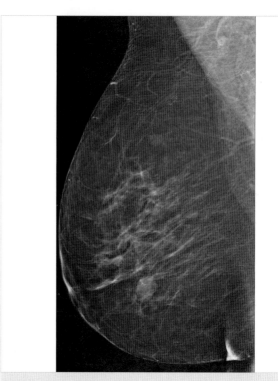

Fig. 13.2 Right mediolateral oblique (RMLO) mammogram.

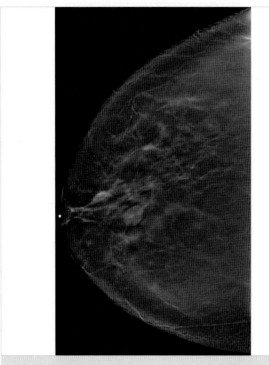

Fig. 13.3 Right craniocaudal digital breast tomosynthesis (RCC DBT), slice 23 of 106.

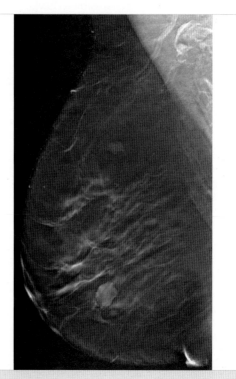

Fig. 13.4 Right mediolateral oblique digital breast tomosynthesis (RMLO DBT), slice 39 of 108.

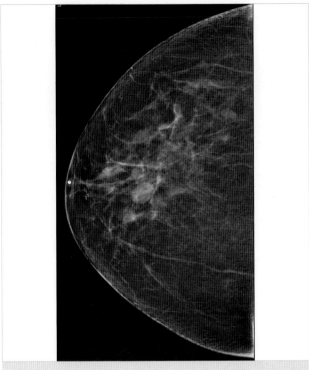

Fig. 13.5 Right craniocaudal (RCC) mammogram comparison.

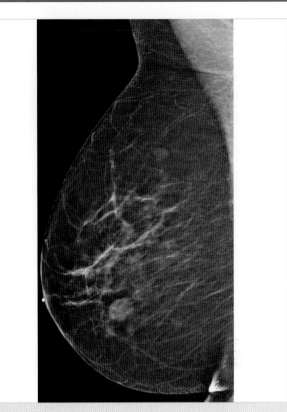

Fig. 13.6 Right mediolateral oblique (RMLO) mammogram comparison.

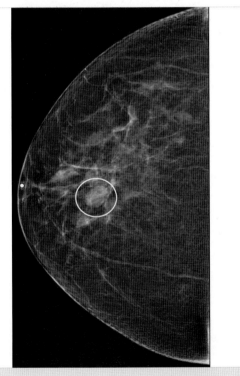

Fig. 13.7 Right craniocaudal (RCC) mammogram with label.

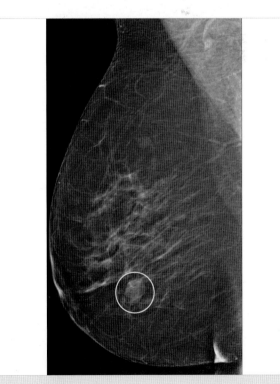

Fig. 13.8 Right mediolateral oblique (RMLO) mammogram with label.

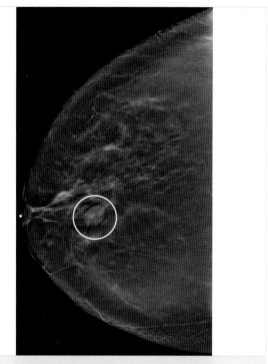

Fig. 13.9 Right craniocaudal digital breast tomosynthesis (RCC DBT), slice 23 of 106 with label.

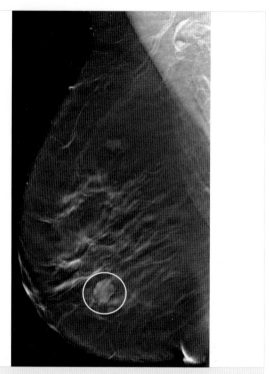

Fig. 13.10 Left mediolateral oblique digial breast tomosynthesis (LMLO DBT), slice 39 of 108 with label.

14 Nonpalpable Mass with Mixed Composition

Lonie R. Salkowski

14.1 Presentation and Presenting Images

(▶ Fig. 14.1, ▶ Fig. 14.2, ▶ Fig. 14.3, ▶ Fig. 14.4)

A 44-year-old female presents for asymptomatic screening mammography.

14.2 Key Images

(▶ Fig. 14.5, ▶ Fig. 14.6, ▶ Fig. 14.7, ▶ Fig. 14.8)

14.2.1 Breast Tissue Density

The breasts are heterogeneously dense, which may obscure small masses.

14.2.2 Imaging Findings

Within the subareolar region of the right breast, there is a partially circumscribed and partially obscured mass with heterogeneous composition. There are elements of fat and fibroglandular tissue within the mass. The anterior, medial/lateral, and superior/inferior margins are well seen on the conventional digital mammograms (▶ Fig. 14.5 and ▶ Fig. 14.6). The posterior margin is obscured. The synthetic mammograms highlight this mass within the breast tissue and make it stand out more than on the conventional mammogram (▶ Fig. 14.3 and ▶ Fig. 14.4). The digital breast tomosynthesis (DBT) images better define all margins of this mass (▶ Fig. 14.7 and ▶ Fig. 14.8). The craniocaudal (CC) DBT is best for demonstrating the posterior margin (▶ Fig. 14.7). The left breast is normal.

14.3 BI-RADS Classification and Action

Category 2: Benign

14.4 Differential Diagnosis

1. **Hamartoma**: This mass is encapsulated which is clearly seen on the DBT images. It also contains adipose and fibroglandular components.

2. *Fibroadenoma*: These masses do not contain adipose components, They are isodense masses that typically present as circumscribed or partially circumscribed masses.
3. *Lipoma*: Lipomas are encapsulated fatty masses; however, they do not contain fibroglandular components.

14.5 Essential Facts

- Hamartomas account for 4.8% of benign breast tumors.
- Most hamartomas are asymptomatic, but, if symptomatic, they present as a palpable lump.
- Histologically hamartomas have all the constituents of normal breast tissue and thus are often reported as normal breast tissue on a biopsy report.
- Hamartomas consist of varying degrees of normal breast tissue elements (benign parenchyma, epithelium, fibrous tissue, and adipose tissue).
- Mammographically hamartomas appear as encapsulated or pseudoencapsulated tumors, but microscopically they are not encapsulated. Rather, the margin is composed of condensed fibrous tissue or collagen around the mass.
- At DBT, a hamartoma has a round or oval shape with a thin, water-density capsule delineating its border.

14.6 Management and Digital Breast Tomosynthesis Principles

- Most encapsulated masses that contain fat, such as hamartomas, lipomas, galactoceles, and lipid cysts, can be classified as benign.
- Hamartomas (also called fibroadenolipomas) contain normal components of breast tissue. They are benign masses; however, due to their breast tissue components, they have the risk of developing breast cancer within them. Suspicious findings within a hamartoma should be evaluated.

14.7 Further Reading

[1] Freer PE, Wang JL, Rafferty EA. Digital breast tomosynthesis in the analysis of fat-containing lesions. Radiographics. 2014; 34(2):343–358
[2] Wahner-Roedler DL, Sebo TJ, Gisvold JJ. Hamartomas of the breast: clinical, radiologic, and pathologic manifestations. Breast J. 2001; 7(2):101–105

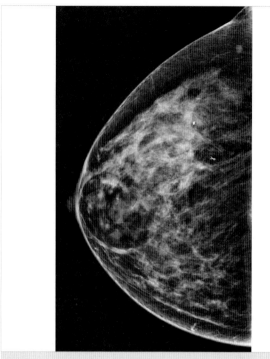

Fig. 14.1 Right craniocaudal (RCC) mammogram.

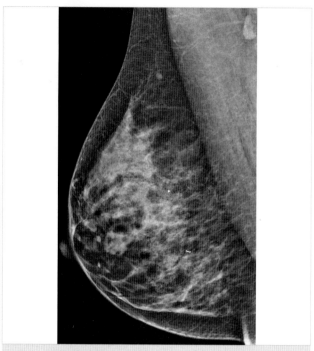

Fig. 14.2 Right mediolateral oblique (RMLO) mammogram.

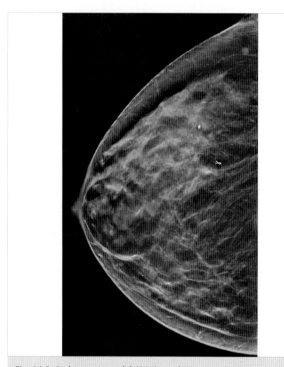

Fig. 14.3 Right craniocaudal (RCC) synthetic mammogram.

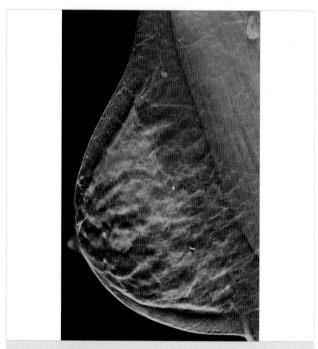

Fig. 14.4 Right mediolateral oblique (RMLO) synthetic mammogram.

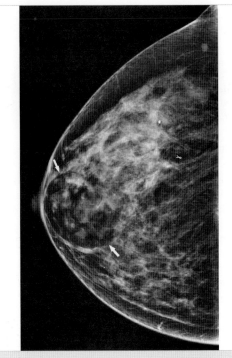

Fig. 14.5 Right craniocaudal (RCC) mammogram with label.

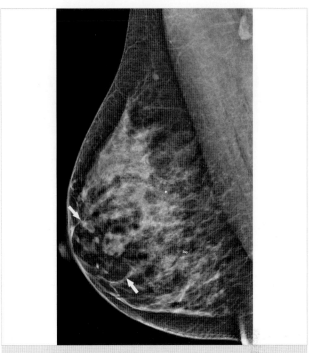

Fig. 14.6 Right mediolateral oblique (RMLO) mammogram with label.

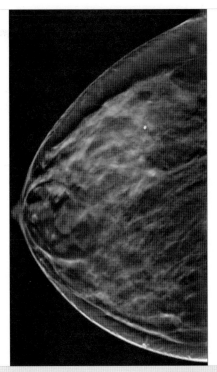

Fig. 14.7 Right craniocaudal digital breast tomosynthesis (RCC DBT), slice 19 of 60.

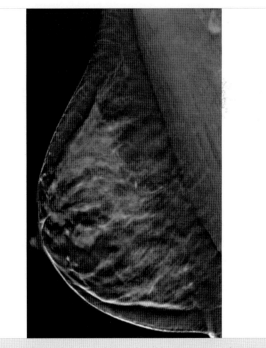

Fig. 14.8 Right mediolateral oblique digital breast tomosynthesis (RMLO DBT), slice 32 of 60.

15 Calcifications

Tanya W. Moseley

15.1 Presentation and Presenting Images

(▸ Fig. 15.1, ▸ Fig. 15.2, ▸ Fig. 15.3, ▸ Fig. 15.4)

A 64-year-old female with a distant history of small lymphocytic lymphoma presents for routine screening mammography.

15.2 Key Images

(▸ Fig. 15.5, ▸ Fig. 15.6, ▸ Fig. 15.7, ▸ Fig. 15.8)

15.2.1 Breast Tissue Density

The breasts are almost entirely fatty.

15.2.2 Imaging Findings

The imaging of the right breast is normal (*not shown*). The left breast demonstrates a group of calcifications (*solid arrow*) in the lower inner quadrant at the 7 o'clock location, 12 cm from the nipple. The left breast tomosynthesis localizes the calcifications to the skin and the inferior-most slice, slice 1 of 60 on the left craniocaudal (LCC) tomosynthesis movie (▸ Fig. 15.7). A mole on the inferior breast, denoted with a circle skin marker (*broken arrow*), is also seen on this slice.

15.3 BI-RADS Classification and Action

Category 2: Benign

15.4 Differential Diagnosis

1. **Skin calcifications**: The tomosynthesis imaging localizes the calcifications to the inferior-most slice of the CC tomosynthesis movie.
2. *Intraparenchymal calcifications*: The calcifications localize to the skin, not within the breast, making this an unlikely possibility.

3. *Artifact*: This finding is reproduced on the both conventional and tomosynthesis imaging. It appears to be within the skin and not on the skin, such as many powders or lotions present.

15.5 Essential Facts

- Before tomosynthesis was available, tangential films were used to diagnose skin lesions and skin calcifications. Now tomosynthesis imaging can easily and quickly localize findings including calcifications to the dermis.
- Skin calcifications may be confused with intraparenchymal calcifications.
- Homer and colleagues described the tattoo sign, which can help radiologists differentiate between dermal and intraparenchymal calcifications.
- Calcifications that maintain a fixed relationship to each other—the tattoo sign—suggest a dermal location.
- Skin calcifications are benign and do not require biopsy.

15.6 Management and Digital Breast Tomosynthesis Principles

- If these calcifications were assessed to be suspicious, an attempt at biopsy would have been unsuccessful. Tomosynthesis evaluation would have avoided an unnecessary biopsy.
- For the person new to tomosynthesis but with the knowledge that the circular marker denoted a mole on the inferior breast, the location of the mole on slice 1 of 60 on the LCC tomosynthesis movie would have alerted him or her to the dermal location of the calcifications.
- Knowing the orientation of the slices makes localizing findings with tomosynthesis easy.
- Tomosynthesis can perform all images that conventional mammography can perform, except a magnification view. The inability to perform magnification views is a limitation of tomosynthesis.

15.7 Further Reading

[1] Homer MJ, D'Orsi CJ, Sitzman SB. Dermal calcifications in fixed orientation: the tattoo sign. Radiology. 1994; 192(1):161–163

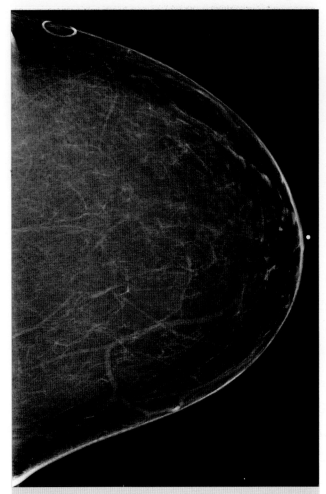

Fig. 15.1 Left craniocaudal (LCC) mammogram.

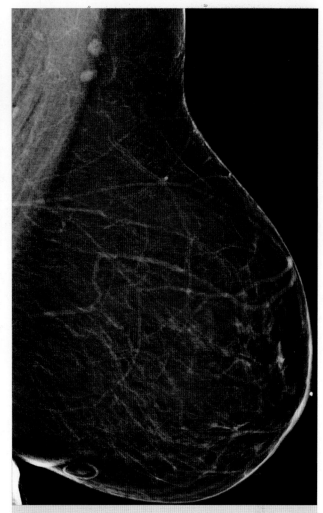

Fig. 15.2 Left mediolateral oblique (LMLO) mammmogram.

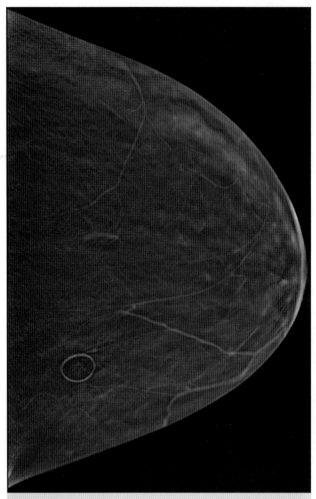

Fig. 15.3 Left craniocaudal digital breast tomosynthesis (LCC DBT), slice 1 of 60.

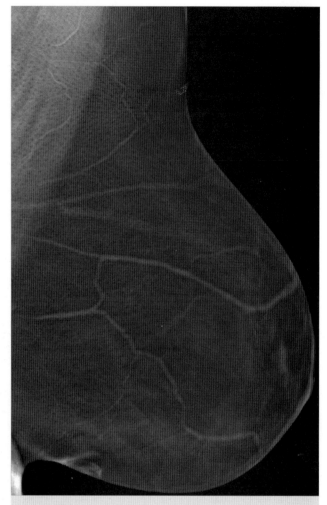

Fig. 15.4 Left mediolateral oblique digital breast tomosynthesis (LMLO DBT), slice 69 of 76.

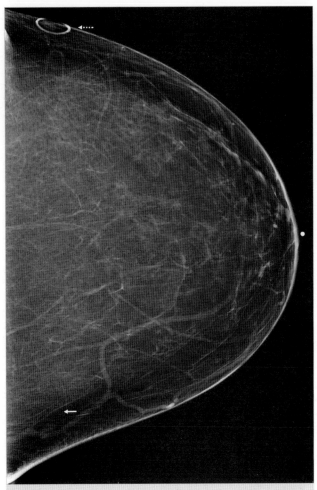

Fig. 15.5 Left craniocaudal (LCC) mammogram with label.

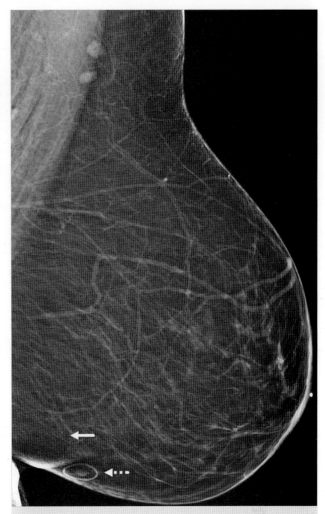

Fig. 15.6 Left mediolateral oblique (LMLO) mammogram with label.

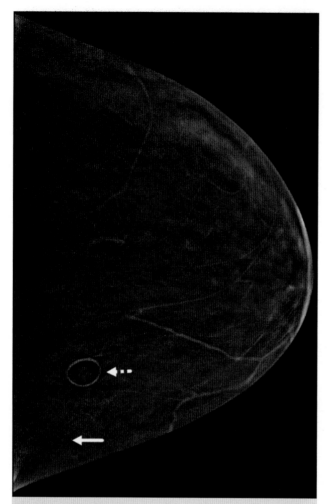

Fig. 15.7 Left craniocaudal digital breast tomosynthesis (LCC DBT), slice 1 of 60 with label.

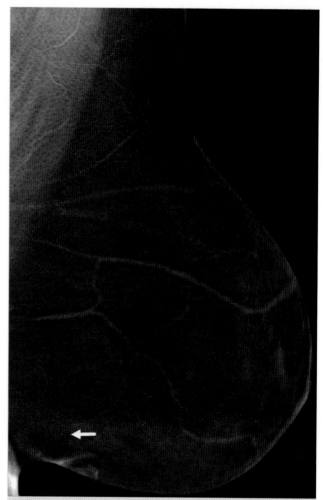

Fig. 15.8 Left mediolateral oblique digital breast tomosynthesis (LMLO DBT), slice 69 of 76 with label.

16 Architectural Distortion

Tanya W. Moseley

16.1 Presentation and Presenting Images

(▶ Fig. 16.1, ▶ Fig. 16.2, ▶ Fig. 16.3, ▶ Fig. 16.4, ▶ Fig. 16.5, ▶ Fig. 16.6)

An 83-year-old female with a history of left breast cancer (invasive ductal carcinoma) treated 15 years ago presents for screening mammography.

16.2 Key Images

(▶ Fig. 16.7, ▶ Fig. 16.8, ▶ Fig. 16.9, ▶ Fig. 16.10, ▶ Fig. 16.11, ▶ Fig. 16.12)

16.2.1 Breast Tissue Density

The breasts are heterogeneously dense, which may obscure small masses.

16.2.2 Imaging Findings

The patient was previously treated for invasive ductal carcinoma with a lumpectomy and radiation therapy. The imaging shows a postsurgical scar (*circle*) with associated architectural distortion, focal skin thickening, and surgical clips in the left breast upper outer quadrant at the 1 o'clock location, 6 cm from the nipple (▶ Fig. 16.7, ▶ Fig. 16.8, ▶ Fig. 16.10, and ▶ Fig. 16.11). There is no mammographic evidence of recurrent disease. The skin is marked with a scar marker (*solid arrow* in ▶ Fig. 16.7 and ▶ Fig. 16.10) and coarse vascular calcifications are noted by the *broken arrow* (▶ Fig. 16.7, ▶ Fig. 16.9, ▶ Fig. 16.10, and ▶ Fig. 16.12).

16.2.3 BI-RADS Classification and Action

Category 2: Benign

16.3 Differential Diagnosis

1. **Postsurgical changes**: The architectural changes at the postsurgical bed seen on the conventional two-dimensional (2D) mammogram or on tomosynthesis images are typical findings.
2. *Recurrent breast cancer*: There is no evidence of a mass, developing asymmetry, or suspicious calcifications in the postsurgical bed on either the conventional 2D mammogram or on tomosynthesis images.
3. *Radial sclerosing lesion*: The clinical history and postsurgical changes make a radial sclerosing lesion a very unlikely diagnosis. Without the clinical history, this could be a reasonable possible diagnosis.

16.3.1 Essential Facts

- Postsurgical scars usually present as an area of architectural distortion with interspersed radiolucency, which represents entrapped fat. Typically scars contract over time. Tomosynthesis reduces overlap and demonstrates entrapped fat within postsurgical scars.
- Radiologists can differentiate between postsurgical changes and recurrent malignancy by having a knowledge of characteristic imaging findings of both entities.
- Postoperative changes usually decrease in size over time. Recurrence may be seen as a new mass, new calcifications, a new asymmetry, or a new area of architectural distortion in the lumpectomy site. Tomosynthesis can help to differentiate between a true mass lesion and a summation artifact resulting from overlapping breast tissue.
- Findings that are equivocal or suspicious for recurrence warrant biopsy. If the findings are sonographically occult, biopsy may be performed using tomosynthesis guidance.
- There are no suspicious findings. The calcifications present in this case are vascular. Tomosynthesis is helpful to demonstrate the orientation and location of the vascular calcifications. The location of the vascular calcifications is importation information if a biopsy is needed.

16.4 Management and Digital Breast Tomosynthesis Principles

- Postsurgical masses, fluid collections, architectural distortions, scars, edema, skin thickening, and calcifications can mimic or mask recurrent malignancy. The three-dimensional imaging capability of tomosynthesis eliminates overlapping tissue providing imaging clarity of findings and the ability to accurately characterize lesions.
- Performing conventional mammography and tomosynthesis imaging in a single compression allows for co-registration of these images, which allows for direct comparison. Any findings seen on the conventional study that are suspicious for new or recurrent malignancy can be either confirmed or excluded on tomosynthesis.
- The inability to perform magnification of suspicious calcifications is a limitation of tomosynthesis, which is overcome by performing these views with conventional mammography.

16.5 Further Reading

[1] Krishnamurthy R, Whitman GJ, Stelling CB, Kushwaha AC. Mammographic findings after breast conservation therapy. Radiographics. 1999; 19(Spec No): S53–S62, quiz S262–S263

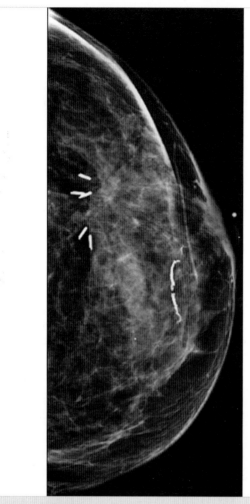

Fig. 16.1 Left craniocaudal (LCC) mammogram.

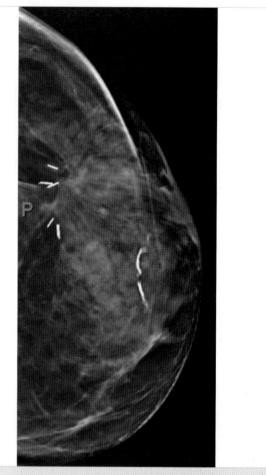

Fig. 16.2 Left craniocaudal digital breast tomosynthesis (LCC DBT), slice 27 of 35.

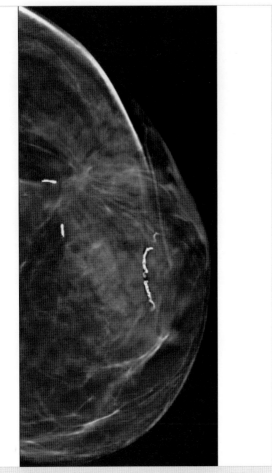

Fig. 16.3 Left craniocaudal sigital breast tomosynthesis (LCC DBT), slice 34 of 35.

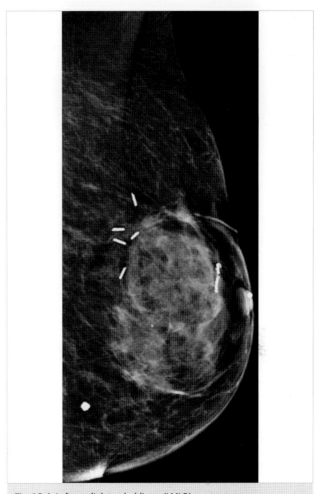

Fig. 16.4 Left mediolateral oblique (LMLO) mammogram.

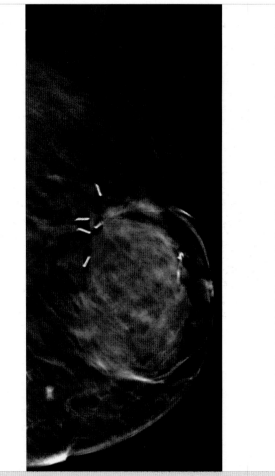

Fig. 16.5 Left mediolateral oblique digital breast tomosynthesis (LMLO DBT), slice 23 of 84.

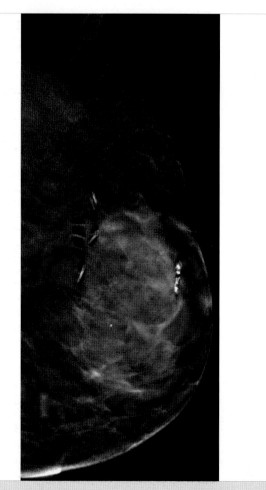

Fig. 16.6 Left mediolateral oblique digital breast tomosynthesis (LMLO DBT), slice 37 of 84.

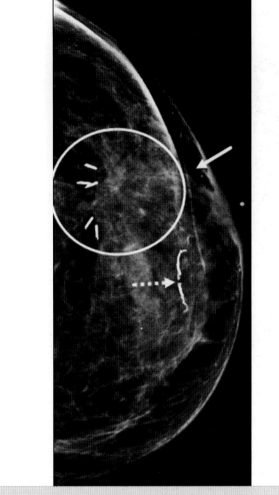

Fig. 16.7 Left craniocaudal (LCC) mammogram with label.

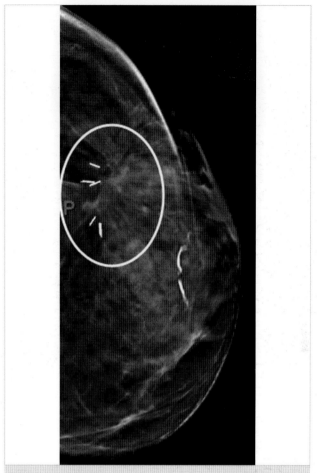

Fig. 16.8 Left craniocaudal digital breast tomosynthesis (LCC DBT), slice 27 of 35 with label.

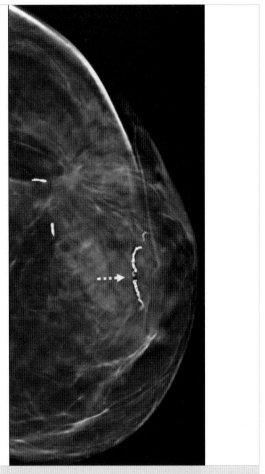

Fig. 16.9 Left craniocaudal digital breast tomosynthesis (LCC DBT), slice 34 of 35 with label.

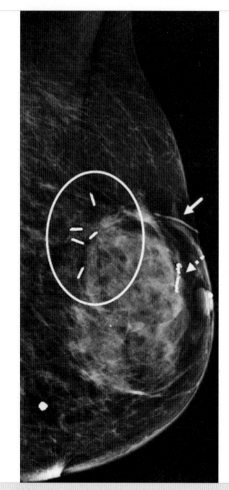

Fig. 16.10 Left mediolateral oblique (LMLO) mammogram with label.

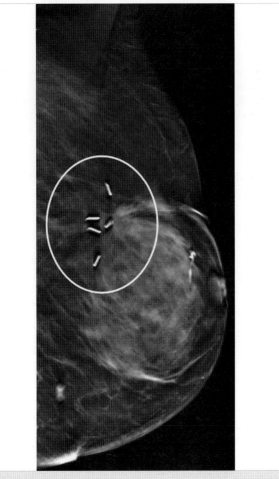

Fig. 16.11 Left mediolateral oblique digital breast tomosynthesis (LMLO DBT), slice 23 of 84 with label.

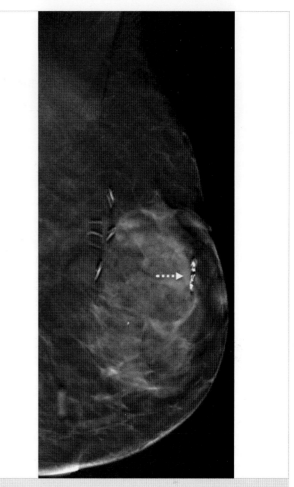

Fig. 16.12 Left mediolateral oblique digital breast tomosynthesis (LMLO DBT), slice 37 of 84 with label.

17 Oval Mass in High-Risk Patient

Lonie R. Salkowski

17.1 Presentation and Presenting Images

(▶ Fig. 17.1, ▶ Fig. 17.2)

A 35-year-old female whose mother and grandmother had premenopausal breast cancer presents for high-risk screening mammography.

17.2 Key images

(▶ Fig. 17.3, ▶ Fig. 17.4, ▶ Fig. 17.5, ▶ Fig. 17.6, ▶ Fig. 17.7, ▶ Fig. 17.8)

17.2.1 Breast Tissue Density

The breasts are heterogeneously dense, which may obscure small masses.

17.2.2 Imaging Findings

Superficially within the upper outer quadrant of the right breast, there is an oval circumscribed mass that is best seen on the craniocaudal (CC) view (▶ Fig. 17.3), and is obscured on the mediolateral oblique (MLO) view (▶ Fig. 17.4). The digital breast tomosynthesis (DBT) images are helpful to isolate this mass from the surrounding tissues (▶ Fig. 17.5 and ▶ Fig. 17.6). On the CC DBT image, there is a suggestion of a fatty cleft (▶ Fig. 17.5). Historical magnetic resonance images (MRI) from the patient demonstrate the classic appearance of a lymph node. The mass is isointense to the glandular tissue on the T1-weighted MRI with a cleft that is the same as the signal intensity of fat (▶ Fig. 17.7). On the T2-wieghted MRI, the mass has increased signal intensity with a central cleft that has decreased signal intensity similar to the surrounding fatty tissue (▶ Fig. 17.8).

17.3 BI-RADS Classification and Action

Category 2: Benign

17.4 Differential Diagnosis

1. **Lymph node**: This mass is circumscribed and contains a fatty hilum, which is supported by the DBT images. Additionally, historical MR images demonstrate the classic appearance of a superficially located lymph node in the upper outer quadrant of the breast.
2. *Fibroadenoma*: Fibroadenomas can occur anywhere in the breast and are very common in patients this age. They can share common characteristics of a lymph node on MR imaging. The presence of a fatty hilum makes a fibroadenoma a less likely diagnosis.
3. *Cyst*: Cysts can have variable appearances. The historical MR imaging favors a lymph node over a cyst.

17.5 Essential Facts

- DBT may help in averting a recall mammogram or a biopsy by better defining a lesion seen on full-field digital mammography (FFDM). In this case, the CC FFDM suggested a lymph node. The MLO view was not helpful. The DBT images were helpful in defining this mass as a lymph node even before exploring the historical MR imaging.
- DBT can be helpful to assess for the presence of a fatty hilum not only in intramammary nodes, but also in axillary nodes. The axilla should be part of the normal search pattern.
- Recall rates have been shown to be significantly decreased with DBT without sacrificing sensitivity.
- Studies have reported that DBT also reduces the false-positive recalls by 40%.

17.6 Management and Digital Breast Tomosynthesis Principles

- It is important to use all historical imaging studies available when evaluating findings at screening mammography. Finding a CT or MR image that can help confirm FFDM or DBT findings helps reduce unnecessary recalls. The electronic medical record (EMR) and picture archiving and communication systems (PACs) have allowed more access to a patient's additional nonbreast imaging studies.
- Some benign-appearing lesions will only be seen on DBT. This is especially reported in dense fibroglandular tissue. A metric needs to be established to know which of these can be dismissed and which may need further evaluation.

17.7 Further Reading

[1] Baker JA, Lo JY. Breast tomosynthesis: state-of-the-art and review of the literature. Acad Radiol. 2011; 18(10):1298–1310

[2] Conant EF. Clinical implementation of digital breast tomosynthesis. Radiol Clin North Am. 2014; 52(3):499–518

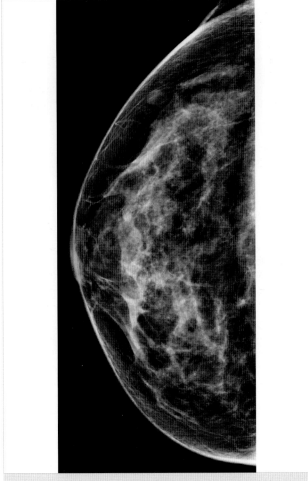

Fig. 17.1 Right craniocaudal (RCC) mammogram.

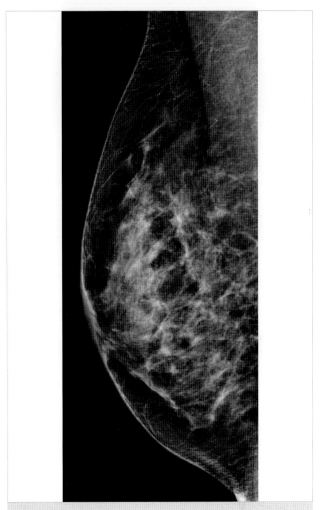

Fig. 17.2 Right mediolateral oblique (RMLO) mammogram.

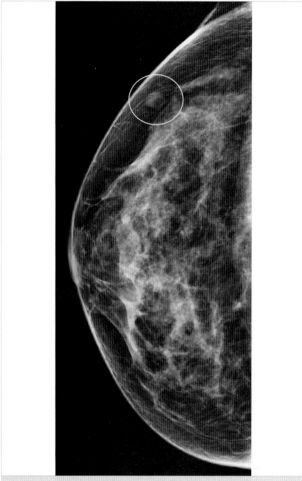

Fig. 17.3 Right craniocaudal (RCC) mammogram with label.

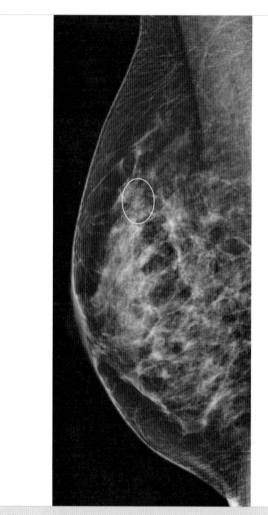

Fig. 17.4 Right mediolateral oblique (RMLO) mammogram with label.

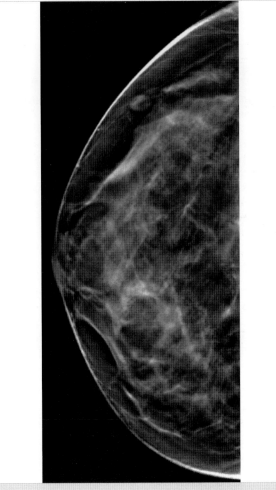

Fig. 17.5 Right craniocaudal digital breast tomosynthesis (RCC DBT), slice 27 of 65.

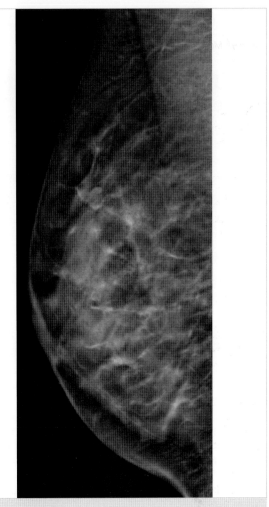

Fig. 17.6 Right mediolateral oblique digital breast tomosynthesis (RMLO DBT), slice 8 of 60.

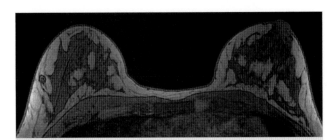

Fig. 17.7 Axial T1-weighted magnetic resonance (MR) image.

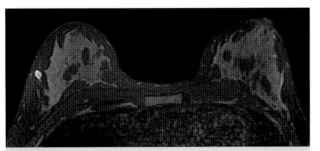

Fig. 17.8 Axial T2-weighted fat-saturation magnetic resonance (MR) image.

18 Resolved Clinical Finding

Tanya W. Moseley

18.1 Presentation and Presenting Images

(▶ Fig. 18.1, ▶ Fig. 18.2, ▶ Fig. 18.3, ▶ Fig. 18.4, ▶ Fig. 18.5, ▶ Fig. 18.6, ▶ Fig. 18.7, ▶ Fig. 18.8)

A 40-year-old female with a history of a palpable right retroareolar mass 2 weeks ago that has since resolved. The referring physician's assessment mentions no palpable abnormalities in either breast. She presents for baseline screening mammography and she requests tomosynthesis.

18.2 Key Images

(▶ Fig. 18.9, ▶ Fig. 18.10)

18.2.1 Breast Tissue Density

There are scattered areas of fibroglandular density.

18.2.2 Imaging Findings

Imaging reveals bilateral retropectoral saline implants (▶ Fig. 18.9 and ▶ Fig. 18.10). Saline implants are relatively radiolucent compared to silicone implants. The implants are behind the pectoralis muscle (*arrow*). The radiopaque smaller circle in the center of the implants represent the valve for implant filling during surgical placement. There are no suspicious masses, architectural distortions, or calcifications in either breast.

18.3 BI-RADS Classification and Action

Category 2: Benign

18.4 Differential Diagnosis

1. ***Retropectoral saline implant and normal mammogram***: The implant is located posterior to, or behind, the pectoralis muscle. Saline implants are easily penetrated by the X-ray beam. There are no mammographic findings seen that correlate to the resolved clinical issue.
2. *Retropectoral silicone implant*: The implant is located posterior to, or behind, the pectoralis muscle. Silicone is dense and not easily penetrated by the X-ray beam. This implant is not dense enough to be silicone.
3. *Prepectoral saline implant*: Prepectoral implants are positioned in front of the pectoralis muscle. The implant, in this example, is behind the pectoralis muscle, or retropectoral.

18.5 Essential Facts

- Tomosynthesis images may be acquired in every conventional mammographic orientation, that is, craniocaudal (CC), mediolateral oblique (MLO), mediolateral (ML), and lateromedial (LM). Tomosynthesis can also perform spot-compression and implant-displaced views, but not magnification views.
- Implants positioned behind the pectoralis muscle have a lower prevalence of capsular contraction than prepectoral implants. It is easier to perform mammograms with retropectoral implants.
- In order to limit radiation exposure in patients with breast implants, we acquire tomosynthesis images only in the implant-displaced views.
- Although this patient informed the referring physician and technologist that the palpable finding had resolved and the referring physician's assessment revealed no palpable abnormalities in either breast, the final report reflected the history, physical examination findings, and the imaging findings that no suspicious right retroareolar findings were seen.

18.5.1 Management and Digital Breast Tomosynthesis Principles

- Tomosynthesis may be safely performed in patients with saline and silicone implants without significant concern for implant rupture. The exact incidence of implant ruptures is unknown. The risk of rupture is directly associated with the age of the implant and inversely related to the thickness of the implant's elastomer shell.
- The amount of breast compression with tomosynthesis is less than the compression with conventional digital mammography. This is important, as discomfort and pain associated with compression for conventional digital mammography is a concern of patients and prevents some patients from remaining compliant with annual mammography. Breast compression may be of even greater concern for patients with implants, who should be assured that tomosynthesis may be safely performed in patients with breast implants.

18.6 Further Reading

[1] Juanpere S, Perez E, Huc O, Motos N, Pont J, Pedraza S. Imaging of breast implants-a pictorial review. Insights Imaging. 2011; 2(6):653–670

[2] Saunders RS, Jr, Samei E, Lo JY, Baker JA. Can compression be reduced for breast tomosynthesis? Monte carlo study on mass and microcalcification conspicuity in tomosynthesis. Radiology. 2009; 251(3):673–682

[3] Yang N, Muradali D. The augmented breast: a pictorial review of the abnormal and unusual. AJR Am J Roentgenol. 2011; 196(4):W451-W460

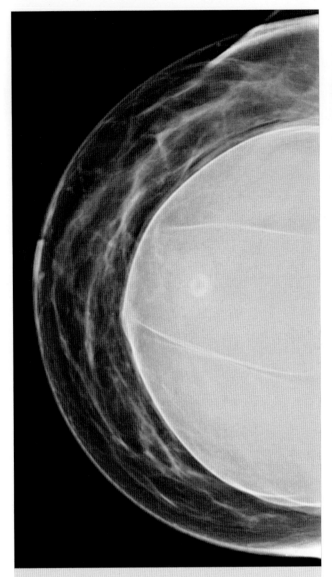

Fig. 18.1 Right craniocaudal (RCC) mammogram.

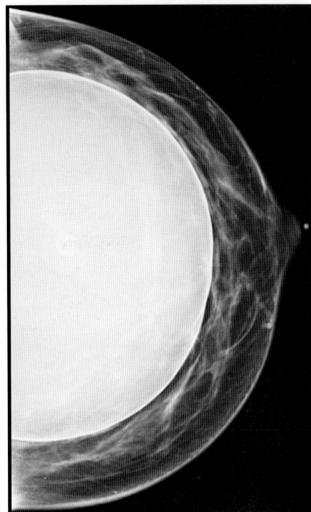

Fig. 18.2 Left craniocaudal (LCC) mammogram.

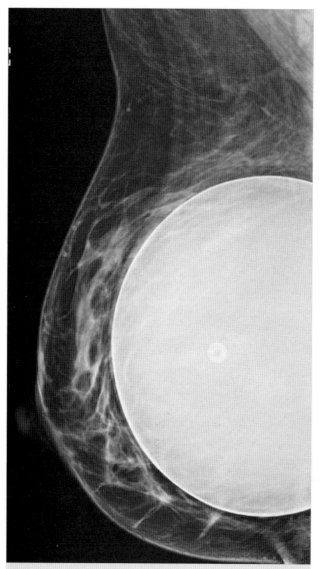

Fig. 18.3 Right mediolateral oblique (RMLO) mammogram.

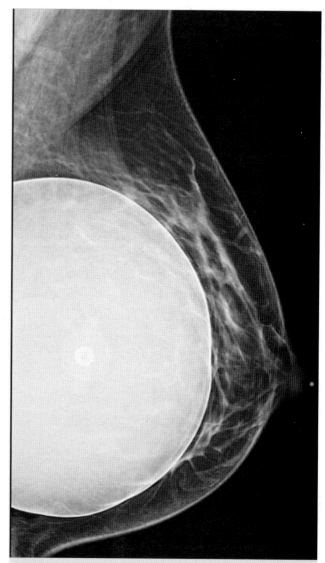

Fig. 18.4 Left mediolateral oblique (LMLO) mammogram.

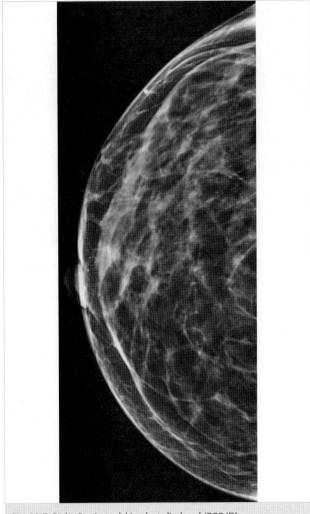

Fig. 18.5 Right Craniocaudal implant-displaced (RCC ID) mammogram.

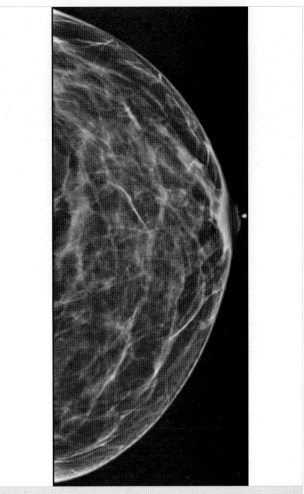

Fig. 18.6 Left Craniocaudal implant-displaced (LCC ID) mammogram.

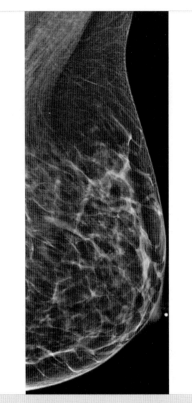

Fig. 18.7 Left mediolateral oblique implant-displaced (RMLO) mammogram.

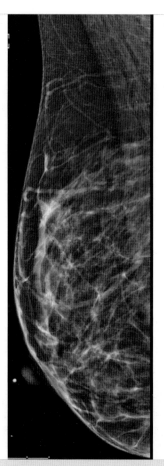

Fig. 18.8 Right mediolateral oblique implant-displaced (LMLO ID) mammogram.

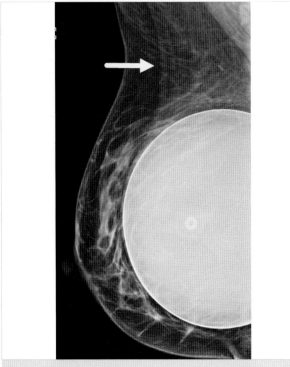

Fig. 18.9 Right mediolateral oblique (RMLO) mammogram with label.

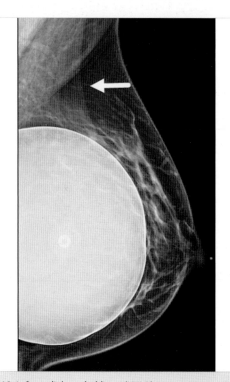

Fig. 18.10 Left mediolateral oblique (LMLO) mammogram with label.

19 Breast Reduction Years Ago

Lonie R. Salkowski

19.1 Presentation and Presenting Images

(▶ Fig. 19.1, ▶ Fig. 19.2, ▶ Fig. 19.3, ▶ Fig. 19.4)

A 52-year-old female with a history of left breast cancer treated with a mastectomy presents for screening mammography.

19.2 Key images

(▶ Fig. 19.5, ▶ Fig. 19.6, ▶ Fig. 19.7, ▶ Fig. 19.8, ▶ Fig. 19.9)

19.2.1 Breast Tissue Density

The breasts are almost entirely fatty.

19.2.2 Imaging Findings

In the posterior central aspect of the right breast, there is a low-density focal asymmetry (▶ Fig. 19.5 and ▶ Fig. 19.6). The digital breast tomosynthesis (DBT) images (▶ Fig. 19.7 and ▶ Fig. 19.8) verify that this focal asymmetry has a very faint rim calcification that partially surrounds a fat-containing mass. There is some faint architectural changes around this mass seen on the DBT images that suggest that this is related to the patient's prior reduction surgery. The outside magnetic resonance (MR) image (▶ Fig. 19.9) confirms that this area is composed of fat.

19.3 BI-RADS Classification and Action

Category 2: Benign

19.4 Differential Diagnosis

1. **Fat necrosis at the surgical scar**: Characteristic findings are present mammographically after reduction surgery. One of these findings is fat necrosis. The degree of fat necrosis can also vary.
2. *Lipoma*: Lipomas are fatty masses that can occur anywhere in the body and have a characteristic thin capsule. The mammographic finding in this case does not share this characteristic finding.
3. *Developing asymmetry*: Patients with breast reduction surgery have the same risk of breast cancer as the rest of the population. New or developing masses need to be distinguished from the development of cancer and postsurgical changes. The surgical history combined with the imaging findings and the prior MRI favor this to be postsurgical changes rather than a developing asymmetry of a possible carcinoma.

19.4.1 Essential Facts

- Fat necrosis can present as oil cysts, spiculated lesions, focal masses, or calcifications.
- During breast-reduction surgery there is redistribution of the breast tissue resulting in characteristic sites of scarring.
- Fat necrosis in breast reduction often occurs along the scar lines.
- The thin capsule of a lipid cyst of fat necrosis is better seen on DBT due to the decrease in summation artifacts. The DBT images can also reveal scar lines that may extend to the skin surface because of this uncovering effect.
- Lipid cysts can have components that are encapsulated fat-containing masses and others that are lined with thin rim-shell calcification.

19.4.2 Management and Digital Breast Tomosynthesis Principles

- Similar fat-necrosis changes can be seen in the breast from a lumpectomy and from reduction surgery. The location and distribution of the findings should help to distinguish the origin. Oncoplastic surgery has become more common in the treatment of breast cancer. Some these patients may have a lumpectomy for their cancer treatment combined with reduction mammoplasty. These scars can be more difficult to follow mammographically.
- Early changes of fat necrosis, especially when appearing as a spiculated lesion or calcifications, can mimic carcinoma. Occasionally these will require a biopsy to confirm benignity.
- All spiculated masses that contain fat should be evaluated and/or strongly correlated with a surgical history before dismissing then as fat necrosis due to surgery. DBT is superior to FFDM for revealing the central fat that can be present in some malignant tumors.

19.5 Further Reading

[1] Freer PE, Wang JL, Rafferty EA. Digital breast tomosynthesis in the analysis of fat-containing lesions. Radiographics. 2014; 34(2):343–358

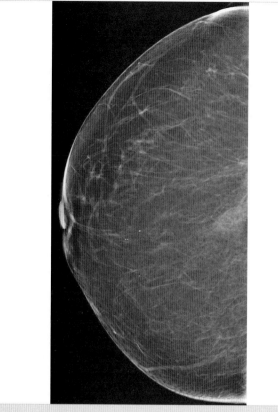

Fig. 19.1 Right craniocaudal (RCC) mammogram.

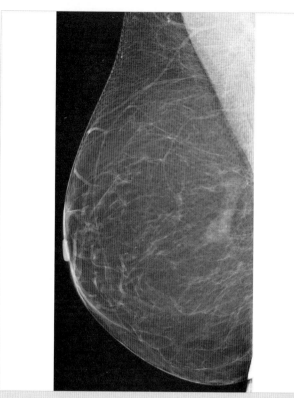

Fig. 19.2 Right mediolateral oblique (RMLO) mammogram.

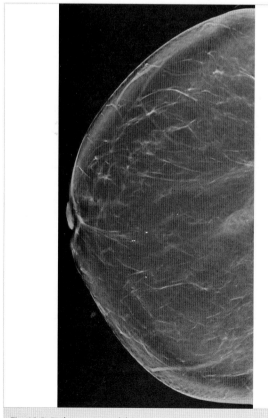

Fig. 19.3 Right craniocaudal (RCC) synthetic mammogram.

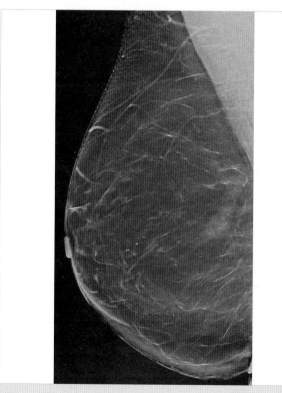

Fig. 19.4 Right mediolateral oblique (RMLO) synthetic mammogram.

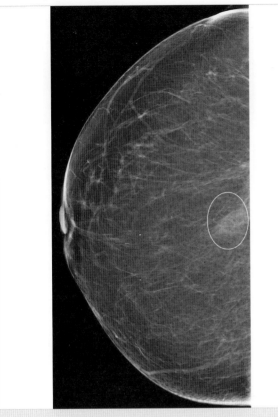

Fig. 19.5 Right craniocaudal (RCC) mammogram with label.

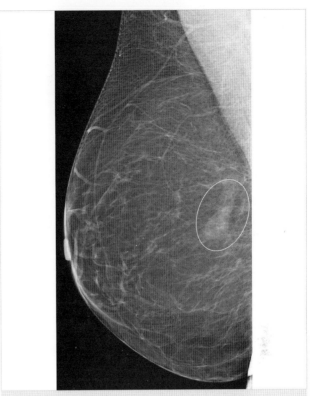

Fig. 19.6 Right mediolateral oblique (RMLO) mammogram with label.

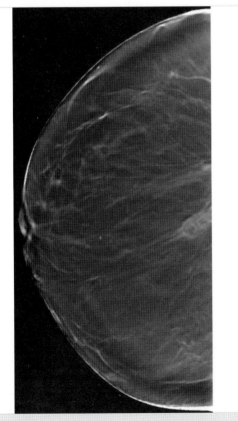

Fig. 19.7 Right craniocaudal digital breast tomosynthesis (RCC DBT), slice 32 of 80.

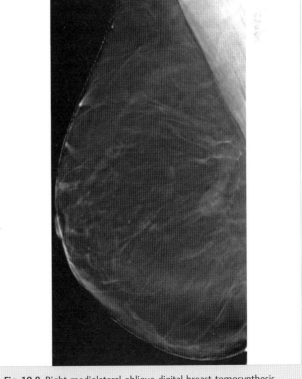

Fig. 19.8 Right mediolateral oblique digital breast tomosynthesis (RMLO DBT), slice 43 of 81.

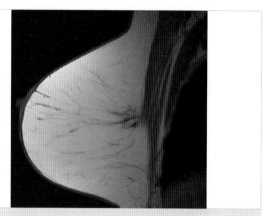

Fig. 19.9 Sagittal T1-weighted non–fat-suppression magnetic resonance (MR) image.

20 Axillary "Calcifications"

Tanya W. Moseley

20.1 Presentation and Presenting Images

(▶ Fig. 20.1, ▶ Fig. 20.2, ▶ Fig. 20.3, ▶ Fig. 20.4)

A 57-year-old female with a history of left ductal carcinoma in situ (DCIS) treated with segmentectomy and radiation therapy presents for routine screening mammography.

20.2 Key Images

(▶ Fig. 20.5, ▶ Fig. 20.6, ▶ Fig. 20.7)

20.2.1 Breast Tissue Density

The breasts are heterogeneously dense, which may obscure small masses.

20.2.2 Imaging Findings

The imaging of the right breast is normal (*not shown*). The left breast demonstrates postsurgical changes with architectural distortion and surgical clips (*solid arrows* in ▶ Fig. 20.6) in the left breast at the 2 to 3 o'clock position and a surgical clip (*broken arrow* in ▶ Fig. 20.6) in the left axilla. Fine radiodense particles project over the left axilla (*circle* in ▶ Fig. 20.6). The left breast tomosynthesis movie demonstrates that the fine densities are in skin folds of the left axilla consistent with deodorant artifact (▶ Fig. 20.7).

20.2.3 BI-RADS Classification and Action

Category 2: Benign

20.3 Differential Diagnosis

1. **Deodorant artifact**: The radiodense particles localize to the skin folds of the axilla. The quality of the radiodense particles also suggest a metallic quality; a metallic compound is a component of deodorant.
2. *Skin calcifications*: The radiodense particles appear on the surface of the skin and are not contained within the skin.
3. *Axillary calcifications* : The radiodense particles are on the surface of the skin and do not localize in the axilla, such as would be seen in nodal calcifications.

20.4 Essential Facts

- Although the finding is not apparent on the left craniocaudal digital breast tomosynthesis (CC DBT) movie, it is well seen on the left mediolateral oblique (MLO) DBT movie. The finding corresponds directly with the lateral-most skin surface and the lateral-most MLO DBT slice (slice 1 of 81 in ▶ Fig. 20.7).
- It is important for patients to thoroughly cleanse the skin of the breast and axilla prior to mammography to prevent artifacts.
- Deodorant artifacts may be mistaken for axillary calcifications and may cause a patient to be recalled.
- Prevention of this artifact is easily remedied by washing the axilla and if not done well, may be identified as an artifact with tomosynthesis imaging.

20.5 Management and Digital Breast Tomosynthesis Principles

- Thorough preparation for conventional mammographic and tomosynthesis imaging involves the removal of deodorant and lotion, which may cause artifacts that mimic calcifications. In some cases, the artifacts mimic suspicious calcifications that may prompt a recall for biopsy.
- Most radiology departments recommend that patients do not wear powder, deodorant, or lotion on the day of mammography.
- Tomosynthesis imaging localizes deodorant to the skin folds rather than the skin. The location of the deodorant is not within the dermis of the axilla but on the skin surface.
- Tomosynthesis evaluation of deodorant artifact can prevent unnecessary biopsies and reduce recall for this benign finding.

20.6 Further Reading

[1] Geiser WR. Artifacts in digital mammography. In: Whitman GJ, Haygood TM, eds. Digital Mammography: A Practical Approach. Cambridge, England: Cambridge University Press; 2012:80

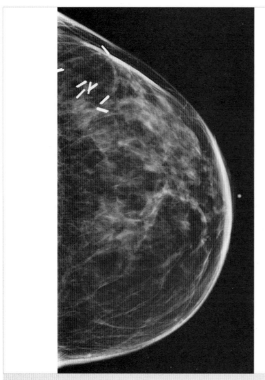

Fig. 20.1 Left craniocaudal (LCC) mammogram.

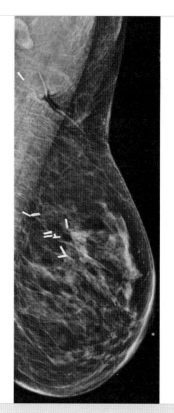

Fig. 20.2 Left mediolateral oblique (LMLO) mammogram.

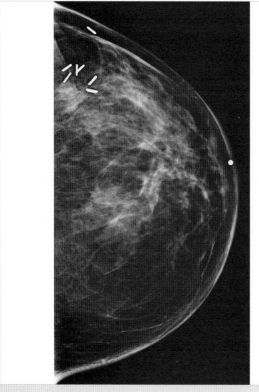

Fig. 20.3 Left craniocaudal (LCC) mammogram comparison.

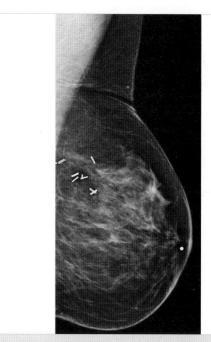

Fig. 20.4 Left mediolateral oblique (LMLO) mammogram comparison.

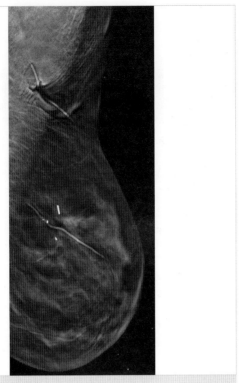

Fig. 20.5 Left mediolateral digital breast tomosymthesis (LMLO DBT), slice 1 of 81.

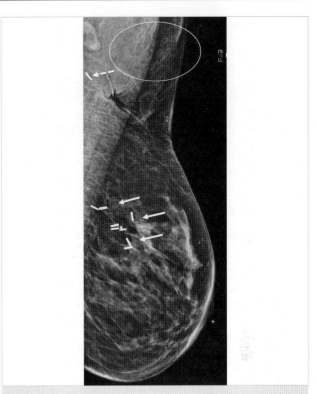

Fig. 20.6 Left mediolateral oblique (LMLO) mammogram with label.

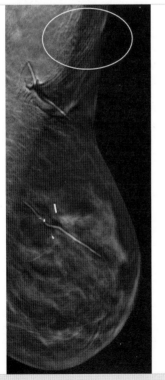

Fig. 20.7 Left mediolateral oblique digital breast tomosynthesis (LMLO DBT), slice 1 of 81 with label.

21 Nonpalpable Mass

Lonie R. Salkowski

21.1 Presentation and Presenting Images

(▶ Fig. 21.1, ▶ Fig. 21.2, ▶ Fig. 21.3, ▶ Fig. 21.4)

A 60-year-old female presents for asymptomatic screening mammography.

21.2 Key images

(▶ Fig. 21.5, ▶ Fig. 21.6, ▶ Fig. 21.7, ▶ Fig. 21.8)

21.2.1 Breast Tissue Density

There are scattered areas of fibroglandular density.

21.2.2 Imaging Findings

Within the subareolar region of the right breast, there appears to be a more focal area of fibroglandular tissue compared to the remaining breast tissue (▶ Fig. 21.5 and ▶ Fig. 21.6). This is seen on the conventional digital mammograms and the synthetic mammograms. The digital breast tomosynthesis (DBT) images (▶ Fig. 21.7 and ▶ Fig. 21.8) reveal that this is part of a mass with circumscribed margins containing fat and fibroglandular components. The left breast is normal (*not shown*).

21.3 BI-RADS Classification and Action

Category 2: Benign

21.4 Differential Diagnosis

1. **Hamartoma**: This mass is present in a fatty to scattered density background. This background can make masses that have a high fat component difficult to identify. The pseudocapsule seen on DBT supports the diagnosis of a hamartoma.
2. *Lipoma* : Lipomas are encapsulated fatty masses; however, they do not contain fibroglandular components.

3. *Normal fibroglandular tissue*: On conventional mammography, this mass appears to blend into the other tissues in the subareolar region. The DBT helps make clear the capsule, which indicates that this mass is a hamartoma.

21.5 Essential Facts

- Hamartomas can be found at any age.
- Hamartomas are often referred to as a 'breast within a breast.'
- The mammographic appearance of hamartomas is variable due to the variation in the amount and types of breast tissue elements that they can contain.
- Typically hamartomas occur as single entities. It is rare for a patient to have multiple hamartomas (unlike fibroadenomas).
- A breast mass that is encapsulated and contains a mixture of adipose and fibroglandular components can be considered benign.

21.6 Management and Digital Breast Tomosynthesis Principles

- The superior marginal detail of DBT allows for more accurate analysis of masses.
- DBT allows for the recognition of benign encapsulated fat-containing masses, when conventional mammography would have dictated the need for further evaluation.
- The ability to scroll through lesions on DBT allows better assessment of margins of masses.
- A mass that fulfills the criteria of a hamartoma, encapsulated and containing fatty and fibrous components, does not need further diagnostic evaluation unless there are findings that could represent an associated suspicious finding. DBT will likely aid in less recall mammography of these benign masses due to the ability to better define the margins of the mass with DBT.

21.7 Further Reading

[1] Conant EF. Clinical implementation of digital breast tomosynthesis. Radiol Clin North Am. 2014; 52(3):499–518
[2] Freer PE, Wang JL, Rafferty EA. Digital breast tomosynthesis in the analysis of fat-containing lesions. Radiographics. 2014; 34(2):343–358

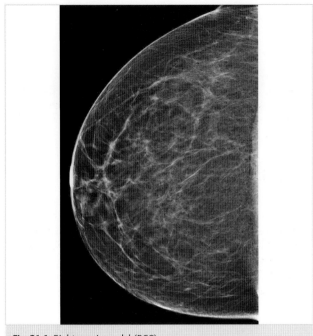

Fig. 21.1 Right craniocaudal (RCC) mammogram.

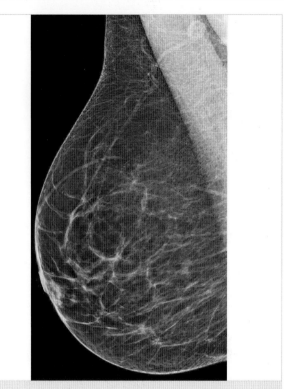

Fig. 21.2 Right mediolateral oblique (RMLO) mammogram.

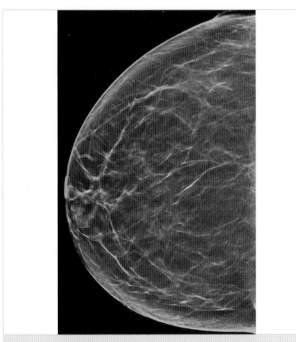

Fig. 21.3 Right craniocaudal (RCC) synthetic mammogram.

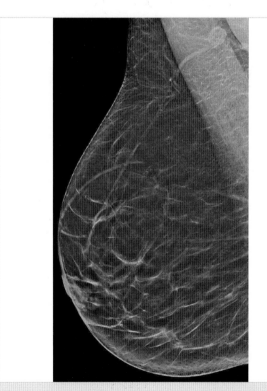

Fig. 21.4 Right mediolateral oblique (RMLO) synthetic mammogram.

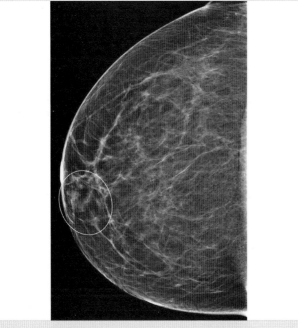

Fig. 21.5 Right craniocaudal (RCC) mammogram with label.

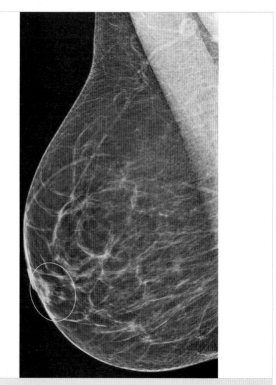

Fig. 21.6 Right mediolateral oblique (RMLO) mammogram with label.

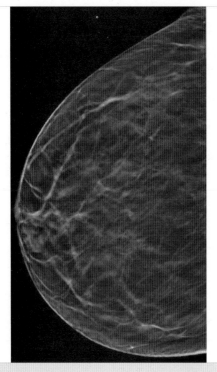

Fig. 21.7 Right craniocaudal digital breast tomosynthesis (RCC DBT), slice 19 of 56.

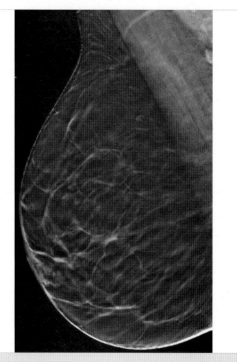

Fig. 21.8 Right mediolateral oblique digital breast tomosynthesis (RMLO DBT), slice 27 of 56.

22 Increased Breast Density

Lonie R. Salkowski

22.1 Presentation and Presenting Images

(▶ Fig. 22.1, ▶ Fig. 22.2, ▶ Fig. 22.3, ▶ Fig. 22.4, ▶ Fig. 22.5, ▶ Fig. 22.6, ▶ Fig. 22.7, ▶ Fig. 22.8)

A 37-year-old female who is breast-feeding presents for her high-risk asymptomatic screening mammogram.

22.1.1 Breast Tissue Density

The breasts are heterogeneously dense, which may obscure small masses.

22.1.2 Imaging Findings

The breast tissue on the patient's current mammogram has increased in density and there also appears to be more of it. The tissue in the upper outer quadrants appears more confluent and there is new tissue present in the left axillary region. Compare the current mammograms (▶ Fig. 22.1, ▶ Fig. 22.2, ▶ Fig. 22.3, and ▶ Fig. 22.4) with those of a year ago (▶ Fig. 22.5, ▶ Fig. 22.6, ▶ Fig. 22.7, and ▶ Fig. 22.8, respectively). All the breast tissue on the current mammograms has the same imaging appearance. No definite masses, architectural distortion, or calcifications are noted. The patient has two biopsy marking clips in the right breast from past magnetic resonance-guided (MR) and ultrasound-guided benign biopsies.

22.2 BI-RADS Classification and Action

Category 2: Benign

22.2.1 Differential Diagnosis

1. **Breast tissue changes due to lactation**: The breast tissue proliferates during lactation. Typically screening is not performed during lactation because of the decrease in sensitivity that the increased breast density introduces. In this case, the patient is high risk and will be breast feeding for several more months.
2. *Incorrect comparative patient mammograms*: When there is a marked contrast between sequential years of mammograms, it is always helpful to ensure that the correct patient's images were placed in the file. In this case, it is the same patient. The biopsy clips aid in identifying that these are indeed of the same patient.
3. *Weight loss*: Weight loss will cause some increase in breast tissue density, but it will not result in proliferation of breast tissue as is seen in this case.

22.3 Essential Facts

- There are few guidelines regarding screening lactating women who are considered high risk for the development of breast cancer with mammography.
- There is diminished sensitivity of mammography during lactation and pregnancy likely secondary to increased parenchymal density in the breast due to hormonal changes.
- If imaging is necessary while a patient is lactating, it is advised that she breast-feed or pump prior to imaging to reduce the overall density of the breast tissue due to retained milk products.
- Pregnancy-associated breast cancer accounts for 0.2 to 3.8% of all newly diagnosed cases of breast cancer.
- Pregnancy-associated breast cancer is the most common malignancy of pregnancy, occurring in 1 in 3000 to 1 in 10,000 pregnancies.

22.4 Management and Digital Breast Tomosynthesis Principles

- Screening mammography is generally not indicated for normal risk patients while pregnant or lactating.
- Ultrasound is typically the first-line imaging modality that is used for symptomatic patients that are pregnant or lactating. The ultrasound findings may determine the need for mammographic imaging.
- DBT imaging has been reported to improve sensitivity and specificity across all breast tissue densities. However, it is unclear if these results can be extrapolated to the breast tissue changes seen in pregnancy and during lactation.

22.5 Further Reading

[1] Conant EF. Clinical implementation of digital breast tomosynthesis. Radiol Clin North Am. 2014; 52(3):499–518
[2] Vashi R, Hooley R, Butler R, Geisel J, Philpotts L. Breast imaging of the pregnant and lactating patient: imaging modalities and pregnancy-associated breast cancer. AJR Am J Roentgenol. 2013; 200(2):321–328

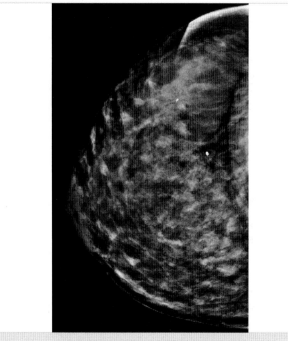

Fig. 22.1 Right craniocaudal (RCC) mammogram.

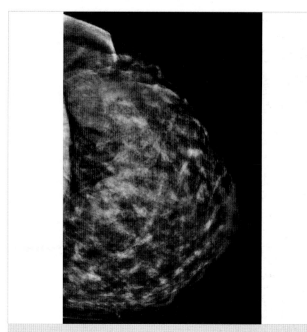

Fig. 22.2 Left craniocaudal (LCC) mammogram.

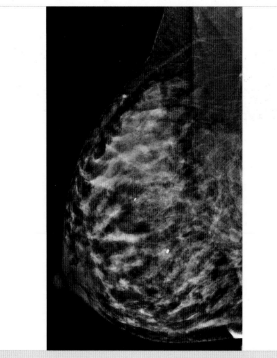

Fig. 22.3 Right mediolateral oblique (RMLO) mammogram.

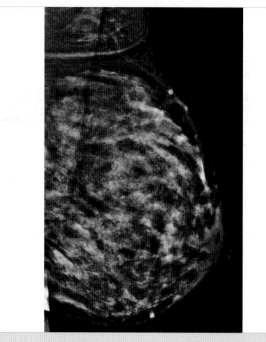

Fig. 22.4 Left mediolateral oblique (LMLO) mammogram.

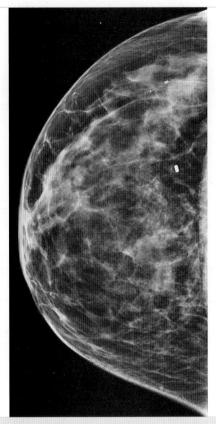

Fig. 22.5 Right craniocaudal (RCC) mammogram 1 year ago.

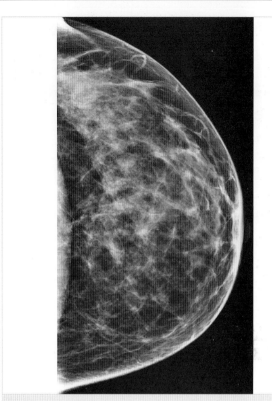

Fig. 22.6 Left craniocaudal (LCC) mammogram 1 year ago.

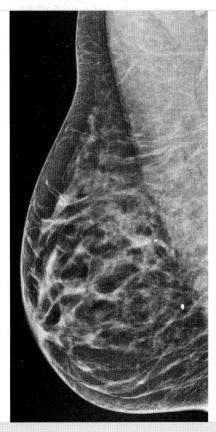

Fig. 22.7 Right mediolateral oblique (RMLO) mammogram 1 year ago.

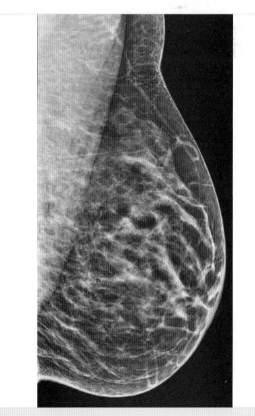

Fig. 22.8 Left mediolateral oblique (LMLO) mammogram 1 year ago.

23 Possible Architectural Distortion

Tanya W. Moseley

23.1 Presentation and Presenting Images

(▶ Fig. 23.1, ▶ Fig. 23.2)

A 59-year-old female with a significant family history of breast cancer and a prior benign right excisional biopsy presents for routine screening mammography.

23.2 Key Images

(▶ Fig. 23.3, ▶ Fig. 23.4)

23.2.1 Breast Tissue Density

There are scattered areas of fibroglandular density.

23.2.2 Imaging Findings

The imaging of the left breast is normal *(not shown)*. The digital mammograms of the right breast shows a possible architectural distortion *(circle)* in the middle depth at the 11 o'clock location, 4 cm from the nipple (▶ Fig. 23.3 and ▶ Fig. 23.4). Scar markers *(arrows)* denote the scarring from the remote excisional biopsy. The tomosynthesis movie demonstrates that the possible architectural distortion is a summation artifact and the result of overlapping breast parenchyma.

23.2.3 BI-RADS Classification and Action

Category 1: Negative

23.3 Differential Diagnosis

1. **Overlapping parenchyma**: Although findings on the conventional mammogram suggested an architectural distortion, tomosynthesis demonstrated that the finding was created by overlapping parenchyma.
2. *Radial scar*: Tomosynthesis did not reveal a persistent architectural distortion nor mass.
3. *Cancer*: Cancers, particularly invasive lobular carcinomas, may present on one view only or as subtle findings. Tomosynthesis makes missing such a finding less likely than on conventional mammography alone.

23.3.1 Essential Facts

- Lesion detection challenges due to overlapping breast parenchyma are a limitation to conventional two-dimensional (2D) analog and digital mammography.

- In this case, if only 2D digital screening mammography had been performed, the patient would have been scheduled for diagnostic mammography and additional views, ultrasound, and possibly a biopsy. Obtaining the 2D digital mammography along with digital breast tomosynthesis (DBT) allowed for direct comparison between the 2D mammogram and DBT images.
- The added DBT images demonstrate that the possible architectural distortion is a summation artifact. No further work-up or biopsy are needed. The patient can return to annual screening mammography, and the radiologist's recall rate is reduced.
- Overlapping breast parenchyma on mammography is one factor that limits interpretation, particularly in patients with denser breast tissue. Overlapping breast parenchyma may obscure cancers, resulting in missed cancer diagnoses. Conversely, overlapping parenchyma, or superimposed normal structures, may create pseudomasses, or summation artifacts, resulting in false-positive diagnoses and unnecessary biopsies.

23.4 Management and Digital Breast Tomosynthesis Principles

- Breast tomosynthesis captures images of the breast at multiple angles during a short scan. The images are then reconstructed into thin slices (1-mm thick) that can be viewed individually or in a tomosynthesis movie. This essentially removes overlapping structures and/or superimposition of structures.
- Many screening callbacks are performed to resolve findings secondary to overlapping parenchyma.
- The addition of tomosynthesis to 2D digital mammography helps identify summation artifacts secondary to overlapping breast parenchyma, thereby decreasing the recall rate for diagnostic mammography and ultrasound and eliminating some unnecessary biopsies.
- Tomosynthesis has been shown to reduce recall rates from 7 to 15%.

23.5 Further Reading

[1] Friedewald SM, Rafferty EA, Rose SL, et al. Breast cancer screening using tomosynthesis in combination with digital mammography. JAMA. 2014; 311 (24):2499–2507

[2] Rose SL, Tidwell AL, Bujnoch LJ, Kushwaha AC, Nordmann AS, Sexton R, Jr. Implementation of breast tomosynthesis in a routine screening practice: an observational study. AJR Am J Roentgenol. 2013; 200(6): 1401–1408

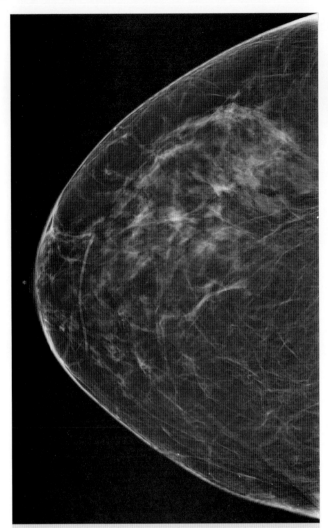

Fig. 23.1 Right craniocaudal (RCC) mammogram.

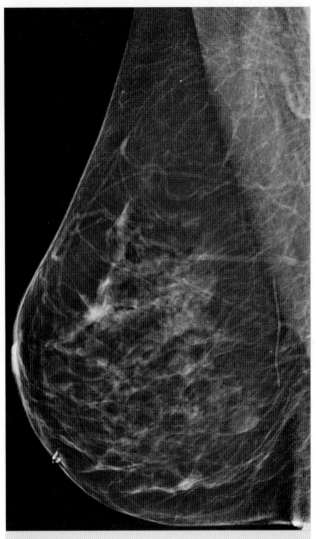

Fig. 23.2 Right mediolateral oblique (RMLO) mammogram.

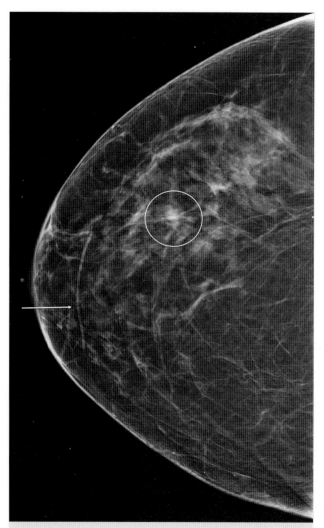

Fig. 23.3 Right craniocaudal (RCC) mammogram with label.

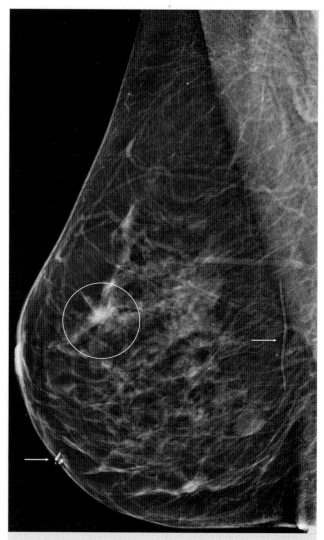

Fig. 23.4 Right mediolateral oblique (RMLO) mammogram with label.

24 Architectural Distortion

Tanya W. Moseley

24.1 Presentation and Presenting Images

(▶ Fig. 24.1, ▶ Fig. 24.2, ▶ Fig. 24.3, ▶ Fig. 24.4, ▶ Fig. 24.5, ▶ Fig. 24.6, ▶ Fig. 24.7, ▶ Fig. 24.8, ▶ Fig. 24.9, ▶ Fig. 24.10, ▶ Fig. 24.11, ▶ Fig. 24.12)

A 48-year-old female treated for right breast cancer 2 years ago presents for screening mammography. The tomosynthesis images obtained when she was diagnosed with breast cancer are included for comparison.

24.2 Key Images

(▶ Fig. 24.13, ▶ Fig. 24.14, ▶ Fig. 24.15, ▶ Fig. 24.16, ▶ Fig. 24.17, ▶ Fig. 24.18, ▶ Fig. 24.19, ▶ Fig. 24.20, ▶ Fig. 24.21, ▶ Fig. 24.22, ▶ Fig. 24.23, ▶ Fig. 24.24)

24.2.1 Breast Tissue Density

The breasts are heterogeneously dense, which may obscure small masses.

24.2.2 Imaging Findings

There is architectural distortion associated with postsurgical clips in the right breast in posterior depth, at 8 to 9 o'clock and 7 cm from the nipple (*box* in ▶ Fig. 24.13, ▶ Fig. 24.14, ▶ Fig. 24.16, and ▶ Fig. 24.21). In this same location, prior imaging shows a 1.7-cm spiculated mass (*circle* in ▶ Fig. 24.18, ▶ Fig. 24.19, and ▶ Fig. 24.20) corresponds to one of the palpable masses (*solid arrow*). The spiculated morphology of this mass is better seen on the tomosynthesis images (▶ Fig. 24.23 and ▶ Fig. 24.24).

The mastopexy scars are seen as straight lines on both the two-dimensional (2D) mammography and on tomosynthesis (*broken arrows* in ▶ Fig. 24.14, ▶ Fig. 24.15, ▶ Fig. 24.16, and ▶ Fig. 24.17). The mastopexy scars are best demonstrated on current right lateromedial (LM) tomosynthesis slice 41 of 84 (▶ Fig. 24.21) and left LM tomosynthesis slice 39 of 85 (▶ Fig. 24.22).

24.3 BI-RADS Classification and Action

Category 2: Benign

24.4 Differential Diagnosis

1. **Postsegmentectomy and mastopexy scars:** There has been interval surgical removal of the spiculated mass. In addition, there are contouring changes of the breast tissue consistent with mastopexy. Many surgical procedures today try to minimize the external scarring; however, the characteristic internal changes are clearly seen on mammography and especially on tomosynthesis. It is important to be aware of these scar characteristics.
2. *Recurrent disease*: There are no findings to suggest recurrence in this case. Recurrence can be as a mass, calcifications, developing asymmetry, or an architectural distortion. It does not need to match the morphology of the original cancer.
3. *Radial scar*: The architectural distortion in this case is most consistent with the history of lumpectomy for breast malignancy.

24.5 Essential Facts

- It is routine practice to compare current and prior mammograms. In fact, fewer abnormal interpretations are made when prior mammograms are available for comparison. Mammogram comparison results in cost savings and reduced morbidity with no further work-up, a reduced callback rate, reduced patient anxiety, reduced false-positives, and fewer biopsies for benign findings.
- The mammogram comparison and tomosynthesis images in this case reveal no findings concerning for new or recurrent malignancy and demonstrate new postsurgical changes of the right breast segmentectomy (*box*) and the bilateral mastopexies (*broken arrows*). The spiculated mass (*circle*) seen on the prior imaging has been surgically removed.
- An imaging finding to be aware of over time with surgical intervention, lumpectomy, or cosmetic surgery is the presence of fat necrosis. It can have variable appearances and can mimic cancer recurrence.

24.5.1 Management and Digital Breast Tomosynthesis Principles

- Although there are no scholarly articles that specifically address the comparison of tomosynthesis imaging over time, the importance of comparison if available is essential to optimal breast imaging interpretation.
- Obtaining the 2D mammograms along with tomosynthesis images allowed direct comparison between them. Having prior tomosynthesis images allowed direct comparison between both 2D mammograms and tomosynthesis images before and after cancer treatment which increases the accuracy of interpretation.

24.6 Further Reading

[1] Friedewald SM, Rafferty EA, Rose SL, et al. Breast cancer screening using tomosynthesis in combination with digital mammography. JAMA. 2014; 311 (24):2499–2507
[2] Rose SL, Tidwell AL, Bujnoch LJ, Kushwaha AC, Nordmann AS, Sexton R, Jr. Implementation of breast tomosynthesis in a routine screening practice: an observational study. AJR Am J Roentgenol. 2013; 200(6):1401–1408

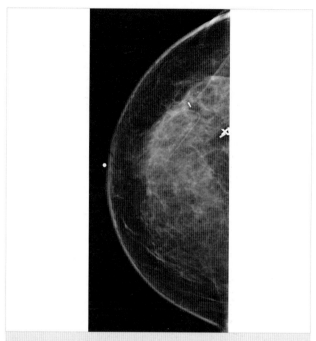

Fig. 24.1 Right craniocaudal (RCC) mammogram.

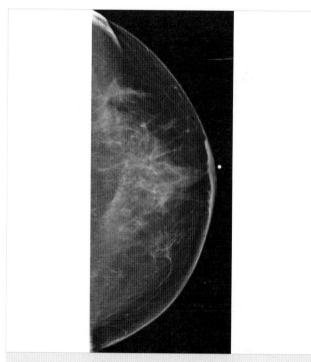

Fig. 24.2 Left craniocaudal (LCC) mammogram.

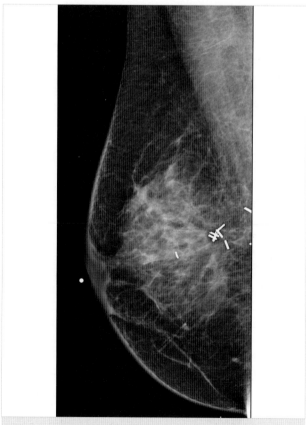

Fig. 24.3 Right mediolateral oblique (RMLO) mammogram.

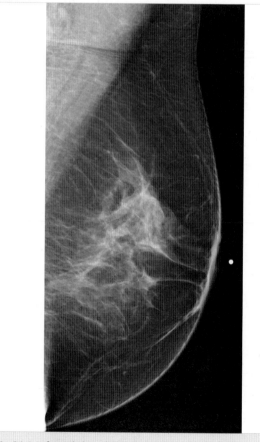

Fig. 24.4 Left mediolateral oblique (LMLO) mammogram.

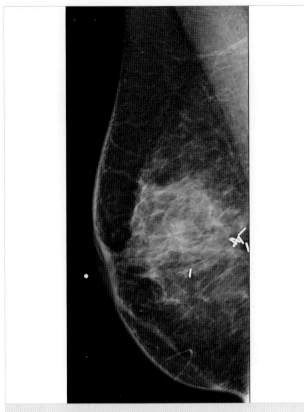

Fig. 24.5 Right lateromedial (RLM) mammogram.

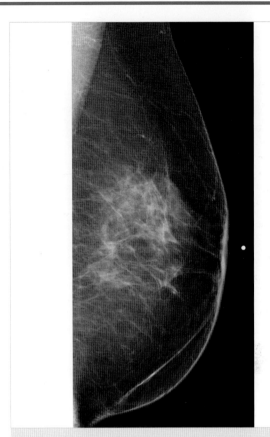

Fig. 24.6 Left lateromedial (LLM) mammogram.

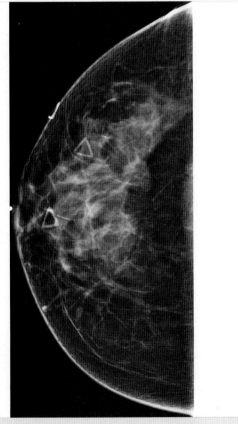

Fig. 24.7 Right craniocaudal (RCC) mammogram comparison.

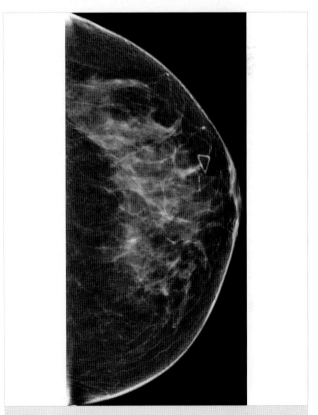

Fig. 24.8 Left craniocaudal (LCC) mammogram comparison.

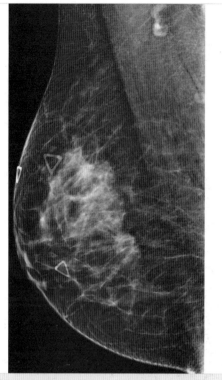

Fig. 24.9 Right mediolateral oblique (RMLO) mammogram comparison.

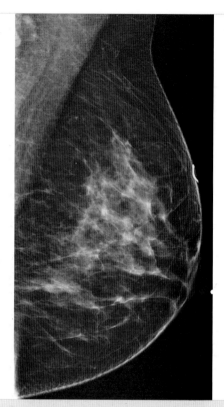

Fig. 24.10 Left mediolateral oblique (LMLO) mammogram comparison.

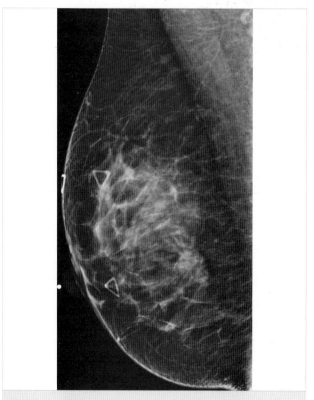

Fig. 24.11 Right lateromedial (RLM) mammogram comparison.

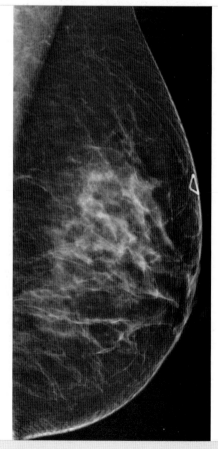

Fig. 24.12 Left lateromedial (LLM) mammogram comparison.

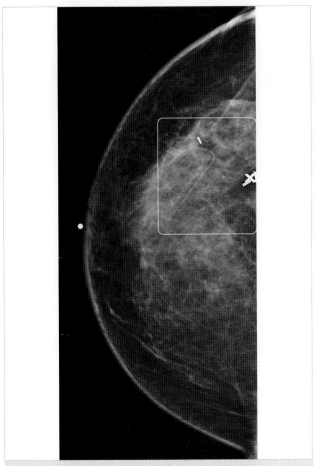

Fig. 24.13 Right craniocaudal (RCC) mammogram with label.

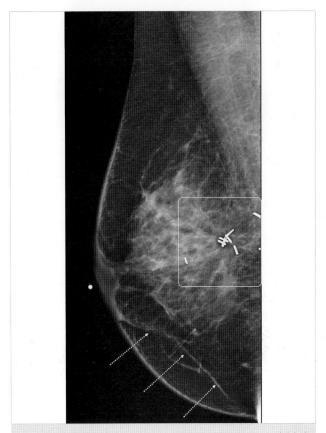

Fig. 24.14 Right mediolateral oblique (RMLO) mammogram with label.

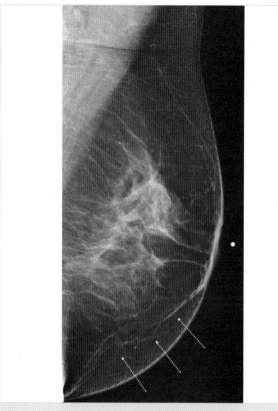

Fig. 24.15 Left mediolateral oblique (LMLO) mammogram with label.

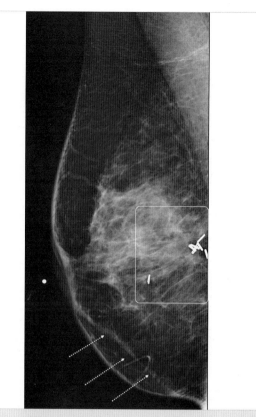

Fig. 24.16 Right lateromedial (RLM) mammogram with label.

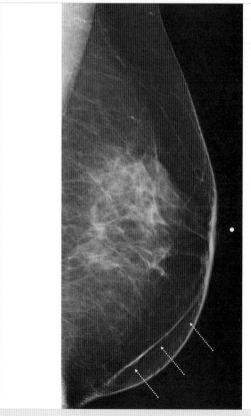

Fig. 24.17 Left lateromedial (LLM) mammogram with label.

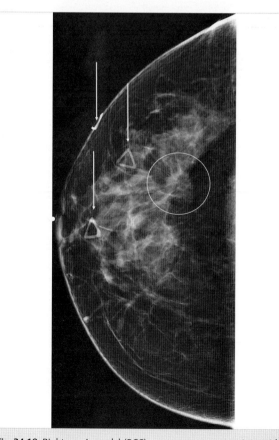

Fig. 24.18 Right craniocaudal (RCC) mammogram comparison with label.

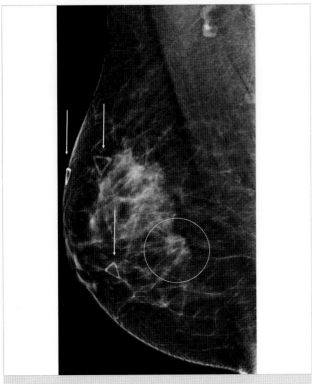

Fig. 24.19 Right mediolateral oblique (RMLO) mammogram comparison with label.

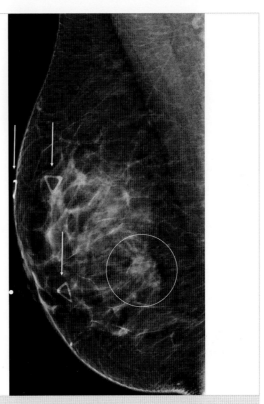

Fig. 24.20 Right lateromedial (RLM) mammogram comparison with label.

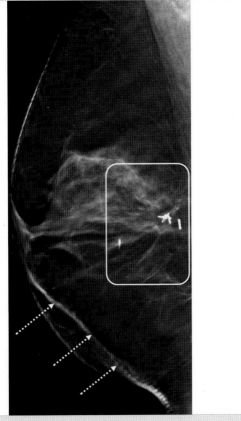

Fig. 24.21 Right lateromedial digital breast tomosynthesis (RLM DBT), slice 41 of 84 with label.

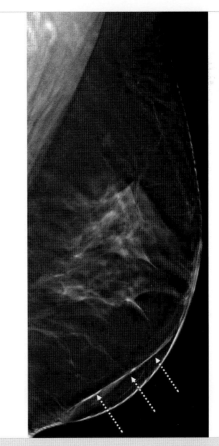

Fig. 24.22 Left lateromedial digital breast tomosynthesis (LLM DBT), slice 39 of 85 with label.

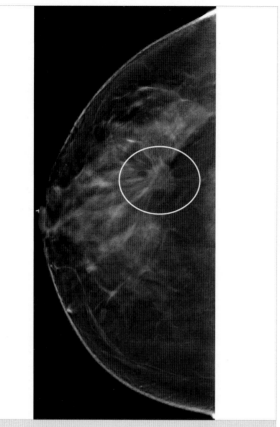

Fig. 24.23 Right craniocaudal digital breast tomosynthesis (RCC DBT), slice 25 of 80 with label, comparison.

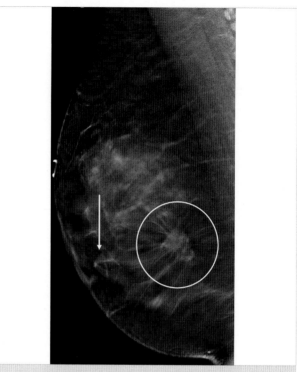

Fig. 24.24 Right lateromedial digital breast tomosynthesis (RLM DBT), slice 45 of 77 with label, comparison

Part III

Cases with Screening Tomosynthesis Evaluation Needing Further Diagnostic Evaluation

25 Mass with Architectural Distortion

Lonie R. Salkowski

25.1 Presentation and Presenting Images

(▶ Fig. 25.1, ▶ Fig. 25.2)

A 49-year-old female who has a sister with breast cancer presents for screening mammography.

25.2 Key Images

(▶ Fig. 25.3, ▶ Fig. 25.4, ▶ Fig. 25.5, ▶ Fig. 25.6)

25.2.1 Breast Tissue Density

There are scattered areas of fibroglandular density.

25.2.2 Imaging Findings

In the upper outer quadrant of the right breast at the 9 o'clock location in the posterior depth, there is a possible focal asymmetry. This is best seen on the digital breast tomosynthesis (DBT) images, especially the mediolateral oblique (MLO) DBT images. There does not initially appear to be a correlate on the corresponding MLO mammogram. The DBT images reveal a mass with indistinct margins at the 9 o'clock location that appears larger on the craniocaudal (CC) DBT images than on the MLO DBT images.

25.3 BI-RADS Classification and Action

Category 0: Mammography: Incomplete. Need additional imaging evaluation and/or prior mammograms for comparison.

25.4 Diagnostic Images

(▶ Fig. 25.7, ▶ Fig. 25.8, ▶ Fig. 25.9)

25.4.1 Imaging Findings

The diagnostic imaging demonstrates a persistent mass on the CC spotcompression mammogram. The ML mammogram suggests a mass at the 9 o'clock location but the density of the breast interferes with further assessment. An ultrasound was performed because the DBT images were convincing that there was a mass present and the margins were indistinct. The ultrasound evaluation revealed an 8-mm anechoic mass with circumscribed margins and posterior acoustic enhancement surrounded by dense breast tissue.

25.5 BI-RADS Classification and Action

Category 2: Benign

25.6 Differential Diagnosis

1. **Simple cyst**: The adjacent dense tissue on conventional mammography and DBT made this mass appear bigger than it is. Ultrasound reveals an anechoic mass with circumscribed margins mostly surrounded by dense tissue.
2. *Solid mass*: Neither conventional mammography nor DBT can tell a fluid-filled (cystic) mass from a solid mass. The ultrasound appearance is highly suggestive of a fluid-filled structure.
3. *Normal fibroglandular tissue*: Conventional mammography was less convincing of the presence of any finding. The ability of DBT to decrease the effects of overlapping tissue can lead to the identification of both malignant and benign findings.

25.7 Essential Facts

- Lesion margins become more apparent with DBT.
- Oval or round masses with gently lobulated margins will be unmasked with DBT when previously concealed on conventional breast imaging. Further studies will be needed to determine whether these masses can be safely followed or ignored.
- Summation artifacts are a known cause of false-positives on screening mammography. DBT can help to minimize this contribution to false-positives by demonstrating that the finding is due to overlapping fibroglandular tissue.

25.8 Management and Digital Breast Tomosynthesis Principles

- There is a learning curve with DBT and readers must reset their threshold for calling back findings on DBT for further evaluation.
- DBT will unmask small circumscribed masses, which are probably cysts or intramammary lymph nodes, that were previously obscured.
- It is uncertain how the unmasking effect of presumably benign findings will affect a clinical practice or how these findings should be managed when only seen on DBT.
- Studies have shown that DBT improves the cancer detection rate and decreases the overall recall rate.

25.9 Further Reading

[1] Baker JA, Lo JY. Breast tomosynthesis: state-of-the-art and review of the literature. Acad Radiol. 2011; 18(10):1298–1310

[2] Roth RG, Maidment AD, Weinstein SP, Roth SO, Conant EF. Digital breast tomosynthesis: lessons learned from early clinical implementation. Radiographics. 2014; 34(4):E89–E102

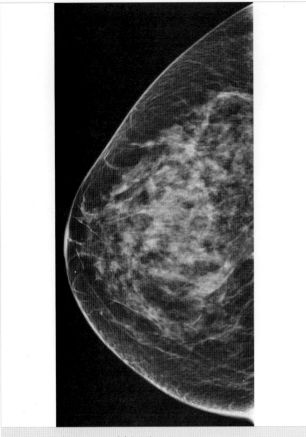

Fig. 25.1 Right craniocaudal (RCC) mammogram.

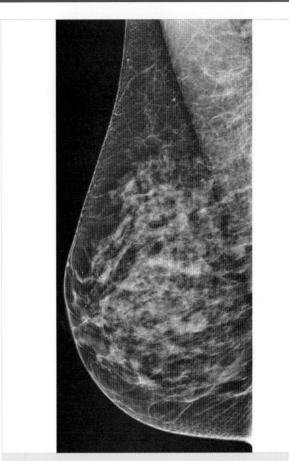

Fig. 25.2 Right mediolateral oblique (RMLO) mammogram.

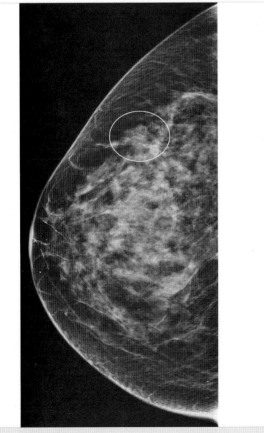

Fig. 25.3 Right craniocaudal (RCC) mammogram with label.

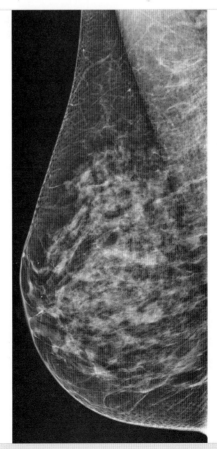

Fig. 25.4 Right mediolateral oblique (RMLO) mammogram.

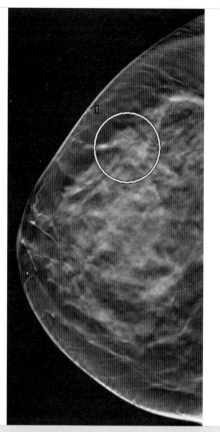

Fig. 25.5 Right craniocaudal digital breast tomosynthesis (RCC DBT), slice 28 of 61, with label.

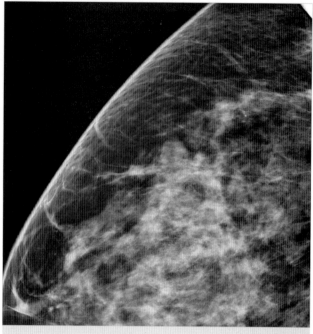

Fig. 25.6 Right craniocaudal (RCC) spot compression mammogram.

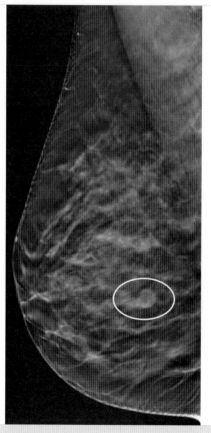

Fig. 25.7 Right craniocaudal (RCC) spot-compression mammogram.

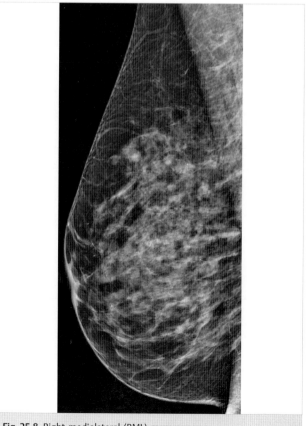

Fig. 25.8 Right mediolateral (RML) mammogram.

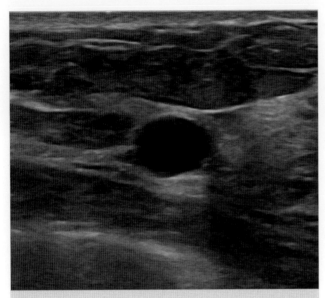

Fig. 25.9 Right breast ultrasound, transverse view.

26 Developing Asymmetry

Lonie R. Salkowski

26.1 Presentation and Presenting Images

(▶ Fig. 26.1, ▶ Fig. 26.2, ▶ Fig. 26.3, ▶ Fig. 26.4)

A 59-year-old female with a history of right breast cancer treated 5 years ago presents for screening mammography.

26.2 Key images

(▶ Fig. 26.5, ▶ Fig. 26.6)

26.2.1 Breast Tissue Density

There are scattered areas of fibroglandular density.

26.2.2 Imaging Findings

In the upper outer quadrant of the left breast at the 1 o'clock location in the posterior depth, there is a focal asymmetry. This is best seen on the digital breast tomosynthesis (DBT) images and especially the mediolateral (MLO) DBT images.

26.3 BI-RADS Classification and Action

Category 0: Mammography: Incomplete. Need additional imaging evaluation and/or prior mammograms for comparison.

26.4 Diagnostic Images

(▶ Fig. 26.7, ▶ Fig. 26.8, ▶ Fig. 26.9, ▶ Fig. 26.10, ▶ Fig. 26.11, ▶ Fig. 26.12)

26.4.1 Imaging Findings

The diagnostic imaging demonstrates a persistent irregular mass with indistinct margins at the 1 o'clock location in the posterior depth. Targeted ultrasound reveals a 4 × 3 × 4 mm irregular mass with indistinct margins and posterior acoustic shadowing. This mass was assessed to be suspicious and a biopsy recommended. The postbiopsy craniocaudal (CC) and mediolateral (ML) mammogram images (▶ Fig. 26.11 and ▶ Fig. 26.12) demonstrate the biopsy clip at the site of the mass seen mammographically.

26.5 BI-RADS Classification and Action

Category 4B: Moderate suspicion for malignancy

26.6 Differential Diagnosis

1. **Fibromatosis**: This mass is irregular with an ultrasound correlate. There is considerable overlap of characteristic imaging findings between fibromatosis and breast cancer, therefore a biopsy is necessary. A biopsy yielding fibromatosis would be concordant with the mammographic, DBT, and ultrasound findings.
2. *Carcinoma:* This mass is irregular in appearance and would require a biopsy to exclude breast cancer as the diagnosis.
3. *Normal breast tissue as a summation artifact:* This small focal asymmetry persists on additional imaging and is new compared to prior exams (*not shown*). Thus, this finding should not be dismissed but rather evaluated.

26.7 Essential Facts

- Fibromatosis is a stromal tumor.
- Fibromatosis is rare, accounting for less than 0.2% of all breast tumors.
- Fibromatosis is benign, but locally aggressive. These tumors require wide local excision to prevent recurrence.
- Fibromatosis tumors typically present mammographically as spiculated masses.
- Fibromatosis significance in breast imaging is that it can mimic breast cancer.
- These tumors are more often located near the chest wall.
- Magnetic resonance (MR) imaging may be helpful to evaluate the extent of the tumor and the possibility of chest-wall invasion if the tumor is not fully seen on the mammogram.

26.8 Management and Digital Breast Tomsynthesis Principles

- Technically DBT reduction of overlapping tissue effects make masses with indistinct or spiculated margins more conspicuous. Thus, fibromatosis, along with cancers, will be more readily apparent on DBT.
- The imaging features of a spiculated locally invasive tumor make it suspicious for malignancy and not distinguishable from breast cancer without a biopsy.

26.9 Further Reading

[1] Glazebrook KN, Reynolds CA. Mammary fibromatosis. AJR Am J Roentgenol. 2009;193(3):856–860

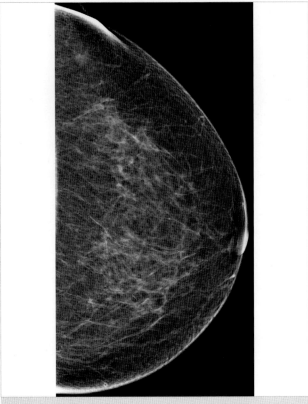

Fig. 26.1 Left craniocaudal (LCC) mammogram.

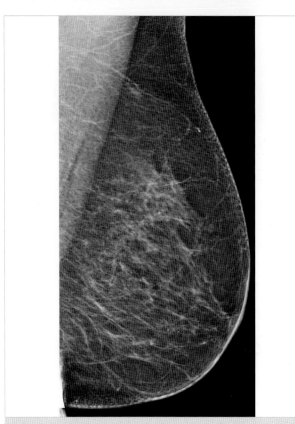

Fig. 26.2 Left mediolateral oblique (LMLO) mammogram.

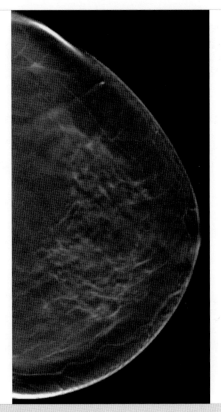

Fig. 26.3 Left craniocaudal digital breast tomosynthesis (LCC DBT), slice 44 of 85.

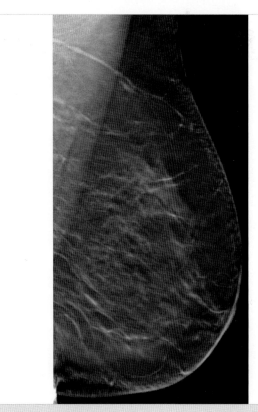

Fig. 26.4 Left mediolateral oblique digital breast tomosynthesis (LMLO DBT), slice 24 of 83.

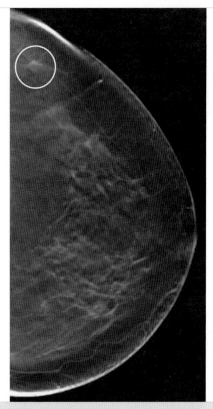

Fig. 26.5 Left craniocaudal digital breast tomosynthesis (LCC DBT) with label.

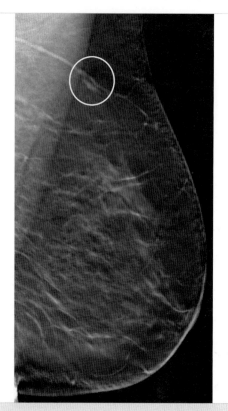

Fig. 26.6 Left mediolateral oblique digital breast tomosynthesis (LMLO DBT) with label.

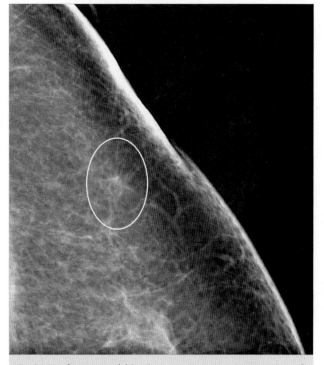

Fig. 26.7 Left craniocaudal (LCC) spot-compression mammogram with label.

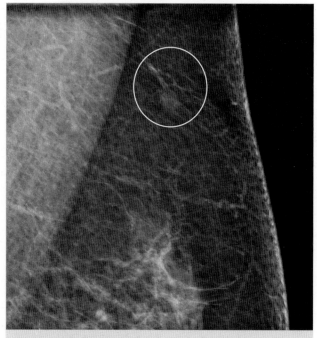

Fig. 26.8 Right mediolateral oblique (RMLO) spot-compression mammogram with label.

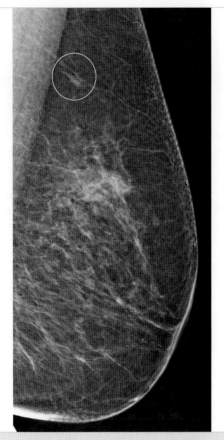

Fig. 26.9 Left mediolateral (LML) mammogram with label.

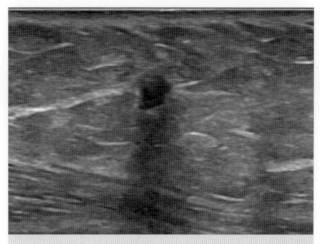

Fig. 26.10 Left breast ultrasound, longitudinal view.

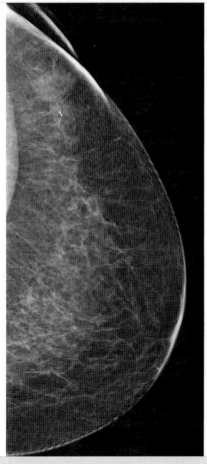

Fig. 26.11 Postbiopsy left craniocaudal (LCC) mammogram.

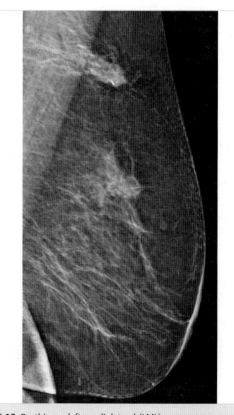

Fig. 26.12 Postbiopsy left mediolateral (LML) mammogram.

27 High-Density Mass

Lonie R. Salkowski

27.1 Presentation and Presenting Images

(▶ Fig. 27.1, ▶ Fig. 27.2)

A 61-year-old female presents for screening mammography.

27.2 Key Images

(▶ Fig. 27.3, ▶ Fig. 27.4)

27.2.1 Breast Tissue Density

There are scattered areas of fibroglandular density.

27.2.2 Imaging Findings

In the upper outer quadrant of the left breast at the 2 o'clock location in the posterior depth, there is a 1.5-cm irregular high-density mass (▶ Fig. 27.3 and ▶ Fig. 27.4). The right mammogram was negative (*not shown*).

27.3 BI-RADS Classification and Action

Category 0: Mammography: Incomplete. Need additional imaging evaluation and/or prior mammograms for comparison.

27.4 Diagnostic Images

(▶ Fig. 27.5, ▶ Fig. 27.6, ▶ Fig. 27.7, ▶ Fig. 27.8, ▶ Fig. 27.9)

27.4.1 Imaging Findings

The diagnostic imaging demonstrates a persistent 1.5-cm irregular high-density mass with indistinct margins at the 2 o'clock location in the posterior depth (▶ Fig. 27.5, ▶ Fig. 27.6, and ▶ Fig. 27.7). The targeted ultrasound reveals a 1.0 × 0.7 × 1.3 cm irregular hypoechoic mass with indistinct margins and posterior acoustic shadowing at 2 o'clock position, 3 cm from the nipple (▶ Fig. 27.8). There is mild vascularity adjacent to the mass but not internally (▶ Fig. 27.9). The ispilateral axillary lymph nodes were normal (*not shown*).

27.5 BI-RADS Classification and Action

Category 4C: High suspicion for malignancy

27.6 Differential Diagnosis

1. **Invasive ductal carcinoma (IDC)**: Core needle biopsy revealed grade 2 IDC with intermediate grade ductal carcinoma in situ (DCIS). The imaging features would support the diagnosis of any invasive carcinoma.
2. *Normal breast tissue*: This mass should not be interpreted as normal breast tissue. The conventional mammogram and DBT both support that this is a mass as defined by its convex margins. A biopsy revealing normal breast tissue would be considered discordant with these findings.
3. *Fibroadenoma*: This mass has an irregular shape with indistinct margins both mammographically and on ultrasound. These imaging findings would not support a benign diagnosis.

27.7 Essential Facts

- Invasive ductal carcinoma is the most common invasive breast cancer (65–75% of cases).
- Most invasive ductal carcinomas are sporadic; only about 10% of cancers are attributable to genetics.
- The incidence of breast cancer increases with age.
- Over half of invasive ductal carcinomas are clinically occult and detected by imaging.
- There is a better prognosis for breast cancers identified at screening compared to interval cancers (cancers detected between screening examinations). This is despite accounting for positive lymph nodes, tumor size, patient age, hormone receptor status, and histological grade. The method of detection (screening or interval) may not have independent prognostic utility, but only that screening leads to earlier detection of cancers.

27.8 Management and Digital Breast Tomosynthesis Principles

- In several studies, digital breast tomosynthesis (DBT) has been shown to decrease the recall rate for further imaging evaluation.
- DBT has shown improved sensitivity and specificity for cancer detection across all breast tissue densities.
- DBT, due to its ability to reduce anatomical noise within a given slice, especially in dense breast tissue, can better assess the size of a tumor and its imaging characteristics. This leads to improved accuracy of diagnosis.
- When full-field digital mammography (FFDM) and DBT are performed in combination, there is an approximate doubling of the radiation dose for FFDM alone.

27.9 Further Reading

[1] Förnvik D, Zackrisson S, Ljungberg O, et al. Breast tomosynthesis: Accuracy of tumor measurement compared with digital mammography and ultrasonography. Acta Radiol. 2010; 51(3):240–247

[2] Shen Y, Yang Y, Inoue LY, Munsell MF, Miller AB, Berry DA. Role of detection method in predicting breast cancer survival: analysis of randomized screening trials. J Natl Cancer Inst. 2005; 97(16):1195–1203

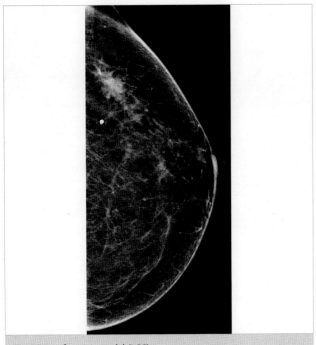

Fig. 27.1 Left craniocaudal (LCC) mammogram.

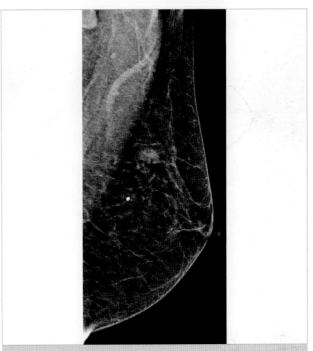

Fig. 27.2 Left mediolateral oblique (LMLO) mammogran.

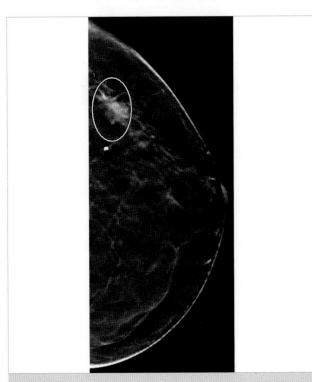

Fig. 27.3 Left craniocaudal digital breast tomosynthesis (LCC DBT), slice 25 of 58.

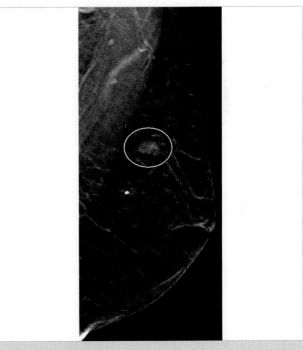

Fig. 27.4 Left mediolateral oblique digital breast tomosynthesis (LMLO DBT), slice 18 of 55.

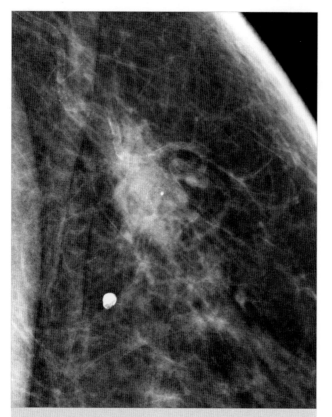

Fig. 27.5 Left craniocaudal (LCC) spot-compression mammogram.

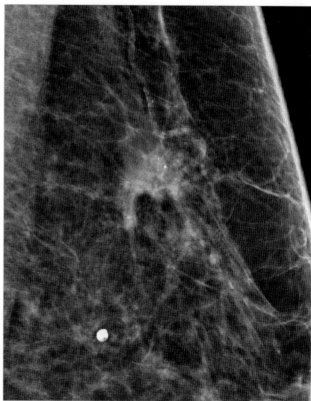

Fig. 27.6 Left mediolateral oblique (LMLO) spot-compression mammogram.

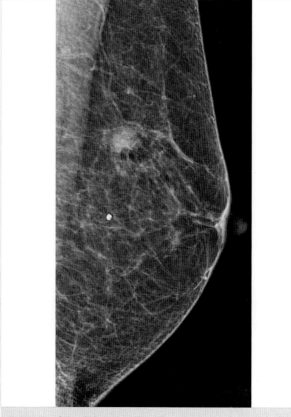

Fig. 27.7 Left mediolateral (LML) mammogram.

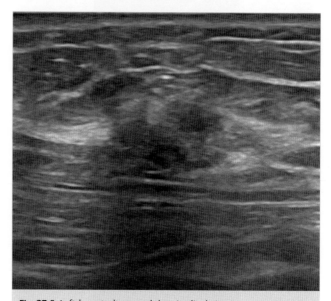

Fig. 27.8 Left breast ultrasound, longitudinal view.

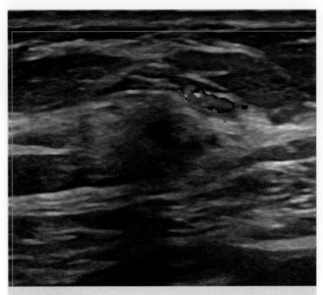

Fig. 27.9 Left breast Doppler ultrasound, transverse view.

28 Mass on Baseline Mammogram

Lonie R. Salkowski

28.1 Presentation and Presenting Images

(▶ Fig. 28.1, ▶ Fig. 28.2)

A 40- year-old female presents for screening mammography.

28.2 Key Images

(▶ Fig. 28.3, ▶ Fig. 28.4)

28.2.1 Breast Tissue Density

There are scattered areas of fibroglandular density.

28.2.2 Imaging Findings

In the upper outer quadrant of the right breast at the 10 o'clock location in the middle depth, there is an oval high-density mass. The digital breast tomosynthesis (DBT) images (▶ Fig. 28.3 and ▶ Fig. 28.4) suggest that the margins of the mass are mostly circumscribed. The left breast imaging (*not shown*) was normal.

28.3 BI-RADS Classification and Action

Category 0: Mammography: Incomplete. Need additional imaging evaluation and/or prior mammograms for comparison.

28.4 Diagnostic Images

(▶ Fig. 28.5, ▶ Fig. 28.6, ▶ Fig. 28.7, ▶ Fig. 28.8, ▶ Fig. 28.9)

28.4.1 Imaging Findings

The diagnostic imaging demonstrates a 1.2-cm oval mass with obscured and circumscribed margins in the right breast in the middle depth. The targeted ultrasound demonstrates a 1.2 × 0.9 × 1.2 cm anechoic oval mass, 7 cm from the nipple, with circumscribed margins, mild posterior acoustic enhancement, and no internal or surrounding vascularity.

28.5 BI-RADS Classification and Action

Category 2: Benign

28.6 Differential Diagnosis

1. **Simple cyst**: This mass on mammography is circumscribed; however, the ultrasound confirms that this is a fluid-containing mass and its imaging features also suggest this is a simple cyst.
2. *Complicated cyst*: Complicated cysts typically have low-level internal echoes and have a look similar to solid masses. This mass has no internal echoes. Sometimes cysts deep in the breast tissue can be difficult to visualize with ultrasound. Thus, it is important that the gain and frequency of the ultrasound machine is properly adjusted to allow for the distinction between cysts and solid masses to be perceived on ultrasound imaging.
3. *Fibroadenoma*: This mass appears fluid-filled thus eliminating fibroadenoma as a diagnosis. On baseline mammograms of young women, the most common masses will be cysts or fibroadenomas.

28.7 Essential Facts

- Recall rates are decreased with DBT compared to full-field digital mammography (FFDM).
- Durand and colleagues (2015) found that baseline recall rates for DBT and FFDM were significantly reduced compared to FFDM alone (20.8% compared with 33.1%, respectively).
- Masses seen on a baseline DBT compared with a baseline FFDM had no significant difference in recall rates.
- There is a significant reduction in recalls for asymmetries seen on baseline FFDM and DBT mammograms compared to asymmetries seen on baseline FFDM alone.

28.8 Management and Digital Breast Tomosynthesis Principles

- The unmasking effect of DBT and the ability to present the slices within a three-dimensional (3D) volume allow for better characterization of the tissue composition and lesions seen within the tissue.
- DBT is superior to FFDM in characterizing the margins of a mass.
- There is not enough experience with DBT to dismiss masses that are completely circumscribed on DBT as benign (BIRADS 2) and in need of no further evaluation.

28.9 Further Reading

[1] Durand MA, Haas BM, Yao X, et al. Early clinical experience with digital breast tomosynthesis for screening mammography. Radiology. 2015; 274(1):85–92
[2] Helvie MA. Digital mammography imaging: breast tomosynthesis and advanced applications. Radiol Clin North Am. 2010; 48(5):917–929

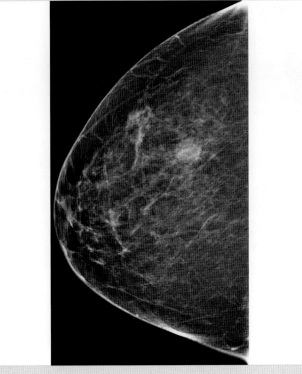

Fig. 28.1 Right craniocaudal (RCC) mammogram.

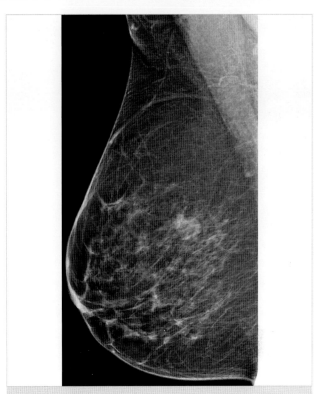

Fig. 28.2 Right mediolateral oblique (RMLO) mammogram.

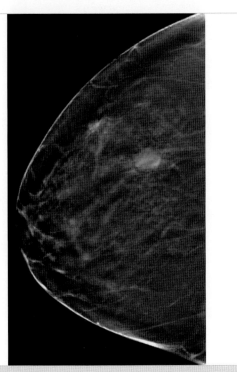

Fig. 28.3 Right craniocaudal digital breast tomosynthesis (RCC DBT), slice 28 of 79.

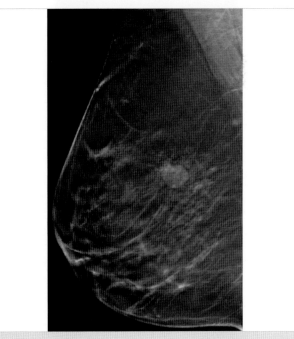

Fig. 28.4 Right mediolateral oblique digital breast tomosynthesis (RMLO DBT), slice 31 of 77.

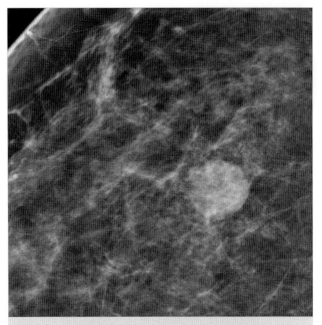

Fig. 28.5 Right craniocaudal (RCC) spot-compression mammogram.

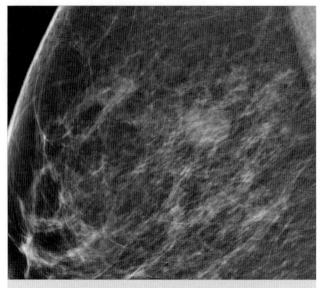

Fig. 28.6 Right mediolateral oblique (RMLO) spot-compression mammogram.

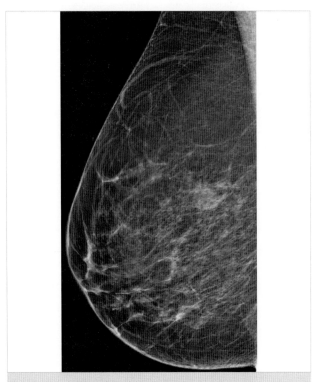

Fig. 28.7 Right mediolateral (RML) mammogram.

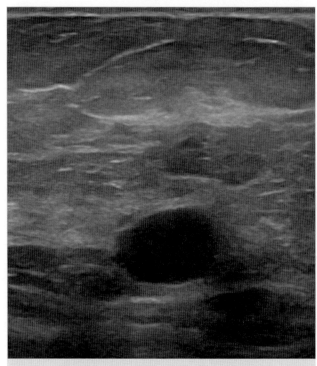

Fig. 28.8 Right breast ultrasound, transverse view.

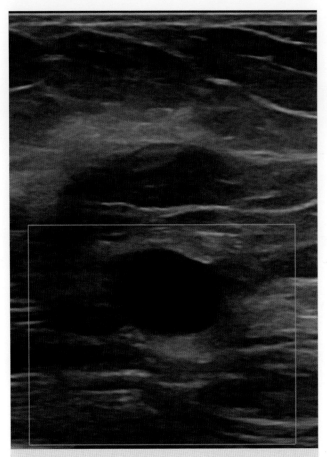

Fig. 28.9 Right breast Doppler ultrasound, sagittal view.

29 Amorphous Calcifications

Lonie R. Salkowski

29.1 Presentation and Presenting Images

(▶ Fig. 29.1, ▶ Fig. 29.2)

A 47-year-old female presents for screening mammography.

29.2 Key Images

(▶ Fig. 29.3, ▶ Fig. 29.4)

29.2.1 Breast Tissue Density

The breasts are extremely dense, which lowers the sensitivity of mammography.

29.2.2 Imaging Findings

In the upper outer quadrant of the right breast at the 10 o'clock location in the anterior depth, there are grouped calcifications. These are very hard to discern on the digital breast tomosynthesis (DBT) images.

29.3 BI-RADS Classification and Action

Category 0: Mammography: Incomplete. Need additional imaging evaluation and/or prior mammograms for comparison.

29.4 Diagnostic Images

(▶ Fig. 29.5, ▶ Fig. 29.6, ▶ Fig. 29.7, ▶ Fig. 29.8, ▶ Fig. 29.9, ▶ Fig. 29.10, ▶ Fig. 29.11, ▶ Fig. 29.12, ▶ Fig. 29.13)

29.4.1 Imaging Findings

The diagnostic imaging demonstrates a 2.5-cm area of segmental amorphous calcifications in the right breast at the 10 o'clock location, 1.5 cm from the nipple. The calcifications do not layer. The morphology of these calcifications warrant a biopsy. The patient reports that she had a biopsy about 6 years ago. These records were located including the stereotactic biopsy images (▶ Fig. 29.9, ▶ Fig. 29.10, and ▶ Fig. 29.11). The specimens from the stereotactic biopsy contain numerous calcifications, which indicate that the area was well-sampled. No biopsy clip was placed according to the procedure report due to bleeding. Comparing the current imaging and the imaging 2 years after the biopsy (▶ Fig. 29.12 and ▶ Fig. 29.13), these calcifications are stable. The biopsy diagnosis 6 years ago was sclerosing adenosis.

29.5 BI-RADS Classification and Action

Category 2: Benign

29.6 Differential Diagnosis

1. ***Sclerosing adenosis***: These calcifications when biopsied revealed sclerosing adenosis. Overall the calcifications are stable with no increase compared to prior examinations. Amorphous calcifications are consistent with sclerosing adenosis.
2. *Ductal carcinoma in situ (DCIS)*: DCIS would be a concordant biopsy result for amorphous calcifications. The fact that these calcifications have been stable and have a benign concordant biopsy result makes DCIS less likely in this case, but it was a concern at initial presentation.
3. *Fibrocystic disease*: Fibrocystic changes can present with various underlying mammographic findings such as cysts, masses, and calcifications. When calcifications are present, these can be seen to layer in cysts, but atypical presentations can occur and thus there is a significant overlap of fibrocystic changes and ADH (atypical ductal hyperplasia) and/or DCIS on the biopsy of grouped calcifications.

29.7 Essential Facts

- Sclerosing adenosis commonly presents as grouped and/or scattered amorphous calcifications. It is often indistinguishable from low-grade DCIS. Biopsy is frequently performed to exclude DCIS.
- Sclerosing adenosis can present mammographically as a mass, an architectural distortion, and calcifications.
- Sclerosing adenosis has many overlapping imaging findings with both invasive and intraductal cancer.
- Sclerosing adenosis is a benign proliferative breast disease.
- In addition to DBT not performing as well in identifying the distribution of calcifications, the low-dose radiation of DBT produces a much noisier projection view compared to full-field digital mammography (FFDM), which has both negative qualitative and quantitative effects on the analysis of calcifications on DBT. This is especially true for those amorphous, or finer, calcifications.

29.8 Management and Digital Breast Tomosynthesis Principles

- Prior imaging studies, especially when accessible, can avert unnecessary biopsies or additional imaging.
- Sclerosing adenosis can exist in the midst of other significant pathology. When assessing the concordance of radiology and pathology, it is important to assess if the imaging findings correlate with the pathology findings. If the lesion is large and only a microscopic area of a certain pathology is found, it is unlikely that the pathology explains the imaging findings. If there is doubt, it is often helpful to discuss or review the slides with the pathologist if this is not a routine practice in a radiology–pathology concordance program.

- When patients have had prior biopsies and no biopsy markers are placed, it is important to correlate prior imaging, procedure information, and medical records to the current mammography and other imaging findings to ensure that the proper management is performed.

29.9 Further Reading

[1] Gill HK, Ioffe OB, Berg WA. When is a diagnosis of sclerosing adenosis acceptable at core biopsy? Radiology. 2003; 228(1):50–57
[2] Uematsu T. The emerging role of breast tomosynthesis. Breast Cancer. 2013; 20(3):204–212

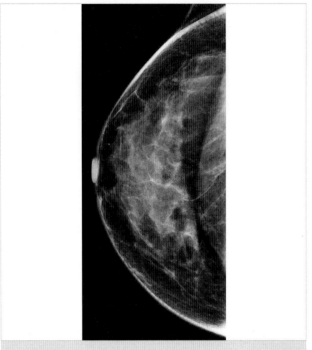

Fig. 29.1 Right craniocaudal (RCC) mammogram.

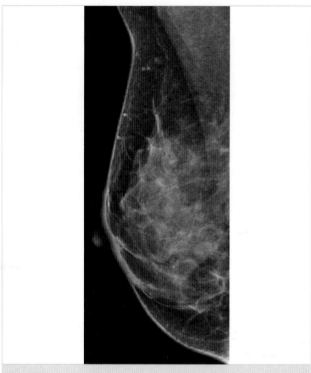

Fig. 29.2 Right mediolateral oblique (RMLO) mammogram.

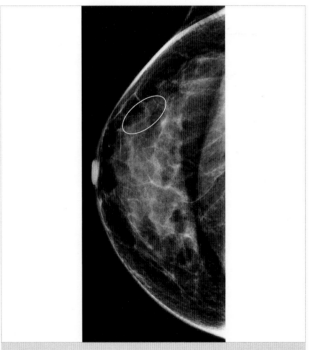

Fig. 29.3 Right craniocaudal (RCC) mammogram with label.

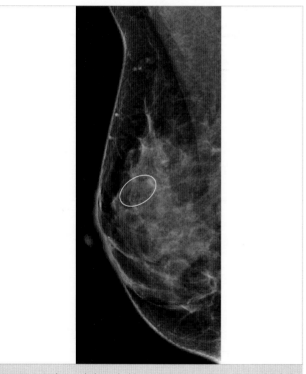

Fig. 29.4 Right mediolateral oblique (RMLO) mammogram with label.

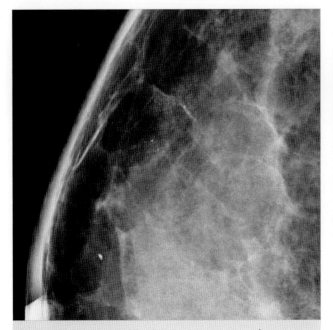

Fig. 29.5 Right craniocaudal (RCC) mammogram, magnification.

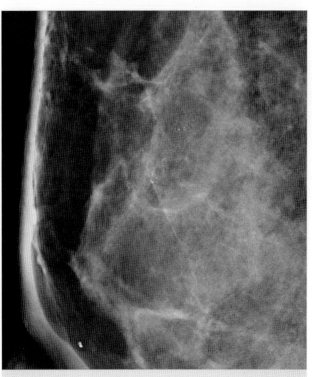

Fig. 29.6 Right mediolateral (RML) mammogram, magnification.

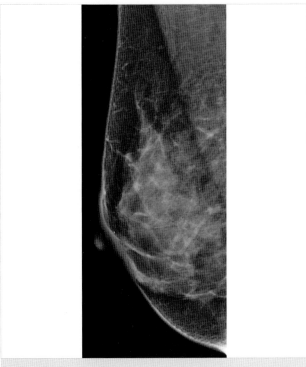

Fig. 29.7 Right mediolateral (RML) mammogram.

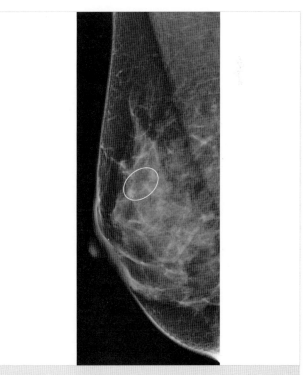

Fig. 29.8 Right mediolateral (RML) mammogram with label.

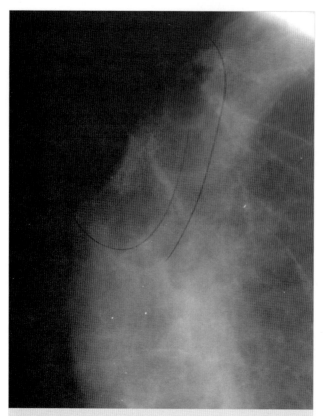

Fig. 29.9 Right craniocaudal (RCC) analog mammogram, spot magnification, 6 years ago.

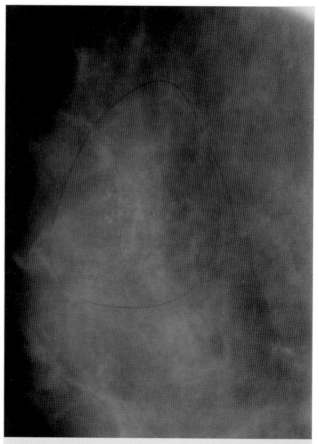

Fig. 29.10 Right mediolateral (RML) analog mammogram, spot magnification, 6 years ago.

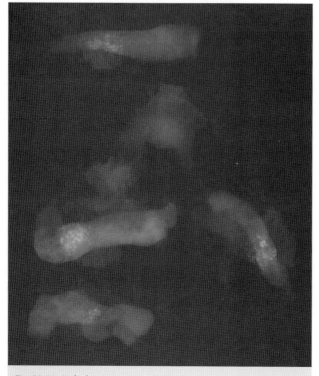

Fig. 29.11 Right breast stereotactic biopsy specimens (analog image).

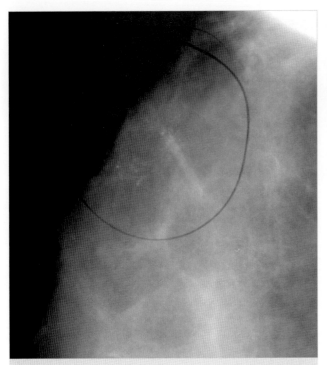

Fig. 29.12 Right craniocaudal (RCC) analog mammogram, spot magnification, 4 years ago.

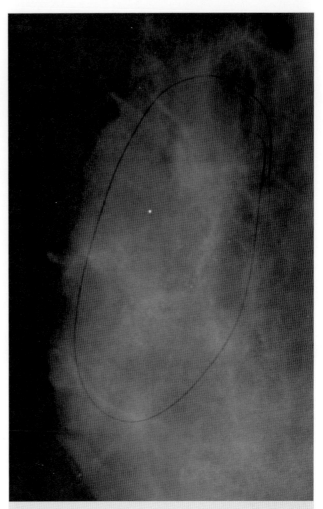

Fig. 29.13 Right mediolateral (RML) analog mammogram, spot magnification, 4 years ago.

30 Obscured Mass within Dense Breast Tissue

Lonie R. Salkowski

30.1 Presentation and Presenting Images

(▶ Fig. 30.1, ▶ Fig. 30.2)

A 52-year-old female presents for screening mammography. She has a history of bilateral breast cancer with her most recent cancer, involving her right breast, treated 5 years ago.

30.2 Key Images

(▶ Fig. 30.3, ▶ Fig. 30.4, ▶ Fig. 30.5, ▶ Fig. 30.6)

30.2.1 Breast Tissue Density

There are scattered areas of fibroglandular density.

30.2.2 Imaging Findings

In the lower outer quadrant of the right breast, there is an oval mass at the edge of the film that has a wire marking the skin incision overlying it. This reflects her prior postsurgical changes and the partial breast irradiation (brachytherapy). On first examination of the digital mammograms of the right breast, there appears to be nothing new. Looking at the tomosynthesis images, an irregular mass with obscured and indistinct margins can be identified at the 12 o'clock location in the posterior depth (▶ Fig. 30.5 and ▶ Fig. 30.6). In retrospect, these areas can be identified on the conventional digital mammograms (▶ Fig. 30.3 and ▶ Fig. 30.4).

30.3 BI-RADS Classification and Action

Category 0: Mammography: Incomplete. Need additional imaging evaluation and/or prior mammograms for comparison.

30.4 Diagnostic Images

(▶ Fig. 30.7, ▶ Fig. 30.8, ▶ Fig. 30.9, ▶ Fig. 30.10, ▶ Fig. 30.11, ▶ Fig. 30.12, ▶ Fig. 30.13)

30.5 Imaging Findings

The indistinct mass is best demonstrated on the diagnostic mediolateral oblique (MLO) spot-compression and left mediolateral (LML) mammograms (▶ Fig. 30.8 and ▶ Fig. 30.9). The surrounding tissues do not interfere as much as they do on the craniocaudal (CC) view (▶ Fig. 30.7), obscuring the mass. There appears to be architectural distortion associated with the 1.1 × 1.5 × 1.2 cm irregular mass with indistinct margins located at 12 o'clock. Targeted ultrasound reveals a 1.2 × 1.3 × 0.9 cm irregular hypoechoic mass with angular margins at the 12 o'clock location, 6 cm from the nipple (▶ Fig. 30.10 and

▶ Fig. 30.11). This mass was biopsied. The ribbon clip is located at the site of the mass (▶ Fig. 30.12 and ▶ Fig. 30.13), which was seen best on the tomosynthesis images (▶ Fig. 30.5 and ▶ Fig. 30.6).

30.6 BI-RADS Classification and Action

Category 4C: High suspicion for malignancy

30.7 Differential Diagnosis

1. **Invasive ductal carcinoma (IDC)**: The imaging characteristics support a diagnosis of cancer. On biopsy, this mass was a grade 2 IDC.
2. *Postoperative scar*: This patient has a history of bilateral treated breast cancers. Her right breast cancer site was marked with a skin marker, which locates it in a different quadrant (lower outer) of the breast than the findings. Thus, this is not a likely diagnosis.
3. *Metastasis*: Metastasis to the breast is rare (0.5 – 6.6% of all breast malignancies). Occasionally it is the presenting lesion of an unknown primary cancer with the most common being lymphoma or melanoma. This patient does not have any other cancers. If a biopsy yielded this pathology, further systemic evaluation of the patient would be required.

30.8 Management and Digital Breast Tomosynthesis Principles

- In this case, digital breast tomosynthesis (DBT) performed better at identifying and localizing the right breast mass.
- Some cancers can be effaced on conventional spot-compression images. It is important that if the DBT imaging is concerning, even with a negative diagnostic conventional mammogram, that an ultrasound be performed. This can aid in diagnosing mammographically occult cancers.
- DBT is helpful with triangulation of lesions, especially within dense breast tissue which may obscure the lesion in one or both projections.
- It is important to remember that not all cancers will be detected on DBT. Evaluation should be directed to the most suspicious imaging findings whether on DBT or full-field digital mammography (FFDM).

30.9 Further Reading

[1] Dershaw DD. Breast imaging and the conservative treatment of breast cancer. Radiol Clin North Am. 2002; 40(3):501–516
[2] Weinstein SP, Orel SG, Pinnamaneni N, et al. Mammographic appearance of recurrent breast cancer after breast conservation therapy. Acad Radiol. 2008; 15(2):240–244

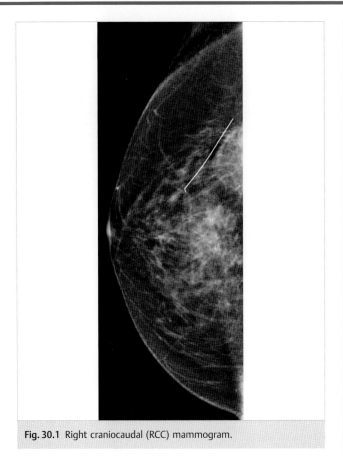

Fig. 30.1 Right craniocaudal (RCC) mammogram.

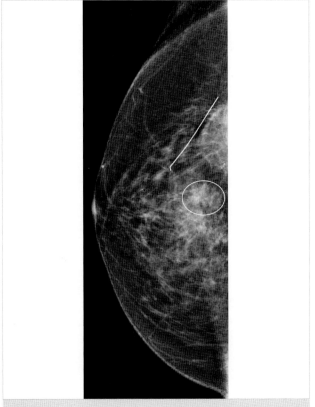

Fig. 30.2 Right mediolateral oblique (RMLO) mammogram.

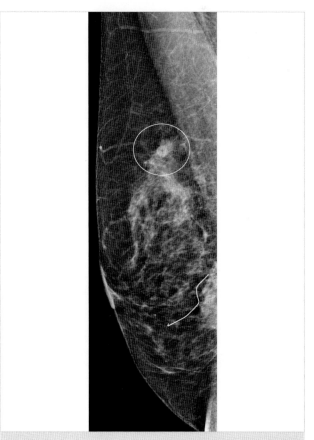

Fig. 30.3 Right craniocaudal (RCC) mammogram with label.

Fig. 30.4 Right mediolateral oblique (RMLO) mammogram with label.

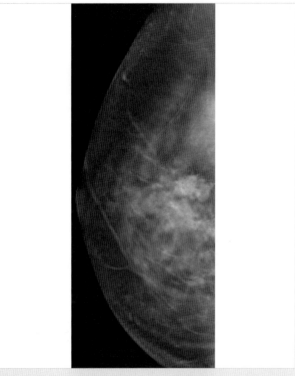

Fig. 30.5 Right craniocaudal digital breast tomosynthesis (RCC DBT), slice 55 of 73.

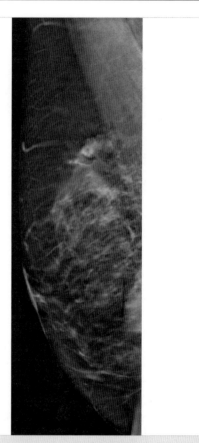

Fig. 30.6 Right mediolateral oblique digital breast tomosynthesis (RMLO DBT), slice 41 of 62.

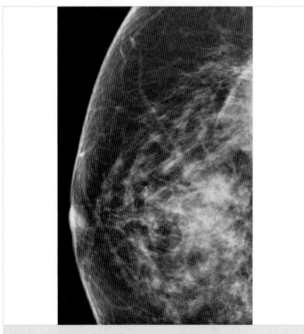

Fig. 30.7 Right craniocaudal (RCC) spot-compression mammogram.

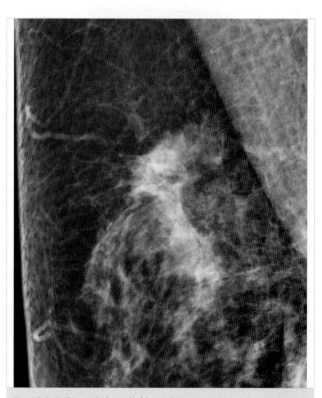

Fig. 30.8 Right mediolateral oblique (RMLO) spot-compression mammogram.

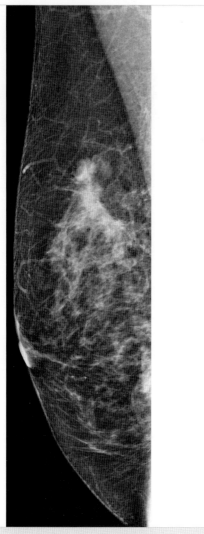

Fig. 30.9 Right mediolateral (RML) mammogram.

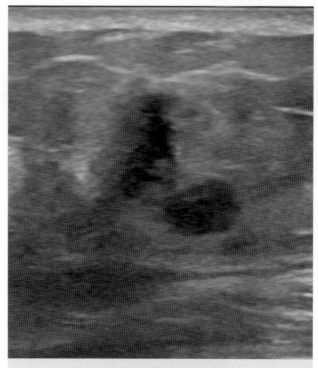

Fig. 30.10 Right breast ultrasound, transverse view.

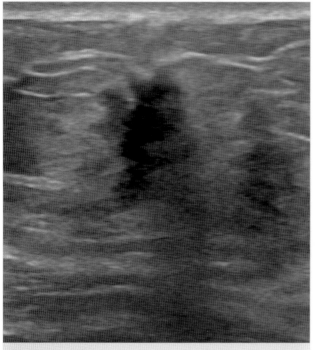

Fig. 30.11 Right breast ultrasound, longitudinal view.

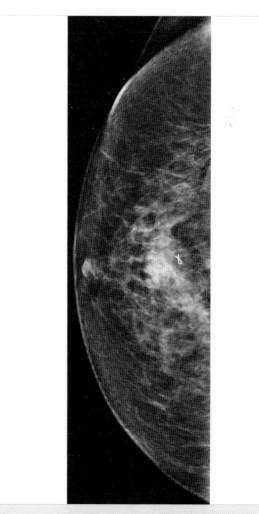

Fig. 30.12 Postbiopsy right craniocaudal (RCC) mammogram.

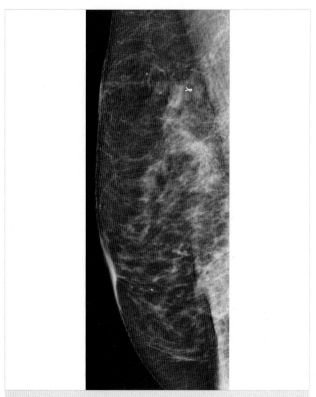

Fig. 30.13 Postbiopsy right mediolateral (RML) mammogram.

31 Mass Only Seen on One View

Lonie R. Salkowski

31.1 Presentation and Presenting Images

(▶ Fig. 31.1, ▶ Fig. 31.2)

A 43-year-old female presents for screening mammography.

31.2 Key Image

(▶ Fig. 31.3)

31.2.1 Breast Tissue Density

There are scattered areas of fibroglandular density.

31.2.2 Imaging Findings

In the posterior and lateral region of the left breast on the craniocaudal (CC) view (▶ Fig. 31.1), there is an oval mass. This is confirmed on the digital breast tomosynthesis (DBT) images, as seen on slice 1 of the DBT images (▶ Fig. 31.3). The DBT images are oriented from superior to inferior; thus, the mass is located in the upper outer quadrant of the left breast. A correlate is not seen on the mediolateral oblique (MLO) mammogram (▶ Fig. 31.2) or MLO DBT image (*not shown*).

31.3 BI-RADS Classification and Action

Category 0: Mammography: Incomplete. Need additional imaging evaluation and/or prior mammograms for comparison.

31.4 Diagnostic Images

(▶ Fig. 31.4, ▶ Fig. 31.5, ▶ Fig. 31.6)

31.4.1 Imaging Findings

The diagnostic imaging demonstrates not one but two masses in the posterior depth of the upper outer quadrant (▶ Fig. 31.4 and ▶ Fig. 31.5). To see these masses on the MLO view (▶ Fig. 31.5), more lateral tissue of the breast was included. For this reason, the nipple is not seen in profile given it was rolled medially. The images confirm that the circumscribed masses are located in the left breast at the 1 o'clock location, 11 cm from the nipple. The ultrasound was performed confirming two masses (▶ Fig. 31.6). The larger mass is 0.9 cm and the adjacent smaller mass is 0.5 cm in size. Both masses are hypoechoic with central echogenic region.

31.5 BI-RADS Classification and Action

Category 2: Benign

31.6 Differential Diagnosis

1. *Lymph node*: By location, a lymph node is the most likely diagnosis. However, the mass does not have the classic appearance to dismiss it as a lymph node on the screening mammogram. The DBT images confirm the circumscribed margins expected of a lymph node but do not offer information about a fatty hilum.
2. *Fibroadenoma*: This can present as a circumscribed mass on mammography, however, it often requires an ultrasound to make this diagnosis. The ultrasound in this case does not support this diagnosis.
3. *Carcinoma*: Breast cancer can occur anywhere in the breast tissue. At the margins of the breast tissue or at the margins of the image are the most common locations in imaging for missed cancers. The initial imaging could not dismiss this as not being a cancer. The subsequent imaging determined it to be benign and not a cancer.

31.7 Essential Facts

- This mass, because it was only seen on the CC view (FFDM and DBT), could be located anywhere along the lateral aspect of the breast. However, the CC DBT image localized the mass to the slice 1. This localizes this mass to the upper outer quadrant.
- DBT allows for triangulation of lesions only seen well on one view.
- The stack of images from DBT is designated as being head to foot or medial to lateral, depending on whether it is a CC or MLO projection. Once the slice number of the stack that the lesion is located within is identified, then the location in the orthogonal plane can be determined. Knowing where to look in the orthogonal view will further assist in characterizing the lesion.

31.8 Management and Digital Breast Tomosynthesis Principles

- DBT triangulation techniques will assist in localizing a lesion prior to a diagnostic ultrasound evaluation. This should improve the success of finding a lesion on ultrasound.
- DBT triangulation localization techniques can help determine if a lesion is within the breast parenchyma or within the skin.
- Although DBT can aid in localizing a lesion in the orthogonal imaging plane, this does not mean that only one DBT view is needed. Studies have shown that DBT in both the CC and MLO projections yield higher accuracy in localizing lesions.

31.9 Further Reading

[1] Conant EF. Clinical implementation of digital breast tomosynthesis. Radiol Clin North Am. 2014; 52(3):499–518
[2] Roth RG, Maidment AD, Weinstein SP, Roth SO, Conant EF. Digital breast tomosynthesis: lessons learned from early clinical implementation. Radiographics. 2014; 34(4):E89–E102

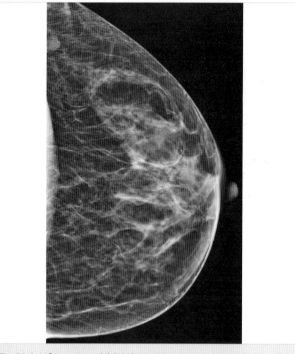

Fig. 31.1 Left craniocaudal (LCC) mammogram.

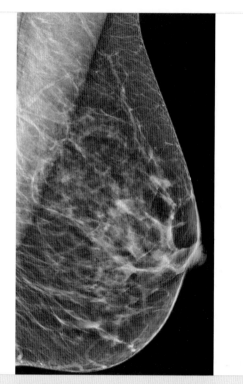

Fig. 31.2 Left mediolateral oblique (LMLO) mammogram.

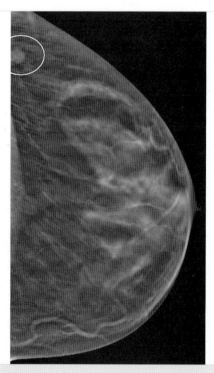

Fig. 31.3 Left craniocaudal digital breast tomosynthesis (LCC DBT), slice 1 of 49.

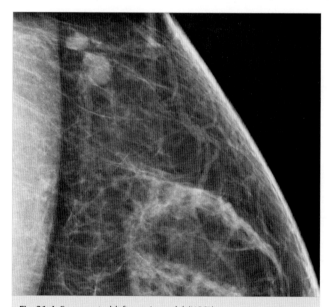

Fig. 31.4 Exaggerated left craniocaudal (XCCL) spot-compression mammogram.

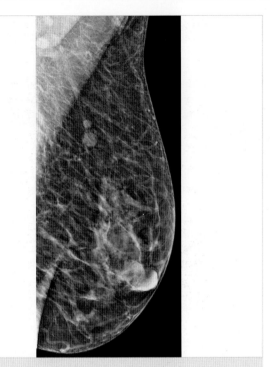

Fig. 31.5 Laterally exaggerated left mediolateral oblique (MLO) mammogram.

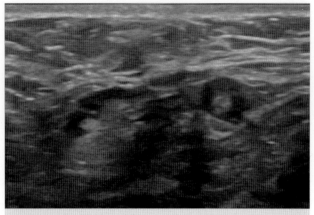

Fig. 31.6 Left breast ultrasound, transverse view.

32 Mass on Baseline Mammogram

Lonie R. Salkowski

32.1 Presentation and Presenting Images

(▶ Fig. 32.1, ▶ Fig. 32.2)

A 43-year-old female presents for baseline screening mammography.

32.2 Key Images

(▶ Fig. 32.3, ▶ Fig. 32.4)

32.2.1 Breast Tissue Density

There are scattered areas of fibroglandular density.

32.2.2 Imaging Findings

Central to the nipple in the anterior depth, there is an oval mass. It appears circumscribed on the craniocaudal (CC) view (▶ Fig. 32.1) and partially obscured on the mediolateral (MLO) view (▶ Fig. 32.2). The digital breast tomosynthesis (DBT) images confirm that this mass is circumscribed (▶ Fig. 32.3 and ▶ Fig. 32.4).

32.3 BI-RADS Classification and Action

Category 0: Mammography: Incomplete. Need additional imaging evaluation and/or prior mammograms for comparison.

32.4 Diagnostic Images

(▶ Fig. 32.5, ▶ Fig. 32.6, ▶ Fig. 32.7, ▶ Fig. 32.8)

32.4.1 Imaging Findings

The diagnostic imaging demonstrates the oval 16 × 11 × 10 mm mass with circumscribed margins at the 9 o'clock location in the anterior depth (▶ Fig. 32.5, ▶ Fig. 32.6, and ▶ Fig. 32.7). The corresponding ultrasound reveals a hypoechoic oval mass that measures 15 × 6 × 15 mm (▶ Fig. 32.8). There is no increase in vascularity.

32.5 BI-RADS Classification and Action

Category 3: Probably benign

32.6 Differential Diagnosis

1. **Fibroadenoma**: This mass is oval and circumscribed and has benign features. With this being a baseline mammogram, it is reasonable to follow benign-appearing masses or offer a biopsy. The patient elected for observation. Her follow-up evaluations at 6 and 12 months revealed no change.
2. *Complicated cyst*: The homogeneous low-level internal echoes that can be present in a complicated cyst can be difficult to distinguish from a solid mass. If there were internal vascularity present, this would exclude a complicated cyst.
3. *Phyllodes tumor*: These tumors are not as common as fibroadenomas, but they can often mimic each other. These typically grow over time and would require intervention if growth were seen during a period of observation.

32.7 Essential Facts

- Fibroadenomas are fibroepithelial tumors with stromal and epithelial elements.
- Fibroadenomas are the most common solid lesions of the breast.
- Most fibroadenomas are unilateral, but up to 20% of patients will have bilateral lesions.
- Recall rates tend to be higher in women receiving a baseline mammogram.
- Due to the increase in specificity without a decrease in sensitivity for patients who have full-field digital mammography (FFDM) with digital breast tomosynthesis (DBT) when receiving a baseline mammogram, there has been a decrease in the recall rate for these patients.
- A reduction in recall rates for DBT were seen irrespective of breast tissue density.

32.8 Management and Digital Breast Tomosynthesis Principles

- DBT can detect many benign lesions (fibroadenomas and cysts). It is uncertain if these lesions can be classified as benign based on their round or oval shape with circumscribed margins. Large-scale studies are needed to determine if these lesions can be dismissed on DBT and, if so, what the strict criteria are to do so.
- A mass with classic benign features on a baseline mammogran can be assigned a BI-RADS 3 category and followed. The typical time course for following is 2 years of stability, with imaging at 6 months, 12 months, and 24 months. However, if this mass is a new finding on a mammogram (one with comparisons), it should be assigned a BI-RADS 4a category and biopsy should be recommended.

32.9 Further Reading

[1] Baker JA, Lo JY. Breast tomosynthesis: state-of-the-art and review of the literature. Acad Radiol. 2011; 18(10):1298–1310
[2] Sumkin JH, Ganott MA, Chough DM, et al. Recall Rate Reduction with Tomosynthesis During Baseline Screening Examinations: An Assessment From a Prospective Trial. Acad Radiol. 2015; 22(12):1477–1482

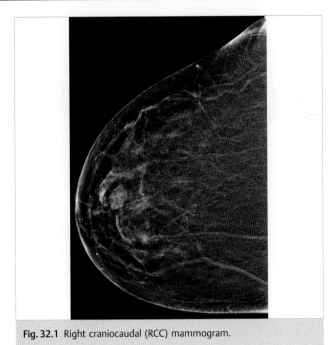

Fig. 32.1 Right craniocaudal (RCC) mammogram.

Fig. 32.3 Right craniocaudal digital breast tomosynthesis (RCC DBT), slice 22 of 67.

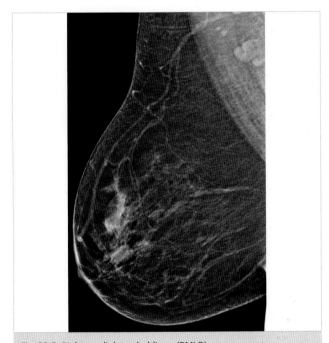

Fig. 32.2 Right mediolateral oblique (RMLO) mammogram.

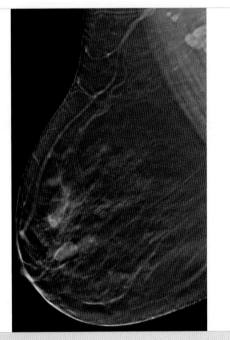

Fig. 32.4 Right mediolateral oblique digital breast tomosynthesis (RMLO DBT), slice 27 of 72.

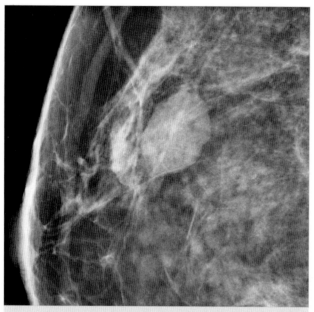

Fig. 32.5 Right craniocaudal (RCC) spot-compression mammogram.

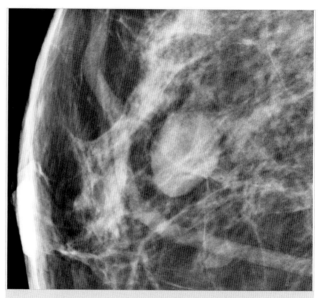

Fig. 32.6 Right mediolateral oblique (RMLO) spot-compression mammogram.

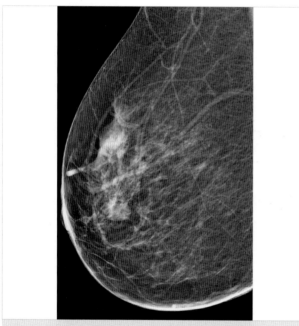

Fig. 32.7 Right mediolateral (RML) mammogram.

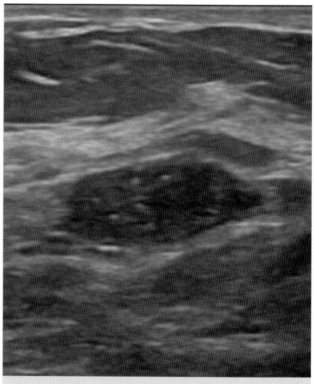

Fig. 32.8 Right breast ultrasound, transverse view.

33 Architectural Distortion

Lonie R. Salkowski

33.1 Presentation and Presenting Images

(▶ Fig. 33.1, ▶ Fig. 33.2, ▶ Fig. 33.3, ▶ Fig. 33.4)

A 54-year-old female who has had prior benign biopsies and surgical excisions of the left breast presents for screening mammography.

33.2 Key Images

(▶ Fig. 33.5, ▶ Fig. 33.6)

33.2.1 Breast Tissue Density

The breasts are heterogeneously dense, which may obscure small masses.

33.2.2 Imaging Findings

There is a subtle area of architectural distortion in the left breast at the 12 o'clock location in the posterior depth, best seen in the digital breast tomosynthesis (DBT) images (▶ Fig. 33.5 and ▶ Fig. 33.6). There is a dumbbell-shaped biopsy clip in the upper outer quadrant from a prior remote benign breast biopsy.

33.3 BI-RADS Classification and Action

Category 0: Mammography: Incomplete. Need additional imaging evaluation and/or prior mammograms for comparison.

33.4 Diagnostic Images

(▶ Fig. 33.7, ▶ Fig. 33.8, ▶ Fig. 33.9, ▶ Fig. 33.10, ▶ Fig. 33.11, ▶ Fig. 33.12)

33.4.1 Imaging Findings

The diagnostic imaging (▶ Fig. 33.7 and ▶ Fig. 33.8) demonstrates persistent very subtle architectural distortion, which is much more evident on the DBT images. A scar marker was placed on the skin incision scar. The surgical site appears to be more lateral to the area of architectural distortion. An ultrasound was performed and identified two areas at the 11 o'clock location. The area 2 cm from the nipple appears as an irregular hypoechoic mass with indistinct margins located within dense fibroglandular tissue (▶ Fig. 33.9). The area 5 cm from the nipple appears to be an irregular mixed echogenicity mass with indistinct margins and with solid and cystic components (▶ Fig. 33.10). Biopsy was performed on both masses identified on ultrasound. The lesion at 2 cm from the nipple was marked with a ribbon biopsy marker, and the lesion at 5 cm from the nipple was marked with a coil biopsy marker (▶ Fig. 33.11 and ▶ Fig. 33.12).

33.5 BI-RADS Classification and Action

Category 4A: Low suspicion for malignancy

33.6 Differential Diagnosis

1. *Radial scar*: The ribbon marker appears closest to the area of architectural distortion mammographically. The diagnosis was radial scar and fibrocystic changes. The diagnosis for the area marked by the coil marker was hyalinized breast stroma.
2. *Surgical scar*: It can be difficult even with DBT in dense breast tissue to differentiate between surgical scars and new findings when they are in close proximity to each other.
3. *Breast cancer*: Breast cancer can present as an architectural distortion. This would have been a concordant diagnosis at biopsy.

33.7 Essential Facts

- Radial scars are benign lesions that are often classified as high risk due to the variety of proliferative lesions that can be associated with them.
- Histologically radial scars have a central sclerotic core from which radiates the proliferative lesions.
- Radial scars range in size form microscopic incidental lesions to larger macroscopic lesions seen mammographically, which are indistinguishable from malignancies.
- Architectural distortion is not a very common imaging finding. Radial scars are the most common benign cause for architectural distortion.

33.8 Management and Digital Breast Tomosynthesis Principles

- Architectural distortion accounts for 12 to 45% of missed breast cancers.
- Architectural distortion is often better seen on DBT than on conventional digital mammography. Radial scars are a subset of the lesions that present as architectural distortion. Controversy remains on whether to manage radial scars with excision or observation; additional data is needed to guide management of radial scars only visible on DBT.
- Architectural distortion is the mammographic finding with the lowest interobserver agreement between radiologists.

33.9 Further Reading

[1] Partyka L, Lourenco AP, Mainiero MB. Detection of mammographically occult architectural distortion on digital breast tomosynthesis screening: initial clinical experience. AJR Am J Roentgenol. 2014; 203(1):216–222

[2] Ray KM, Turner E, Sickles EA, Joe BN. Suspicious Findings at Digital Breast Tomosynthesis Occult to Conventional Digital Mammography: Imaging Features and Pathology Findings. Breast J. 2015; 21(5):538–542

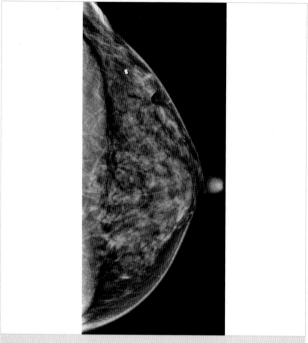

Fig. 33.1 Left cranicaudal (LCC) mammogram.

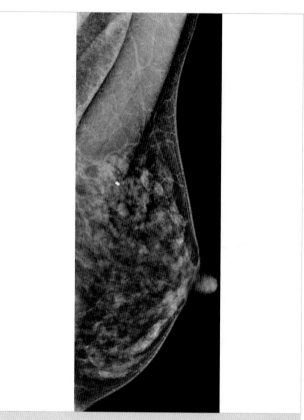

Fig. 33.2 Left mediolateral oblique (LMLO) mammogram.

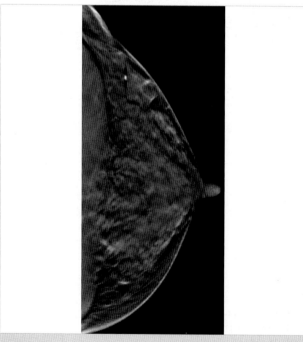

Fig. 33.3 Left craniocaudal digital breast tomosynthesis (LCC DBT), slice 20 of 42.

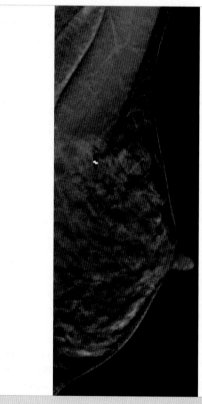

Fig. 33.4 Left mediolateral oblique digital breast tomosynthesis (LMLO DBT), slice 8 of 38.

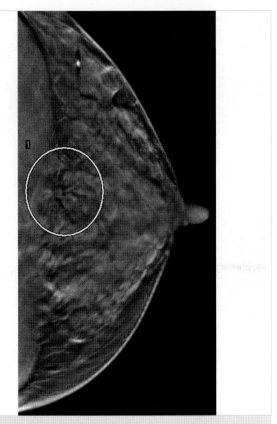

Fig. 33.5 Left craniocaudal digital breast tomosynthesis (LCC DBT), slice 20 of 42.

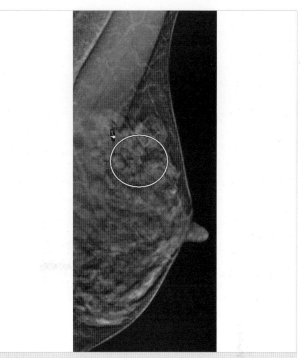

Fig. 33.6 Left mediolateral oblique digital breast tomosynthesis (LMLO DBT), slice 8 of 38.

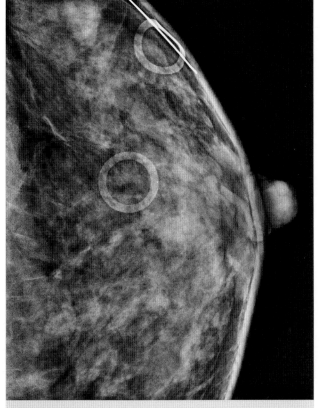

Fig. 33.7 Left craniocaudal (LCC) spot-compression mammogram.

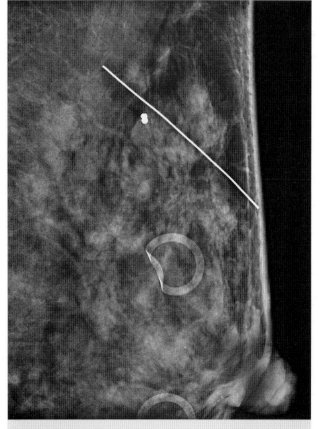

Fig. 33.8 Left mediolateral oblique (LMLO) spot-compression mammogram.

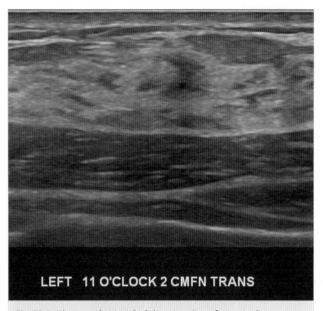

LEFT 11 O'CLOCK 2 CMFN TRANS

Fig. 33.9 Ultrasound, 11 o'clock location, 2 cm from nipple.

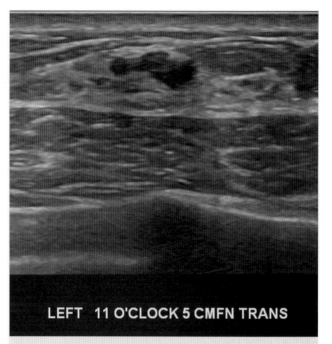

LEFT 11 O'CLOCK 5 CMFN TRANS

Fig. 33.10 Ultrasound, 11 o'clock location, 5 cm from nipple.

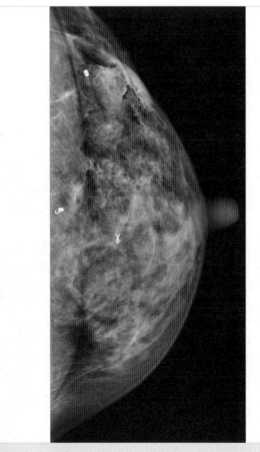

Fig. 33.11 Postbiopsy left craniocaudal (LCC) mammogram.

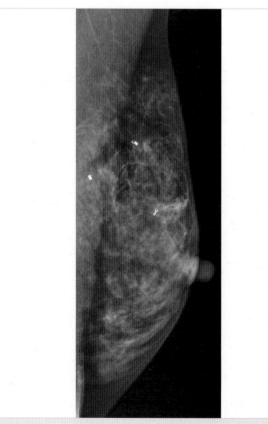

Fig. 33.12 Postbiopsy left mediolateral (LML) mammogram.

34 Grouped Amorphous Calcifications

Lonie R. Salkowski

34.1 Presentation and Presenting Images

(▶ Fig. 34.1, ▶ Fig. 34.2)

A 49-year-old female presents for screening mammography.

34.2 Key Images

(▶ Fig. 34.3, ▶ Fig. 34.4)

34.2.1 Breast Tissue Density

There are scattered areas of fibroglandular density.

34.2.2 Imaging Findings

There is a group of calcifications in the right breast at the 9 o'clock location in the posterior depth. These calcifications are very faint and difficult to see on the digital breast tomosynthesis (DBT) images. In the area of the calcifications, the DBT does not reveal any associated mass.

34.3 BI-RADS Classification and Action

Category 0: Mammography: Incomplete. Need additional imaging evaluation and/or prior mammograms for comparison.

34.4 Diagnostic Images

(▶ Fig. 34.5, ▶ Fig. 34.6, ▶ Fig. 34.7, ▶ Fig. 34.8, ▶ Fig. 34.9)

34.4.1 Imaging Findings

The diagnostic imaging demonstrates a 1.5-cm group of amorphous calcifications in the posterior depth at the 9 o'clock location. They do not layer on the lateral magnification view. There is no associated mass. These calcifications were sampled using stereotactic biopsy. Multiple cores contained the calcifications of interest.

34.5 BI-RADS Classification and Action

Category 4A: Low suspicion for malignancy

34.6 Differential Diagnosis

1. **Flat epithelial atypia (FEA)**: FEA presents as grouped amorphous calcifications. By imaging, it is not discernable from any other cause for amorphous calcifications. Amorphous calcifications represent malignancy in 13 to 25% of biopsies.

A biopsy is warranted. The fine nature of these amorphous calcifications may be at the limit of DBTs sensitivity in the reconstruction images.

2. *Ductal carcinoma in situ (DCIS)*: DCIS has variable presentations. Low-grade DCIS is most commonly associated with amorphous calcifications.
3. *Fibrocystic changes*: Amorphous calcifications can be associated with cysts seen in fibrocystic changes.

34.7 Essential Facts

- FEA is the term used when the epithelial layer of the duct is replaced by one to several layers of cuboidal to columnar cells with low-grade atypia.
- Intraluminal secretions are common in FEA and have a tendency to calcify.
- FEA is considered a high-risk lesion.
- FEA is frequently associated with atypical ductal hyperplasia (ADH), lobular neoplasia, low-grade DCIS, and tubular carcinoma.
- FEA is considered by many to be a precursor to low-grade DCIS.
- Most recommend excision of FEA diagnosed at core needle biopsy.
- Full-field digital mammography (FFDM) is more sensitive than DBT to the detection of calcifications.

34.8 Management and Digital Breast Tomosynthesis Principles

- Slabbing of DBT slices (that is, combining slices, yielding a set of thicker images) may help in perceiving the distribution of calcifications.
- The fineness of amorphous calcifications may limit their perception in the reconstructed DBT planes, thus the importance in calcification assessment of also obtaining a full-field digital mammogram (FFDM) or synthesized mammogram when DBT studies are obtained.
- There is lack of data on the upgrade rates of FEA; there is controversy as to whether FEA is a precursor to low-grade DCIS or low-grade invasive carcinoma.
- DBT's viewing of images in slices may impede the perception of the distribution, or clustering, of calcifications.
- There is limited literature on the evaluation of calcifications on DBT. Studies are needed to assess the observed morphology of calcifications on DBT and their benign or malignant outcomes.

34.9 Further Reading

[1] Molleran V. Postbiopsy management. Semin Roentgenol. 2011; 46(1):40–50
[2] Spangler ML, Zuley ML, Sumkin JH, et al. Detection and classification of calcifications on digital breast tomosynthesis and 2D digital mammography: a comparison. AJR Am J Roentgenol. 2011; 196(2):320–324

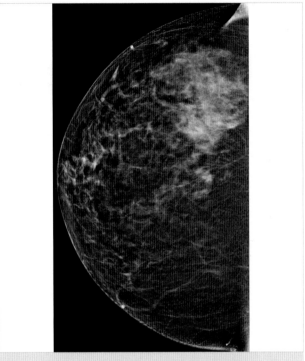

Fig. 34.1 Right craniocaudal (RCC) mammogram.

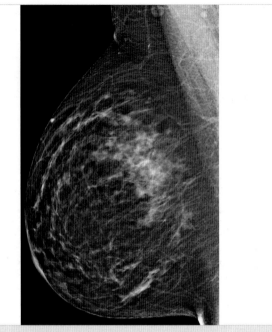

Fig. 34.2 Right mediolateral oblique (RMLO) mammogram.

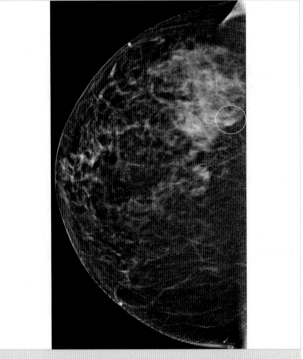

Fig. 34.3 Right craniocaudal (RCC) mammogram with label.

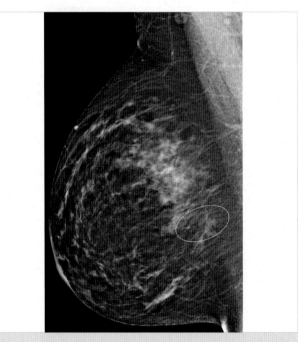

Fig. 34.4 Right mediolateral oblique (RMLO) mammogram with label.

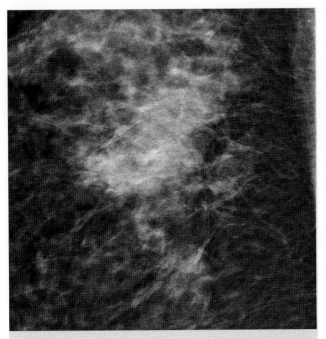

Fig. 34.5 Right craniocaudal (RCC) mammogram, spot magnification.

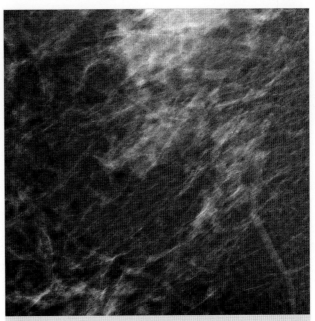

Fig. 34.6 Right mediolateral (RML) mammogram, spot magnification.

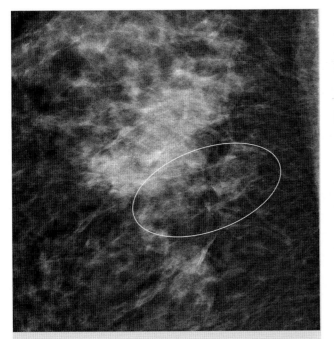

Fig. 34.7 Right craniocaudal (RCC) mammogram, spot magnification with label.

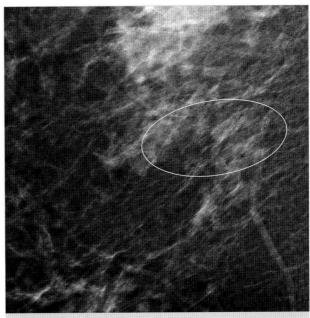

Fig. 34.8 Right mediolateral (RML) mammogram, spot magnification with label.

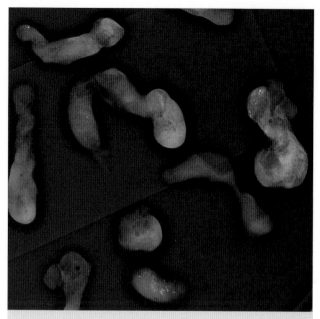

Fig. 34.9 Radiograph of biopsy specimen.

35 Architectural Distortion Only Seen on Tomosynthesis

Lonie R. Salkowski

35.1 Presentation and Presenting Images

(▶ Fig. 35.1, ▶ Fig. 35.2)

A 44-year-old female with a history of right breast cancer treated 3 years ago presents for screening mammography.

35.2 Key Images

(▶ Fig. 35.3, ▶ Fig. 35.4)

35.2.1 Breast Tissue Density

The breasts are heterogeneously dense, which may obscure small masses.

35.2.2 Imaging Findings

In the superior aspect of the left breast, there is an area of architectural distortion that is seen on the mediolateral oblique (MLO) view (▶ Fig. 35.3) and best seen on the MLO digital breast tomosynthesis (DBT) slice 30 of 58 (▶ Fig. 35.4). Therefore this area of architectural distortion should be around the 11 to 12 o'clock location. No definitive correlate can be seen on the craniocaudal (CC) view (▶ Fig. 35.5).

35.3 BI-RADS Classification and Action

Category 0: Mammography: Incomplete. Need additional imaging evaluation and/or prior mammograms for comparison.

35.4 Diagnostic Images

(▶ Fig. 35.5, ▶ Fig. 35.6, ▶ Fig. 35.7, ▶ Fig. 35.8, ▶ Fig. 35.9, ▶ Fig. 35.10, ▶ Fig. 35.11, ▶ Fig. 35.12, ▶ Fig. 35.13)

35.4.1 Imaging Findings

The diagnostic imaging demonstrates persistent architectural distortion in the upper half of the left breast. The repeat CC view did not reveal any correlate to this (▶ Fig. 35.5). Based on the information from the DBT imaging performed at screening, the ultrasound was directed to the 11 to 12 o'clock location. At the 11 o'clock location, 4 cm from the nipple, there is a mass with indistinct margins and posterior acoustic shadowing (▶ Fig. 35.10 and ▶ Fig. 35.11). This lesion was referred for biopsy. The images demonstrate a ribbon clip placed at the site of the biopsy performed by ultrasound (▶ Fig. 35.12 and ▶ Fig. 35.13).

35.5 BI-RADS Classification and Action

Category 4B: Moderate suspicion for malignancy

35.6 Differential Diagnosis

1. *Radial scar*: The mammographic and sonographic features are consistent with the diagnosis of a radial scar, which can mimic cancer.
2. *Breast cancer*: Architectural distortion has a high probability of cancer when identified mammographically.
3. *Sclerosing adenosis*: Architectural distortion is one of the three presenting features of sclerosing adenosis, with the other two being a mass and calcifications. If the biopsy was largely composed of sclerosing adenosis in proportion to the size of the imaging finding, and not just an incidental finding, it could be considered a concordant diagnosis.

35.7 Essential Facts

- A radial scar and complex sclerosing lesion are similar. A complex sclerosing lesion is larger than a radial scar (> 1 cm) and has more proliferative tissue.
- Most radial scars are asymptomatic.
- Radial scars are mostly identified at screening mammography or as an incidental finding on biopsy for another reason.
- Radial scars on mammography present as distortion with long thin spicules emanating from a central region without a "mass."
- On ultrasound, radial scars are commonly irregular hypoechoic masses with posterior shadowing.

35.8 Management and Digital Breast Tomosynthesis Principles

- Radial scars mimic cancer on mammography and ultrasound, and thus warrant a biopsy.
- Architectural distortion when present on mammography represents cancer in 75% of cases.
- A radial scar or a complex sclerosing lesion are the most common nonmalignant pathologic findings of architectural distortion.
- Architectural distortion without an ultrasound correlate has only a 30% chance of being cancer according to the study by Bahl and colleagues (2015). This 30% risk is too high to avert a biopsy.

35.9 Further Reading

[1] Bahl M, Baker JA, Kinsey EN, Ghate SV. Architectural Distortion on Mammography: Correlation With Pathologic Outcomes and Predictors of Malignancy. AJR Am J Roentgenol. 2015; 205(6):1339–1345

[2] Shaheen R, Schimmelpenninck CA, Stoddart L, Raymond H, Slanetz PJ. Spectrum of diseases presenting as architectural distortion on mammography: multimodality radiologic imaging with pathologic correlation. Semin Ultrasound CT MR. 2011; 32(4):351–362

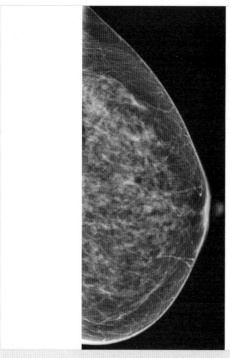

Fig. 35.1 Left craniocaudal (LCC) mammogram.

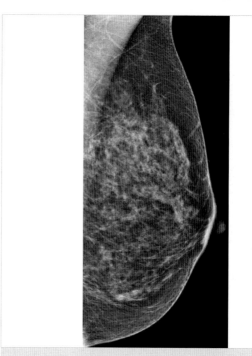

Fig. 35.2 Left mediolateral oblique (LMLO) mammogram.

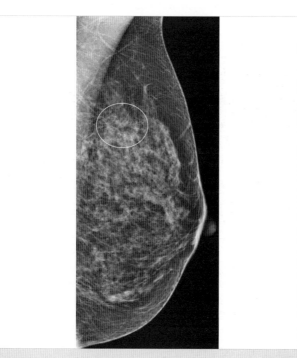

Fig. 35.3 Left mediolateral oblique (LMLO) mammogram with label.

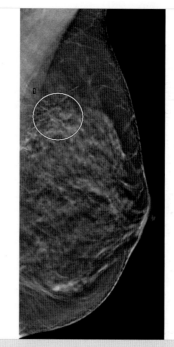

Fig. 35.4 Left mediolateral oblique digital breast tomosynthesis (LMLO DBT), slice 30 of 58.

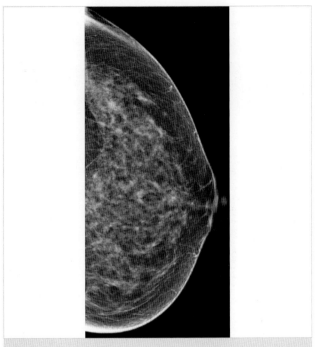

Fig. 35.5 Diagnostic left craniocaudal (LCC) mammogram.

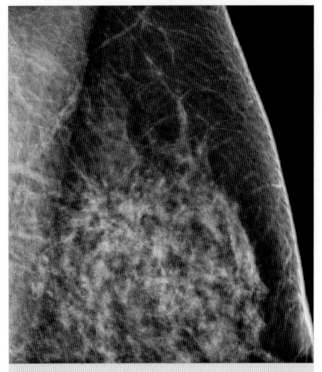

Fig. 35.6 Left mediolateral oblique (LMLO) spot-compression mammogram.

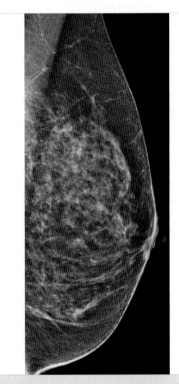

Fig. 35.7 Left mediolateral (LML) mammogram.

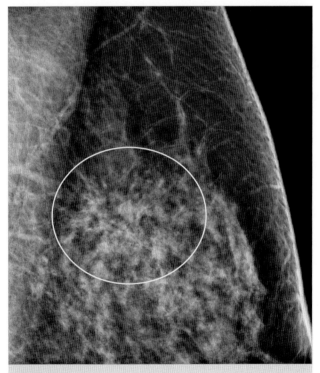

Fig. 35.8 Left mediolateral oblique (LMLO) spot-compression mammogram with label.

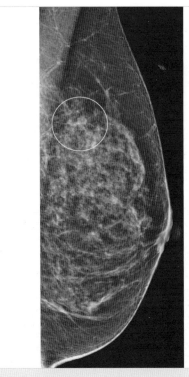

Fig. 35.9 Left mediolateral (LML) mammogram with label.

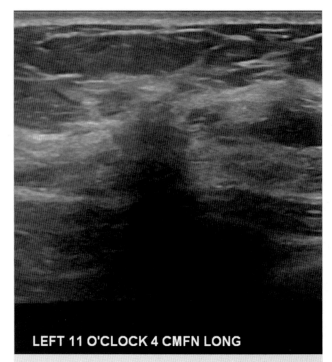

LEFT 11 O'CLOCK 4 CMFN LONG

Fig. 35.10 Left breast ultrasound, longitudinal view.

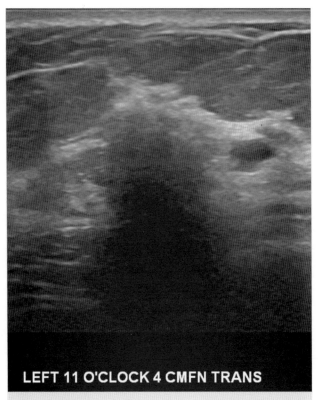

LEFT 11 O'CLOCK 4 CMFN TRANS

Fig. 35.11 Left breast ultrasound, transverse view.

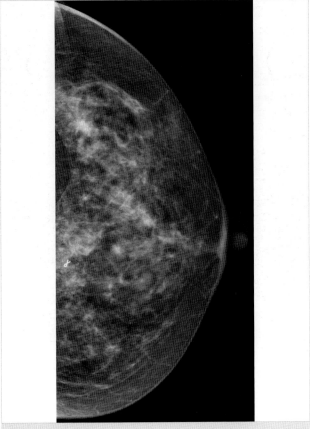

Fig. 35.12 Postbiopsy left craniocaudal (LCC) mammogram.

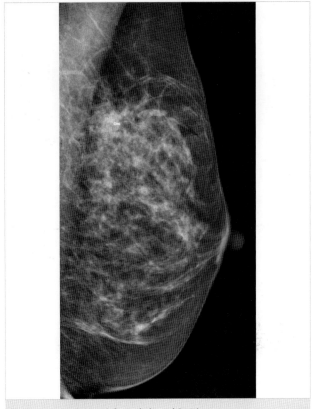

Fig. 35.13 Postbiopsy left mediolateral (LML) mammogram.

36 Small Spiculated Mass

Lonie R. Salkowski

36.1 Presentation and Presenting Images

(▶ Fig. 36.1, ▶ Fig. 36.2)

A 71-year-old female presents for screening mammography.

36.2 Key Images

(▶ Fig. 36.3, ▶ Fig. 36.4, ▶ Fig. 36.5, ▶ Fig. 36.6)

36.2.1 Breast Tissue Density

There are scattered areas of fibroglandular density.

36.2.2 Imaging Findings

Within the scattered fibroglandular tissue of the right breast, there is a possible small mass with architectural distortion in the middle depth at the 2 o'clock location. This mass was not initially seen on the full-field digital mammography (FFDM); however, it was seen on the craniocaudal digital breast tomosynthesis (CC DBT) (▶ Fig. 36.5) and then later localized on the mediolateral oblique digital breast tomosynthesis (MLO DBT) (▶ Fig. 36.6), and then in both projections on the FFDM (▶ Fig. 36.3 and ▶ Fig. 36.4).

36.3 BI-RADS Classification and Action

Category 0: Mammography: Incomplete. Need additional imaging evaluation and/or prior mammograms for comparison.

36.4 Diagnostic Images

(▶ Fig. 36.7, ▶ Fig. 36.8, ▶ Fig. 36.9, ▶ Fig. 36.10, ▶ Fig. 36.11, ▶ Fig. 36.12, ▶ Fig. 36.13, ▶ Fig. 36.14)

36.4.1 Imaging Findings

The diagnostic imaging demonstrates a 5-mm oval mass with spiculated margins at the 2 o'clock location, 4 cm from the nipple. On the diagnostic mammograms, it is seen best on the CC spot-compression view (▶ Fig. 36.7). The corresponding ultrasound reveals a 5-mm oval hypoechoic mass with spiculated margins and an echogenic halo (▶ Fig. 36.12). There was no increase in vascularity (*not shown*). This mass was biopsied with ultrasound guidance. The postbiospy mammogram (▶ Fig. 36.13 and ▶ Fig. 36.14) demonstrates the biopsy clip within the small mass that was noted on the initial screening examination.

36.5 BI-RADS Classification and Action

Category 4B: Moderate suspicion for malignancy

36.6 Differential Diagnosis

1. **Carcinoma**: Although small, this mass has the characteristic spiculated mass features of a carcinoma. The biopsy of this mass revealed a grade 2 invasive ductal carcinoma.
2. *Radial scar*: A radial scar typically presents as an architectural distortion. The DBT images suggest that this lesion is a mass, which would favor a diagnosis of cancer over that of a radial scar.
3. *Summation artifact*: This mass, seen better on the DBT images, did persist on the diagnostic images and ultrasound. Therefore, this mass would not qualify as superimposition of tissues and warrants further tissue sampling.

36.7 Essential Facts

- The background anatomical noise of the breast tissue can decrease the detection of masses on FFDM. DBT can unmask a mass. In this case, the patient's underlying breast tissue has scattered areas of higher density, a pattern of density distribution of the breast tissue that can easily obscure a small mass. DBT was more effective at unmasking this 5-mm mass.
- Cancer size can be more accurately assessed by DBT compared with conventional mammography.
- DBT is less sensitive to the surrounding breast tissue density compared with FFDM when assessing tumor size.
- Accurate measurements of the cancer aid in the preoperative staging of breast cancer.
- Current studies suggest that the additional cancers that are detected on DBT are mostly invasive, and not in situ, malignancies.

36.8 Management and Digital Breast Tomosynthesis Principles

- Studies suggest that DBT significantly improved diagnostic accuracy for noncalcified lesions compared with supplemental diagnostic mammography.
- Studies suggest that screening DBT appears to have improved specificity for noncalcified masses. Some suggest that the diagnostic mammogram can be bypassed in these cases and one should go directly to ultrasound. However, prior to bypassing a diagnostic mammogram, further larger studies are needed to support this change in management.

36.9 Further Reading

[1] Förnvik D, Zackrisson S, Ljungberg O, et al. Breast tomosynthesis: Accuracy of tumor measurement compared with digital mammography and ultrasonography. Acta Radiol. 2010; 51(3):240–247

[2] Zuley ML, Bandos AI, Ganott MA, et al. Digital breast tomosynthesis versus supplemental diagnostic mammographic views for evaluation of noncalcified breast lesions. Radiology. 2013; 266(1):89–95

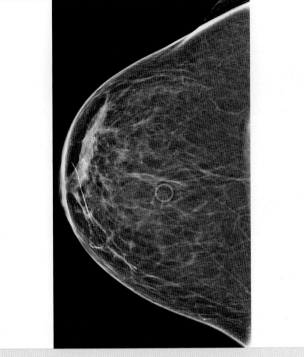

Fig. 36.1 Right craniocaudal (RCC) mammogram.

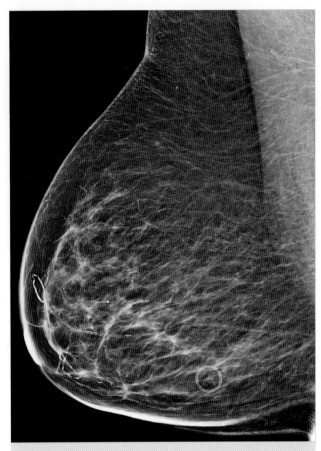

Fig. 36.2 Right mediolateral oblique (RMLO) mammogram.

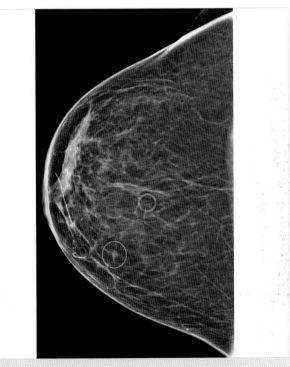

Fig. 36.3 Right craniocaudal (RCC) mammogram with label.

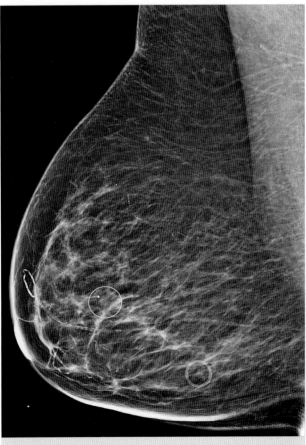

Fig. 36.4 Right mediolateral oblique (RMLO) mammogram with label.

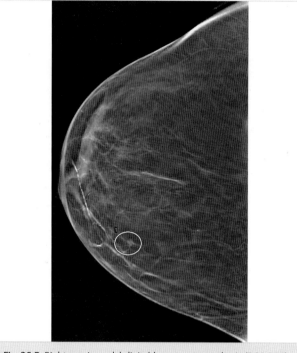

Fig. 36.5 Right craniocaudal digital breast tomosynthesis (RCC DBT), slice 37 of 65.

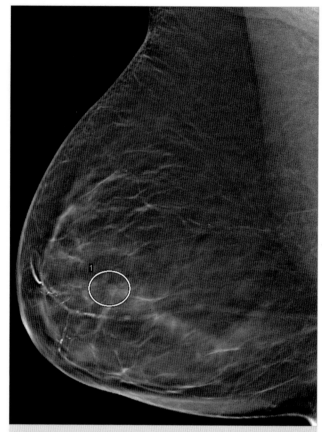

Fig. 36.6 Right mediolateral oblique digital breast tomosynthesis (RMLO DBT), slice 47 of 69.

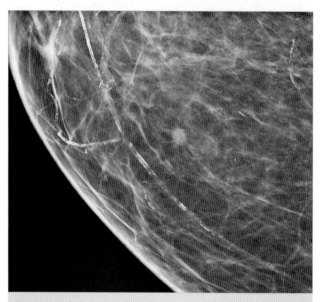

Fig. 36.7 Right craniocaudal (RCC) spot-compression mammogram.

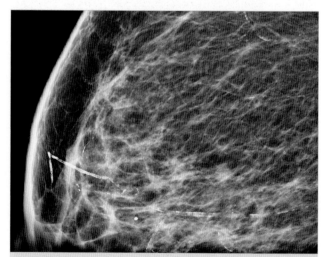

Fig. 36.8 Right mediolateral oblique (RMLO) spot-compression mammogram.

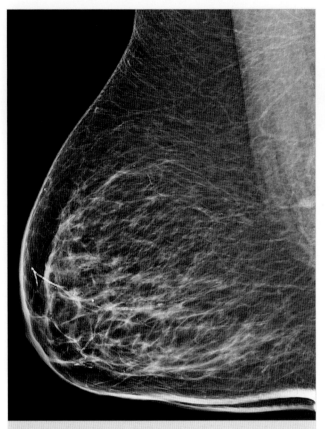

Fig. 36.9 Right mediolateral (RML).

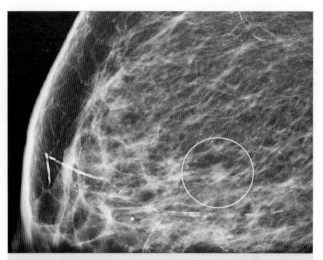

Fig. 36.10 Right mediolateral oblique (RMLO) spot-compression mammogram with label.

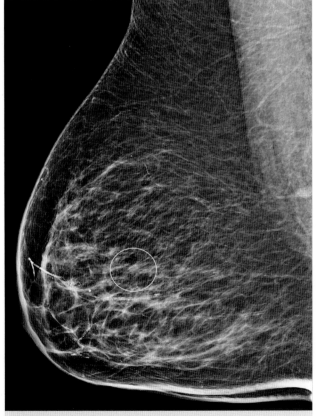

Fig. 36.11 Right mediolateral (RML) mammogram with label.

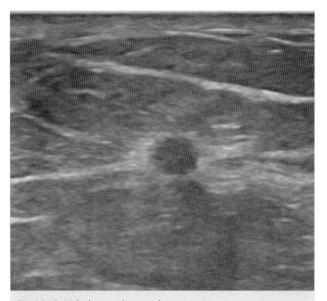

Fig. 36.12 Right breast ultrasound, transverse.

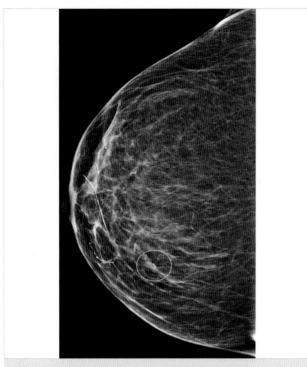

Fig. 36.13 Postbiopsy right craniocaudal (RCC) mammogram.

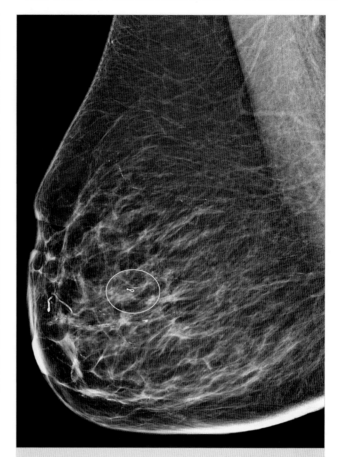

Fig. 36.14 Postbiopsy right mediolateral (RML) mammogram.

37 Mass on High-Risk Screening Mammogram

Tanya W. Moseley

37.1 Presentation and Presenting Images

(▶ Fig. 37.1, ▶ Fig. 37.2, ▶ Fig. 37.3, ▶ Fig. 37.4, ▶ Fig. 37.5, ▶ Fig. 37.6, ▶ Fig. 37.7)

A 36-year-old female with a strong family history of breast cancer presents for high-risk screening mammography.

37.2 Key Images

(▶ Fig. 37.8, ▶ Fig. 37.9, ▶ Fig. 37.10, ▶ Fig. 37.11, ▶ Fig. 37.12, ▶ Fig. 37.13)

37.2.1 Breast Tissue Density

There are scattered areas of fibroglandular density

37.2.2 Imaging Findings

There is a 1.3-cm oval mass (*circle* in ▶ Fig. 37.8 and ▶ Fig. 37.9) in the retroareolar region of the right breast. Additionally, there is 1.5-cm asymmetry located 9 cm from the nipple in the inferior aspect of the left breast, seen only on the mediolateral oblique (MLO) view (*box* in ▶ Fig. 37.10).

The right craniocaudal (RCC) views (▶ Fig. 37.8 and ▶ Fig. 37.5, conventional mammogram and tomosynthesis movie, respectively) are ill-positioned with the nipple not in profile. On these views, it is easy to mistake the mass (*circle*) for the nipple (*arrow*) (▶ Fig. 37.8). Only the conventional imaging was repeated, to reduce the amount of radiation exposure (▶ Fig. 37.11).

The left breast asymmetry does not persist on tomosynthesis. The right breast mass is demonstrated on tomosynthesis (▶ Fig. 37.12 and ▶ Fig. 37.13) as a well-circumscribed mass in the retroareolar region. Ultrasound is recommended for further evaluation.

37.3 BI-RADS Classification and Action

Category 0: Mammography: Incomplete. Need additional imaging evaluation and/or prior mammograms for comparison.

37.4 Diagnostic Images

(▶ Fig. 37.14, ▶ Fig. 37.15, ▶ Fig. 37.16, ▶ Fig. 37.17)

37.4.1 Imaging Findings

Ultrasound of the right breast reveals a well-circumscribed oval hypoechoic mass in the retroareolar region (▶ Fig. 37.16 and ▶ Fig. 37.17) that corresponds to the mammographic and tomosynthesis findings.

37.5 BI-RADS Classification and Action

Category 2: Benign

37.6 Differential Diagnosis

1. *Fibroadenoma*: Cystic and solid masses may have the same appearance on mammography. Sonography can reliably differentiate between cystic and solid masses. This is a solid, well-circumscribed oval hypoechoic mass on ultrasound.
2. *Cyst*: This mass does not have the sonographic characteristics of a cyst.
3. *Breast cancer (invasive ductal carcinoma [IDC])*: High-grade carcinomas and medullary carcinomas can mimic complicated cysts. These carcinomas may be markedly hypoechoic and have a round shape.

37.7 Essential Facts

- Cystic and solid masses may have the same appearance on mammography, but sonography can reliably differentiate between cystic and solid masses.
- Sonography may be used to guide a biopsy of indeterminate and suspicious lesions. If ultrasound had not identified this mass and biopsy was deemed necessary, tomosynthesis-directed stereotactic biopsy could also have been performed.
- Fibroadenomas are very common benign masses. Options for diagnosis are image-guided biopsy, excision, or sequential follow-up imaging that demonstrates stability for 2 years. Any lesion that is being followed must adhere to strict criteria and not have a positive predictive value (PPV) greater than 2%, thus not satisfying the BIRADS 3 assessment category.

37.8 Management and Digital Breast Tomosynthesis Principles

- Tomosynthesis is not just helpful in finding abnormalities in patients with denser breast tissue but also in patients with scattered breast parenchyma.
- The detection of lesions obscured by overlapping breast tissue is a limitation of conventional mammography. Imagers may have difficulty identifying abnormalities. In some cases, lesions may go undetected.
- Tomosynthesis helps imagers to identify true mass lesions and to dismiss pseudomasses or summation artifacts.
- Radiologists must avoid dismissing well-circumscribed masses as benign. Additional studies evaluating circumscribed cancers on tomosynthesis need to be performed to identify commonalities among these malignant lesions that would help with their identification as malignant.

- Positioning is just as important on tomosynthesis as it is on conventional mammography. The first RCC view in this case (conventional mammogram and tomosynthesis movie) is ill-positioned with the nipple not in profile. In fact, this view is more of a right laterally exaggerated craniocaudal (XCCL) view than a CC view. The mass (*circle*) could have been mistaken for the nipple (*arrow*). Only the conventional imaging was repeated to reduce the amount of radiation exposure.

37.9 Further Reading

[1] Rafferty EA, Park JM, Philpotts LE, et al. Assessing radiologist performance using combined digital mammography and breast tomosynthesis compared with digital mammography alone: results of a multicenter, multireader trial. Radiology. 2013; 266(1):104–113

[2] Rose SL, Tidwell AL, Bujnoch LJ, Kushwaha AC, Nordmann AS, Sexton R, Jr. Implementation of breast tomosynthesis in a routine screening practice: an observational study. AJR Am J Roentgenol. 2013; 200(6):1401–1408

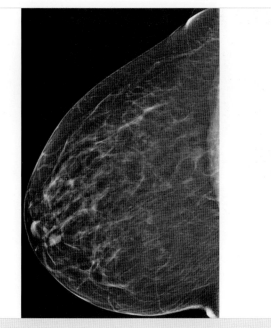

Fig. 37.1 Right craniocaudal (RCC) mammogram.

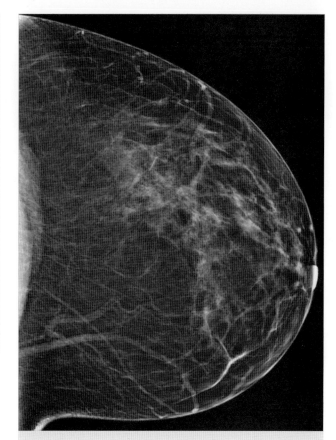

Fig. 37.2 Left craniocaudal (LCC)mammogram.

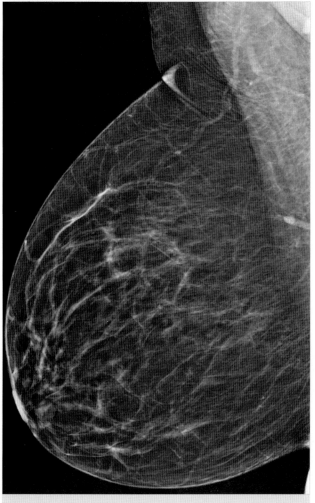

Fig. 37.3 Right mediolateral oblique (RMLO) mammogram.

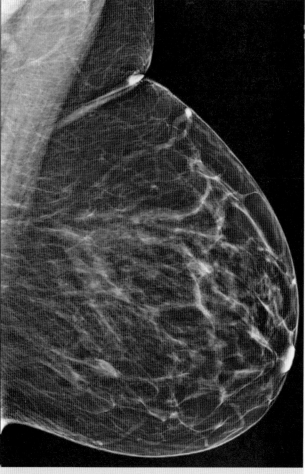

Fig. 37.4 Left mediolateral oblique (LMLO) mammogram.

161

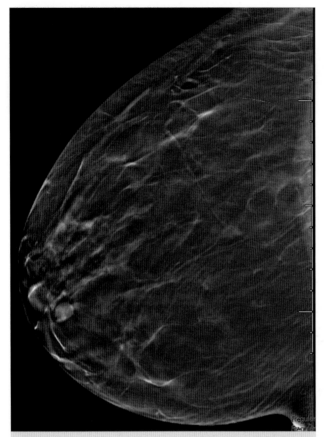

Fig. 37.5 Right craniocaudal digital breast tomosynthesis (RCC DBT), slice 14 of 76.

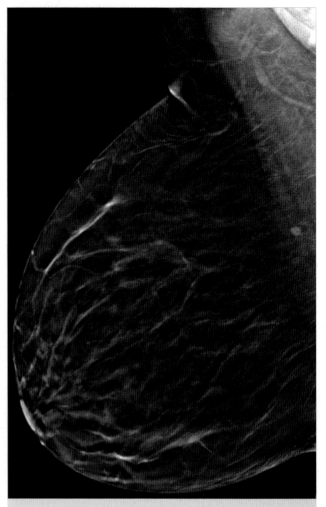

Fig. 37.6 Right mediolateral digital breast tomosynthesis (RMLO DBT), slice 24 of 76.

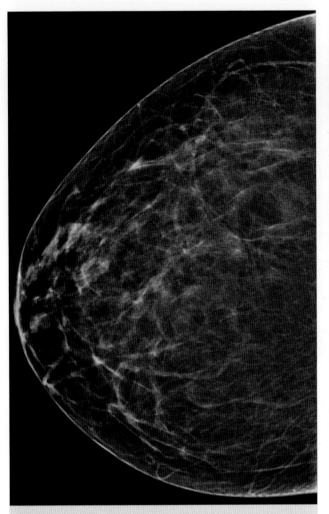

Fig. 37.7 Repeated right craniocaudal (RCC) mammogram for positioning.

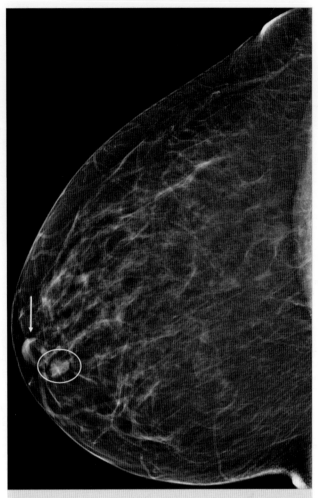

Fig. 37.8 Right craniocaudal (RCC) mammogram with label.

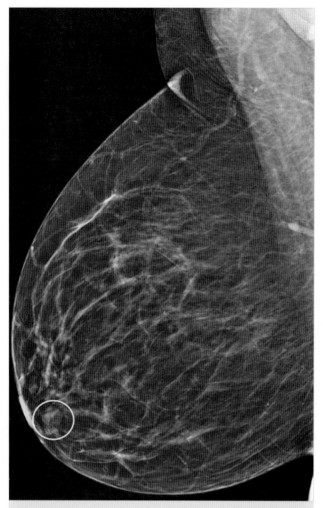

Fig. 37.9 Right mediolateral oblique (RMLO) mammogram with label.

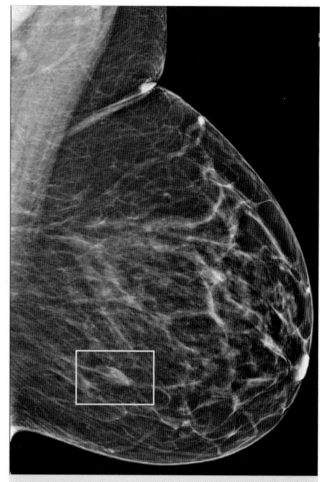

Fig. 37.10 Left mediolateral oblique (LMLO) mammogram with label.

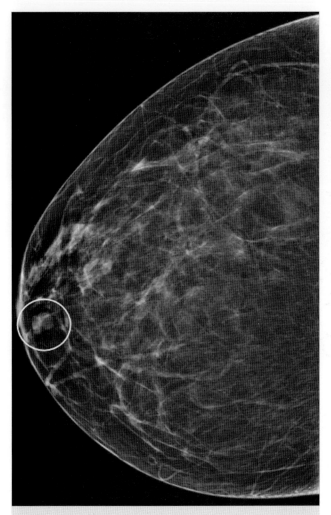

Fig. 37.11 Repeated right craniocaudal (RCC) mammogram with label.

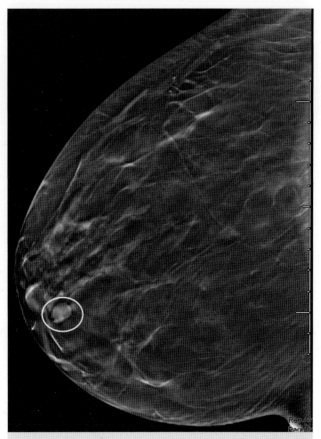

Fig. 37.12 Right craniocaudal digital breast tomosynthesis (RCC DBT), slice 14 of 76 with label.

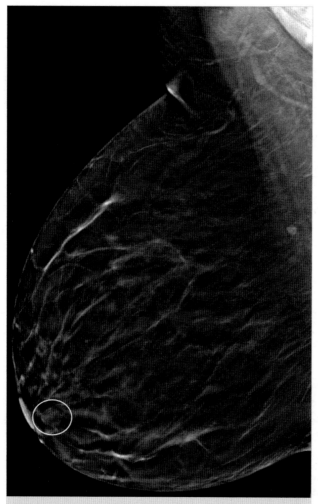

Fig. 37.13 Right mediolateral oblique digital breast tomosynthesis (RMLO DBT), slice 24 of 76 with label.

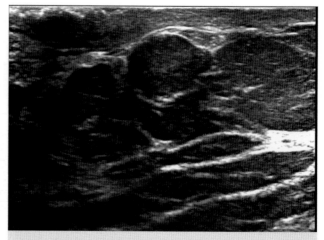

Fig. 37.14 Right breast ultrasound, transverse view.

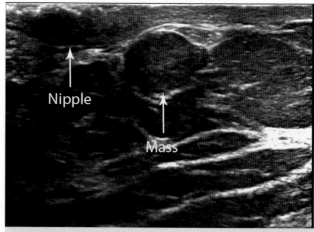

Fig. 37.16 Right breast ultrasound, transverse view with label.

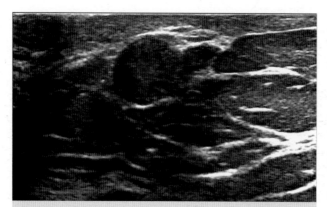

Fig. 37.15 Right breast ultrasound, longitudinal view.

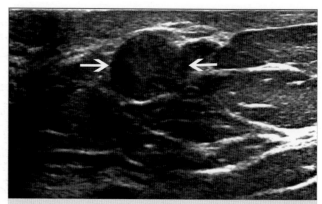

Fig. 37.17 Right breast ultrasound, longitudinal view with label.

38 Architectural Distortion Best Seen on Digital Breast Tomosynthesis

Lonie R. Salkowski

38.1 Presentation and Presenting Images

(▶ Fig. 38.1, ▶ Fig. 38.2)

A 53-year-old female presents for screening mammography.

38.2 Key Images

(▶ Fig. 38.3, ▶ Fig. 38.4)

38.2.1 Breast Tissue Density

The breasts are heterogeneously dense, which may obscure small masses.

38.2.2 Imaging Findings

In the lower inner quadrant of the left breast, there is a subtle area of architectural distortion on the mediolateral oblique (MLO) view (▶ Fig. 38.2). However, it is best seen in the tomosynthesis images (▶ Fig. 38.3 and ▶ Fig. 38.4). The right breast was normal (*not shown*).

38.3 BI-RADS Classification and Action

Category 0: Mammography: Incomplete. Need additional imaging evaluation and/or prior mammograms for comparison.

38.4 Diagnostic Images

(▶ Fig. 38.5, ▶ Fig. 38.6, ▶ Fig. 38.7, ▶ Fig. 38.8, ▶ Fig. 38.9, ▶ Fig. 38.10, ▶ Fig. 38.11)

38.4.1 Imaging Findings

The diagnostic imaging demonstrates persistent architectural distortion. However, it is best seen on the left mediolateral oblique (LMLO) spot-compression image (▶ Fig. 38.6). On this image, longer spicules that draw into a central region can be seen. A focally defined mass is not seen. The ultrasound reveals an irregular mixed hypoechoic mass with angular and indistinct margins located at 7 o'clock 4 cm from the nipple. This 2.1 × 1.3 × 1.3 cm mass has mild posterior acoustic shadowing

(▶ Fig. 38.8 and ▶ Fig. 38.9). This mass was biopsied with ultrasound guidance. The postbiopsy mammogram demonstrates the biopsy marker clip (ribbon-shaped) in the expected location.

38.5 BI-RADS Classification and Action

Category 5: Highly suggestive of malignancy

38.6 Differential Diagnosis

1. ***Breast cancer (invasive lobular carcinoma)***: The architectural distortion was best seen on digital breast tomosynthesis (DBT). The additional mammographic images were supportive in the mediolateral oblique (MLO) spot-compression view. The ultrasound confirmed an irregular mass for which biopsy was strongly recommended.
2. *Radial scar*: Radial scars are known to be elusive on conventional mammographic imaging. The DBT images demonstrate architectural distortion. The diagnostic ultrasound reveals a larger mass than is typical for a radial scar. If an image-guided biopsy yielded a radial scar for this lesion, a surgical consult for excision would be warranted.
3. *Normal breast tissue*: The DBT images are too worrisome to stop and call this a summation artifact. Findings at DBT without a fully supportive diagnostic mammography evaluation warrant an ultrasound. The ultrasound does not demonstrate normal breast tissue.

38.7 Essential Facts

- DBT allows the breast to be viewed in a three-dimensional format allowing for stacks of in-focus planes, or slices, to be viewed thus reducing the impact of superimposed breast tissue.
- Some DBT–only findings can be effaced on conventional diagnostic imaging.
- Architectural distortion and lesion margins are more apparent on DBT.
- Architectural distortion is the most common DBT finding that is mammographically occult.
- Invasive lobular carcinomas have a high frequency of being seen on DBT and of being occult to very subtle on full-field digital mammography (FFDM).

38.8 Management and Digital Breast Tomosynthesis Principles

- Architectural distortion on DBT is the most frequently missed sign of breast cancer, and so result in false-negatives on screening mammography.
- The incidence of malignancy for architectural distortion on DBT without a mammographic finding ranges from 21 to 36%.
- Worrisome DBT findings that are not reproduced on conventional mammography warrant evaluation with ultrasound. These cases often are found to be cancers that would otherwise be overlooked mammographically.
- Worrisome DBT findings without an ultrasound correlate warrant either a wire-localization or tomosynthesis-guided biopsy due to the high incidence of malignancy.

38.9 Further Reading

[1] Conant EF. Clinical implementation of digital breast tomosynthesis. Radiol Clin North Am. 2014; 52(3):499–518

[2] Ray KM, Turner E, Sickles EA, Joe BN. Suspicious Findings at Digital Breast Tomosynthesis Occult to Conventional Digital Mammography: Imaging Features and Pathology Findings. Breast J. 2015; 21(5):538–542

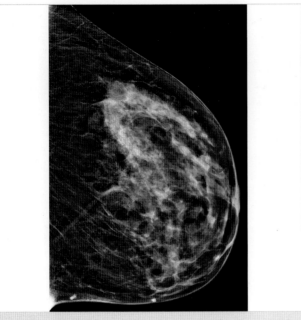

Fig. 38.1 Left craniocaudal (LCC) mammogram.

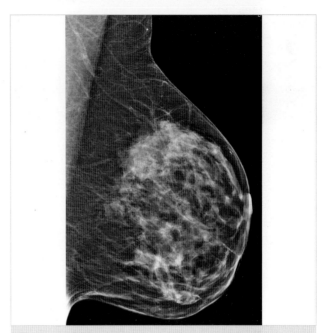

Fig. 38.2 Left mediolateral oblique (LMLO) mammogram.

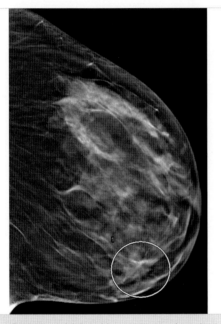

Fig. 38.3 Left craniocaudal digital breast tomosynthesis (LCC DBT), slice 21 of 74.

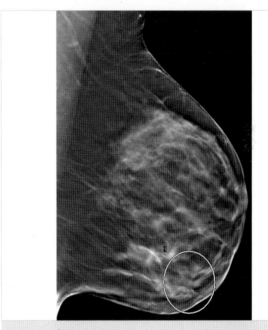

Fig. 38.4 Left mediolateral oblique digital breast tomosynthesis (LMLO DBT), slice 32 of 75.

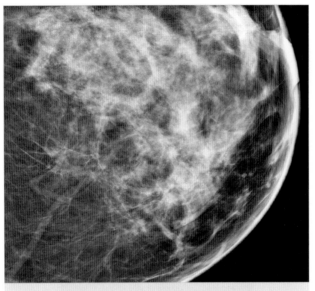

Fig. 38.5 Left craniocaudal (LCC) spot-compression mammogram.

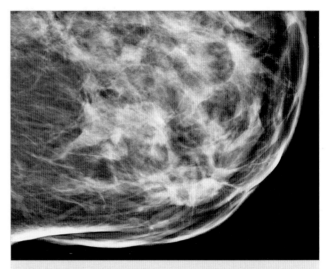

Fig. 38.6 Left mediolateral oblique (LMLO) spot-compression mammogram.

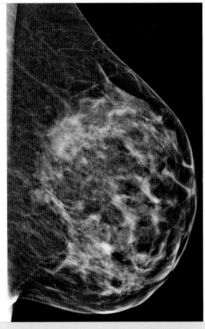

Fig. 38.7 Left mediolateral (LML) mammogram.

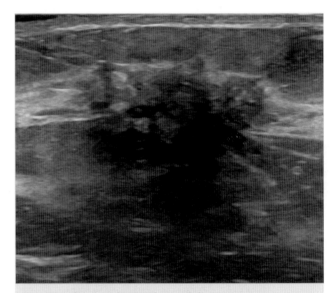

Fig. 38.8 Left breast ultrasound, antiradial.

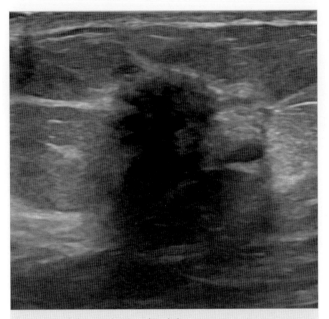

Fig. 38.9 Left breast ultrasound, radial.

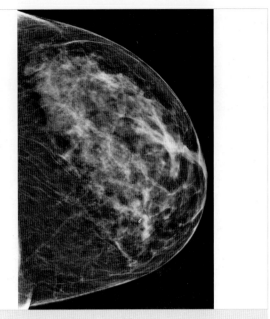

Fig. 38.10 Postbiopsy left craniocaudal (LCC) mammogram.

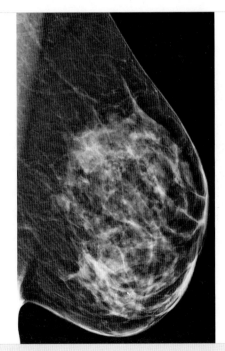

Fig. 38.11 Postbiopsy left mediolateral (LML) mammogram.

39 Focal Asymmetry

Tanya W. Moseley

39.1 Presentation and Presenting Images

(▶ Fig. 39.1, ▶ Fig. 39.2, ▶ Fig. 39.3, ▶ Fig. 39.4)

A 44-year-old female presents for routine screening mammography.

39.2 Key Images

(▶ Fig. 39.5, ▶ Fig. 39.6)

39.2.1 Breast Tissue Density

The breasts are heterogeneously dense, which may obscure small masses.

39.2.2 Imaging Findings

There is a 1.2-cm focal asymmetry (*circle* in ▶ Fig. 39.5 and ▶ Fig. 39.6) in the upper outer quadrant of the left breast at the 2 o'clock location, 6 cm from the nipple. There are no suspicious findings on the right breast, and there are no prior mammograms of the left breast available for comparison.

39.3 BI-RADS Classification and Action

Category 0: Mammography: Incomplete. Need additional imaging evaluation and/or prior mammograms for comparison.

39.4 Diagnostic Images

39.4.1 Imaging Findings

At diagnostic imaging, only tomosynthesis was performed. The tomosynthesis movie demonstrated that the finding in the left breast is not a true lesion but is the result of overlapping breast parenchyma.

39.5 BI-RADS Classification and Action

Category 2: Benign

39.6 Differential Diagnosis

1. **Summation artifact**: This finding resolves on the diagnostic tomosynthesis movie, consistent with a pseudomass or summation artifact.

2. *Asymmetry:* This finding is seen on two views. An asymmetry is a one-view finding.
3. *Developing asymmetry:* There were no prior images for comparison so one cannot ascertain if this finding has increased in conspicuity or size over time.

39.7 Essential Facts

- In this case the screening mammography was done without tomosynthesis. If a combination study with conventional mammography and tomosynthesis had been performed, this patient would not have been recalled for additional imaging because the finding would have resolved on tomosynthesis.
- There are four types of asymmetries described in the ACR BI-RADS Atlas, 5th edition: asymmetry, focal asymmetry, developing asymmetry, and global asymmetry.
  ○ An asymmetry is a finding seen on only one mammographic view.
  ○ A focal asymmetry is a nonmass lesion visible on at least two mammographic views that occupies less than a quadrant.
  ○ A developing asymmetry is a focal asymmetry that is new, larger, or more conspicuous than noted previously. The risk of malignancy is 15% at screening mammography and 25% at diagnostic mammography, making this a suspicious finding.
  ○ A global asymmetry is a nonmass lesion visible on at least two mammographic views that occupies at least a quadrant.

39.8 Management and Digital Breast Tomosynthesis Principles

- Tomosynthesis helps imagers to identify true mass lesions and to dismiss pseudomasses or summation artifacts.
- The detection of lesions obscured by overlapping breast tissue is a limitation to conventional mammography.
- Overlapping breast tissue can obscure cancers resulting in a missed cancer diagnosis. Also, overlapping breast tissue can create summation artifacts or pseudomasses resulting in a false-positive diagnosis and a biopsy of a benign finding.
- Tomosynthesis reduces the effects of overlapping breast tissue, thus reducing callbacks and biopsies.

39.9 Further Reading

[1] Leung JWT, Sickles EA. Developing asymmetry identified on mammography: correlation with imaging outcome and pathologic findings. AJR Am J Roentgenol. 2007; 188(3):667–675

[2] Sickles EA, D'Orsi CJ, Bassett LW, et al. ACR BI-RADS Mammography. In: ACR BI-RADS Atlas, 5th edition. Reston, VA: American College of Radiology; 2013

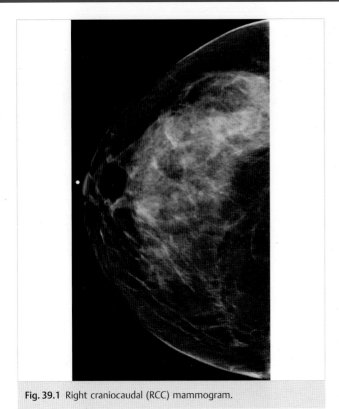

Fig. 39.1 Right craniocaudal (RCC) mammogram.

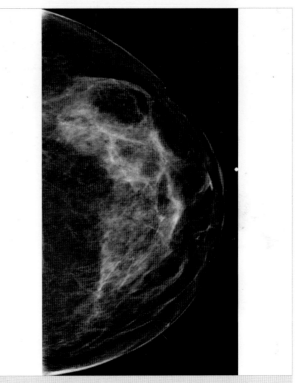

Fig. 39.2 Left craniocaudal (LCC) mammogram.

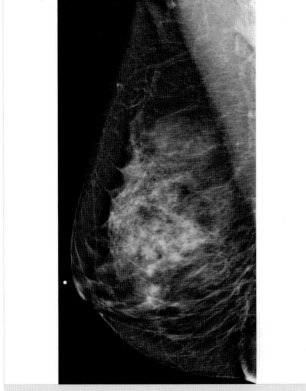

Fig. 39.3 Right mediolateral oblique (RMLO) mammogram.

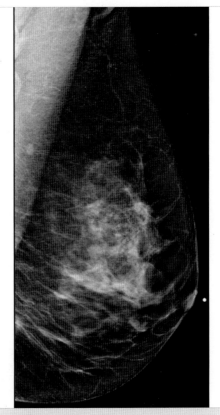

Fig. 39.4 Left mediolateral oblique (LMLO) mammogram.

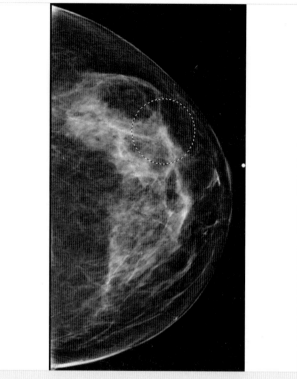

Fig. 39.5 Left craniocaudal (LCC) mammogram with label.

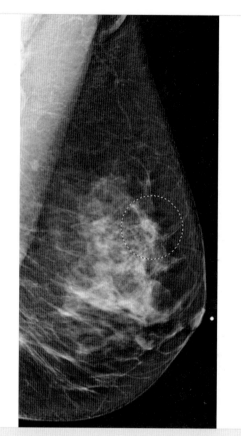

Fig. 39.6 Left mediolateral oblique (LMLO) mammogram with label.

40 Obscured Mass

Lonie R. Salkowski

40.1 Presentation and Presenting Images

(▸ Fig. 40.1, ▸ Fig. 40.2)

A 52-year-old female with a personal history of right breast cancer treated with lumpectomy and radiation therapy 4 years prior presents for screening mammography.

40.2 Key Images

(▸ Fig. 40.3, ▸ Fig. 40.4)

40.2.1 Breast Tissue Density

There are scattered areas of fibroglandular density.

40.2.2 Imaging Findings

In the upper inner quadrant at the 10 o'clock location in the middle depth of the left breast, there is a small obscured mass. The complexity of the breast tissue pattern makes it difficult to localize this mass from the background on the conventional digital mammograms (▸ Fig. 40.1 and ▸ Fig. 40.2). The tomosynthesis images, help to identify and localize this small mass (▸ Fig. 40.3 and ▸ Fig. 40.4).

40.3 BI-RADS Classification and Action

Category 0: Mammography: Incomplete. Need additional imaging evaluation and/or prior mammograms for comparison.

40.4 Diagnostic Images

(▸ Fig. 40.5, ▸ Fig. 40.6, ▸ Fig. 40.7, ▸ Fig. 40.8, ▸ Fig. 40.9, ▸ Fig. 40.10, ▸ Fig. 40.11, ▸ Fig. 40.12)

40.4.1 Imaging Findings

The diagnostic imaging demonstrates a persistent 6-mm irregular mass with spiculated margins. It is best seen on the craniocaudal (CC) view (▸ Fig. 40.5), and remains mostly obscured on the mediolateral oblique (MLO) spot-compression view (▸ Fig. 40.6 and ▸ Fig. 40.8). A targeted ultrasound (▸ Fig. 40.9) reveals a corresponding 6-mm irregular hypoechoic mass with angular margins and mild posterior shadowing located at 10 o'clock, 5 cm from the nipple. An ultrasound-

guided biopsy was performed and the postprocedure mammograms reveal the coil biopsy marker clip in the area of the mammographic mass (▸ Fig. 40.10 and ▸ Fig. 40.11). This mass was eventually localized by a wire for surgical excision. The specimen radiograph demonstrates a small spiculated mass with the localization wire and coil marker clip adjacent to it (▸ Fig. 40.12).

40.5 BI-RADS Classification and Action

Category 4C: High suspicion for malignancy

40.6 Differential Diagnosis

1. ***Breast cancer (invasive ductal carcinoma):*** The margins of the mass as seen on DBT and ultrasound suggest a suspicious finding. Cancer is highly suspected.
2. *Sclerosing adenosis (SA)*: Sclerosing adenosis is known to mimic cancer. When assessing biopsy concordance, the size of the lesion seen on imaging should be reflective of the lesion size on pathology. A microscopic focus of SA in the background of other breast tissue would not be concordant, and excision should be recommended.
3. *Focal fibrosis (FF)*: Similar to SA, FF can also mimic cancer, as an architectural distortion or an irregular mass. Similar to SA, a pathologic diagnosis based on an image-guided biopsy should reflect the size of the lesion on imaging to be considered concordant.

40.7 Essential Facts

- DBT is very helpful in localizing a lesion seen in one projection to the orthogonal image. In this case, the lesion is well seen on the FFDM CC view, where there little if any overlap of tissues in the medial aspect of the breast. However, on the FFDM MLO view, there are many similar-appearing densities in the breast at the depth of the lesion seen on the FFDM CC view.
- A lesion seen in only one DBT projection still affords the potential for localization. The side-to-side (MLO projection) or head-to-foot (CC projection) location within the DBT stack will aid in directing diagnostic mammography and/or an ultrasound examination.
- A developing asymmetry is a focal asymmetry that is new or increasing in size compared to prior imaging studies.
- DBT may increase the perception of developing asymmetries due to its unmasking ability.

40.8 Management and DBT Principles

- Developing asymmetries are often subtle mammographic findings.
- Developing asymmetries can often present as only a one-view finding. Traditional triangulation techniques are helpful to localize a lesion. DBT may provide added benefit in triangulating a lesion in two orthogonal planes to optimize characterization, ultrasound evaluation, and biopsy.
- Lesions that are only seen on one view are difficult to evaluate. A nontargeted ultrasound exam may find one or several lesions. The risk is that one or none of these might be the lesion seen mammographically.

40.9 Further Reading

[1] Price ER, Joe BN, Sickles EA. The developing asymmetry: revisiting a perceptual and diagnostic challenge. Radiology. 2015; 274(3):642–651

[2] Roth RG, Maidment AD, Weinstein SP, Roth SO, Conant EF. Digital breast tomosynthesis: lessons learned from early clinical implementation. Radiographics. 2014; 34(4):E89–E102

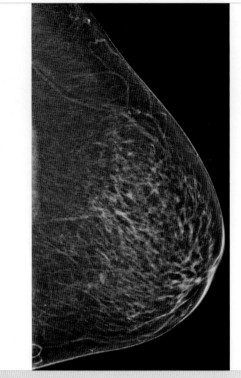

Fig. 40.1 Left craniocaudal (LCC) mammogram.

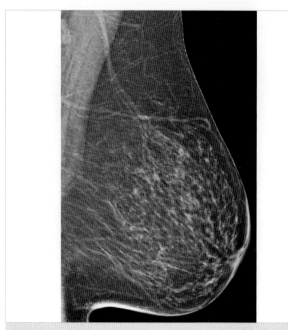

Fig. 40.2 Left mediolateral oblique (LMLO) mammogram.

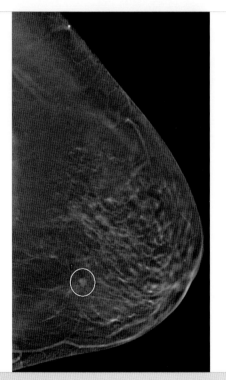

Fig. 40.3 Left craniocaudal digital breast tomosynthesis (LCC DBT), slice 53 of 81, with label.

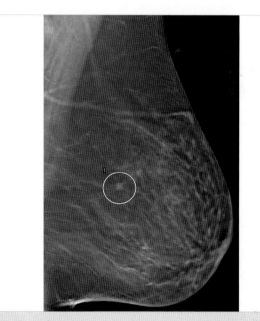

Fig. 40.4 Left mediolateral digital breast tomosynthesis (LMLO DBT), slice 62 of 85, with label.

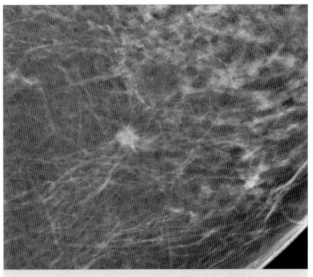

Fig. 40.5 Left craniocaudal (LCC) spot-compression mammogram.

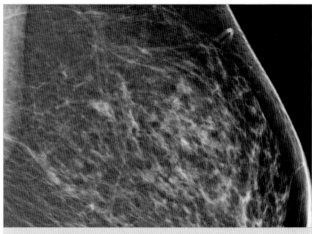

Fig. 40.6 Left mediolateral oblique (LMLO) spot-compression mammogram.

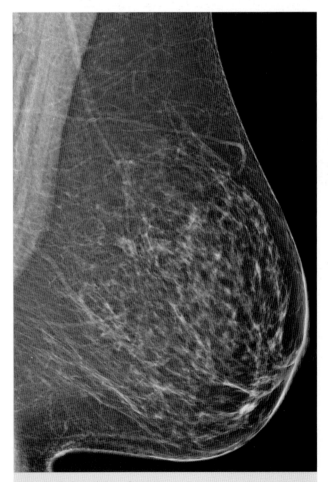

Fig. 40.7 Left mediolateral (LML).

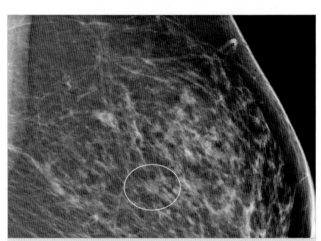

Fig. 40.8 Left mediolateral oblique (LMLO) spot-compression mammogram with label.

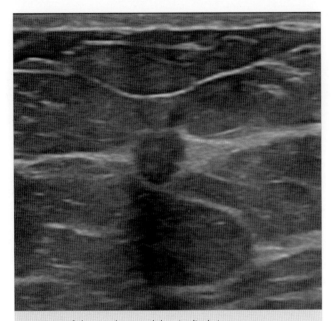

Fig. 40.9 Left breast ultrasound, longitudinal view.

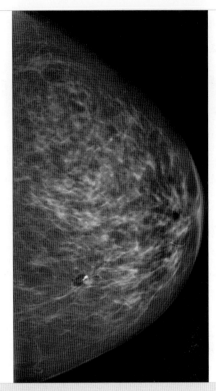

Fig. 40.10 Postbiopsy left craniocaudal (LCC) mammogram.

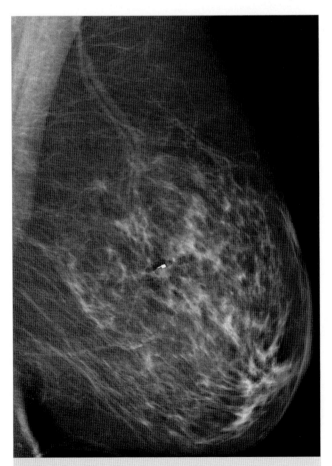

Fig. 40.11 Postbiopsy left medioalateral (LML) mammogram.

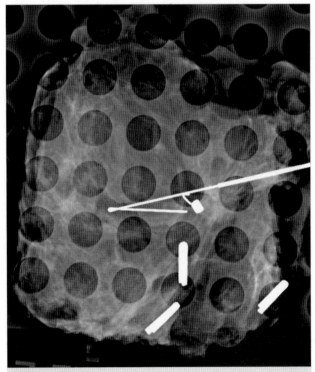

Fig. 40.12 Radiograph of surgical specimen.

41 Subtle Mass

Lonie R. Salkowski

41.1 Presentation and Presenting Images

(▶ Fig. 41.1, ▶ Fig. 41.2, ▶ Fig. 41.3, ▶ Fig. 41.4)

A 76-year-old female presents for screening mammography. She was treated for right breast ductal carcinoma in situ (DCIS) 10 years ago with a lumpectomy and hormonal therapy and had a repeat lumpectomy for DCIS 2 years ago.

41.2 Key Images

(▶ Fig. 41.5, ▶ Fig. 41.6)

41.2.1 Breast Tissue Density

There are scattered areas of fibroglandular density.

41.2.2 Imaging Findings

Central to the nipple, there are the expected postlumpectomy changes as demonstrated by architectural distortion and surgical clips. The wire on the skin surface denotes the skin incision site (just inferior to the areola). Within the lumpectomy bed, there is a new group of masses (▶ Fig. 41.1 and ▶ Fig. 41.2; DBT images ▶ Fig. 41.5 and ▶ Fig. 41.6) when compared to the prior mammography (▶ Fig. 41.3 and ▶ Fig. 41.4).

41.3 BI-RADS Classification and Action

Category 0: Mammography: Incomplete. Need additional imaging evaluation and/or prior mammograms for comparison.

41.4 Diagnostic Images

(▶ Fig. 41.7, ▶ Fig. 41.8, ▶ Fig. 41.9, ▶ Fig. 41.10, ▶ Fig. 41.11, ▶ Fig. 41.12, ▶ Fig. 41.13)

41.4.1 Imaging Findings

The diagnostic imaging demonstrates a 1.2 × 1.1 × 1.9 cm oval mass with circumscribed margins central to the nipple within the lumpectomy bed (▶ Fig. 41.7, ▶ Fig. 41.8, and ▶ Fig. 41.9). The targeted ultrasound demonstrates the shadowing scar from the prior lumpectomy (▶ Fig. 41.10) and a mass along the lateral side of the scar. The longitudinal ultrasound image (▶ Fig. 41.11) demonstrates an anechoic oval mass with a thickened wall and/or a mural mass. There is no increase in vascularity (*not shown*). The mammographic finding is composed of two similar adjacent masses measuring 7 mm and 5 mm at greatest dimensions. These masses underwent an ultrasound-guided biopsy. The postbiopsy mammogram demonstrates the new ribbon clip (*black arrow*) in the center of the prior lumpectomy site (▶ Fig. 41.12 and ▶ Fig. 41.13).

41.5 BI-RADS Classification and Action

Category 4B: Moderate suspicion for malignancy

41.6 Differential Diagnosis

1. ***Recurrent cancer (DCIS)*** : The patient had a prior recurrence of DCIS, which was treated with lumpectomy alone. The patient declined radiation therapy. A new mass within the lumpectomy bed has a high suspicion of recurrence. The biopsy of this mass revealed recurrent low-grade DCIS.
2. *Fat necrosis*: Fat necrosis can have various forms and can present several years after a lumpectomy. This finding is too radiopaque (even on DBT) to represent an oil cyst. There are no associated dystrophic or rim calcifications. This lesion warrants a biopsy and not dismissal as fat necrosis.
3. *Seroma*: It is unlikely for a seroma to develop at a lumpectomy site several years after the surgery. Seromas present early after surgery and over time decrease in size.

41.7 Essential Facts

- Postsurgical beds can be very complex and even subtle changes in them can be an indication of a possible recurrence of cancer.
- Mammographic findings after breast-conserving therapy can be varied and present as masses (hematomas, fat necrosis, fibrosis), fluid collections (seromas, abscess), increased breast density (edema, radiation changes), skin thickening, architectural distortion, and calcifications. These findings should show evolution to stability.
- Changes in the lumpectomy bed that should raise suspicion are increasing asymmetry, an enlarging mass, increasing edema or skin thickening, or development of suspicious calcifications.
- Recurrence of cancer at the treatment site is generally treatment failure, that is, an inability to eradicate the original cancer.
- Recurrences more than 10 years after treatment are more likely to be outside of the treated area and represent new malignancies.

41.8 Management and Digital Breast Tomosynthesis Principles

- Changes in the lumpectomy site after stabilization raise concern for tumor recurrence.
- Recurrences are rare within the first 2 years of treatment.

- Digital breast tomosynthesis (DBT) may be helpful in resolving the differences between a lumpectomy scar and a local recurrence of cancer on imaging.
- Patients who have not received radiation following breast-conserving therapy, especially for DCIS, have an increased local recurrence rate. The mammographic signs of recurrence may appear earlier than those treated with radiation.
- Careful inspection should be made at the lumpectomy site on DBT for any subtle changes.

41.9 Further Reading

[1] Chansakul T, Lai KC, Slanetz PJ. The postconservation breast: part 1, Expected imaging findings. AJR Am J Roentgenol. 2012; 198(2):321–330

[2] Chansakul T, Lai KC, Slanetz PJ. The postconservation breast: part 2, Imaging findings of tumor recurrence and other long-term sequelae. AJR Am J Roentgenol. 2012; 198(2):331–343

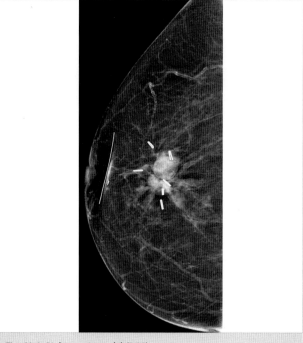

Fig. 41.1 Right craniocaudal (RCC) mammogram.

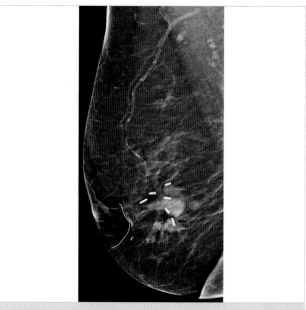

Fig. 41.2 Right mediolateral oblique (RMLO) mammogram.

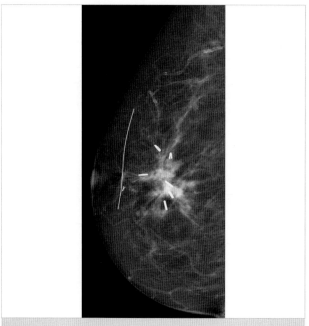

Fig. 41.3 Right craniocaudal (RCC) mannogram 1 year ago.

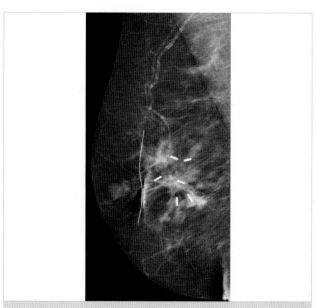

Fig. 41.4 Right mediolateral oblique (RMLO) mammogram 1 year ago.

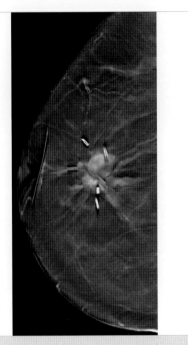

Fig. 41.5 Right cranocaudal digital breast tomosynthesis (RCC DBT), slice 22 of 68.

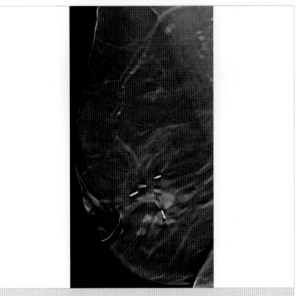

Fig. 41.6 Right mediolateral oblique digital breast tomosynthesis (RMLO DBT), slice 26 of 75.

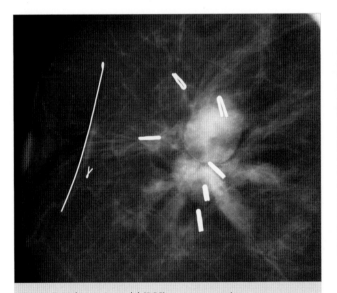

Fig. 41.7 Right craniocaudal (RCC) spot-compression mammogram.

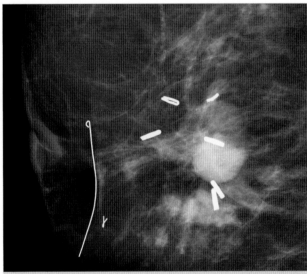

Fig. 41.8 Right mediolateral oblique (RMLO) spot-compression mammogram.

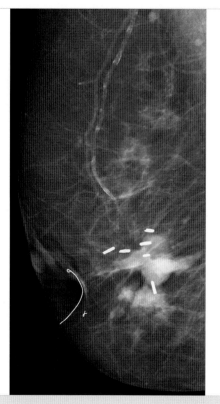

Fig. 41.9 Right mediolateral (RML) mammogram.

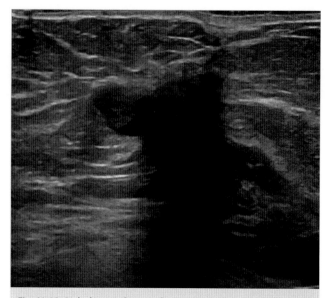

Fig. 41.10 Right breast ultrasound, transverse view.

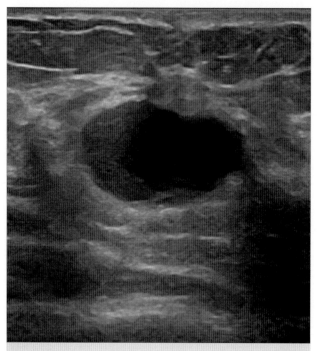

Fig. 41.11 Right breast ultrasound, longitudinal view.

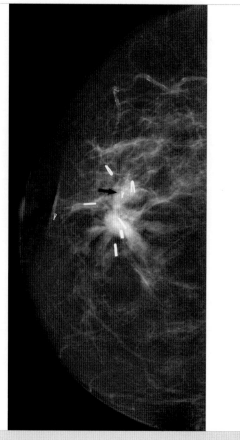

Fig. 41.12 Postbiopsy right craniocaudal (RCC) mammogram with label.

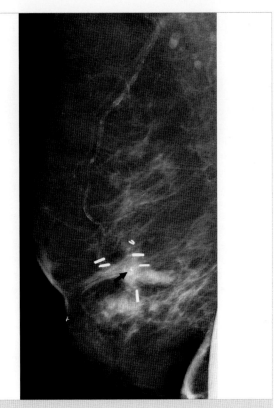

Fig. 41.13 Postbiopsy right mediolateral (RML) mammogram with label.

42 Coarse Heterogeneous Calcifications

Lonie R. Salkowski

42.1 Presentation and Presenting Images

(▶ Fig. 42.1, ▶ Fig. 42.2)

A 52-year-old female with a personal history of left breast cancer treated with lumpectomy, radiation therapy, and chemotherapy presents for screening mammography.

42.2 Key Images

(▶ Fig. 42.3, ▶ Fig. 42.4, ▶ Fig. 42.5, ▶ Fig. 42.6)

42.2.1 Breast Tissue Density

The breasts are heterogeneously dense, which may obscure small masses.

42.2.2 Imaging Findings

There is a group of calcifications in the right breast at the 1 o'clock location in the posterior depth (▶ Fig. 42.3 and ▶ Fig. 42.4). These calcifications are seen on the DBT images (▶ Fig. 42.5 and ▶ Fig. 42.6). In the area of the calcifications, the DBT does not reveal any associated mass.

42.3 BI-RADS Classification and Action

Category 0: Mammography: Incomplete. Need additional imaging evaluation and/or prior mammograms for comparison.

42.4 Diagnostic Images

(▶ Fig. 42.7, ▶ Fig. 42.8, ▶ Fig. 42.9, ▶ Fig. 42.10, ▶ Fig. 42.11, ▶ Fig. 42.12)

42.4.1 Imaging Findings

The diagnostic imaging demonstrates a 1.5-cm group of coarse heterogeneous calcifications at the 1 o'clock location in the posterior depth (▶ Fig. 42.7, ▶ Fig. 42.8 and ▶ Fig. 42.9) They do not layer on the mediolateral magnification view (▶ Fig. 42.8). There is no associated mass. These calcifications were sampled using stereotactic biopsy. Multiple cores contain the calcifications of interest (▶ Fig. 42.10). The postprocedure images reveal removal of many of the calcifications and the presence of the biopsy marker clip (bar-shaped) anterior and superior to the epicenter of the biopsy (▶ Fig. 42.11 and ▶ Fig. 42.12).

42.5 BI-RADS Classification and Action

Category 4B: Moderate suspicion for malignancy

42.6 Differential Diagnosis

1. ***Ductal carcinoma in situ (DCIS)***: Coarse heterogeneous calcifications can be suggestive of DCIS; there is an increased likelihood if they are in a linear or segmental distribution.
2. *Fibroadenoma*: Fibroadenomas can be seen mammographically as only calcifications. A biopsy with sufficient sampling of the calcifications and a pathologic diagnosis of a fibroadenoma associated with the calcifications could be considered concordant.
3. *Invasive carcinoma*: Typically coarse heterogeneous calcifications that present as an invasive cancer are associated with a spiculated or indistinct mass. The DBT did not reveal a mass associated with these calcifications.

42.7 Essential Facts

- Coarse heterogeneous calcifications have a 15% positive predictive value (PPV) of malignancy.
- Beyond morphology, the distribution of calcifications is an important predictor of malignancy. Grouped calcifications have a PPV of malignancy just over 30%, compared to linear and segmental calcifications, which have PPVs of 60% and 62%, respectively.
- The X-ray source, motion, pixel size, and reconstruction algorithms of a digital breast tomosynthesis (DBT) system will affect its detection of calcifications.
- DBT has good in-plane resolution (direction perpendicular to the X-ray plane), but its out-of-plane resolution is poor. The relatively poor z-depth resolution of DBT contributes to the blurring of calcifications.
- Full-field digital mammography (FFDM) has a higher in-plane resolution compared to current DBT.

42.8 Managing and Digital Breast Tomosynthesis Principles

- To improve the sensitivity and specificity of DBT for calcifications, it may require a hybrid approach to reading mammograms. The FFDM would be used to assess calcifications and the DBT would provide more information about masses, asymmetries, and architectural distortion.
- Larger studies are needed to determine the success of DBT compared to FFDM for detection (sensitivity) and characterization (specificity) of microcalcifications. Current studies suggest that FFDM outperforms DBT.

42.9 Further Reading

[1] Helvie MA. Digital mammography imaging: breast tomosynthesis and advanced applications. Radiol Clin North Am. 2010; 48(5):917–929
[2] Sickles EA, D'Orsi CJ, Bassett LW, et al. ACR BI-RADS Mammography. In: ACR BI-RADS Atlas, 5th edition. Reston, VA: American College of Radiology; 2013

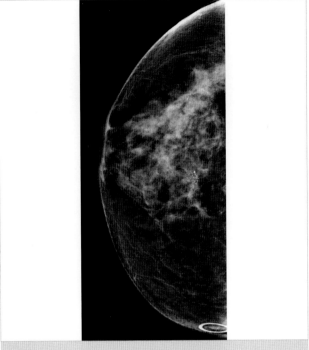

Fig. 42.1 Right craniocaudal (RCC) mammogram.

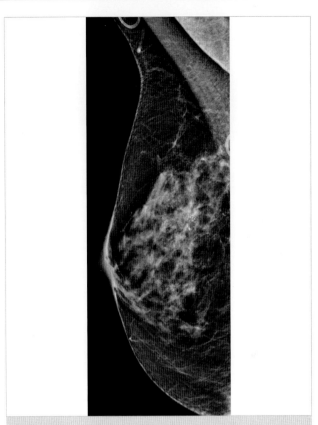

Fig. 42.2 Right mediolateral oblique (RMLO) mammogram.

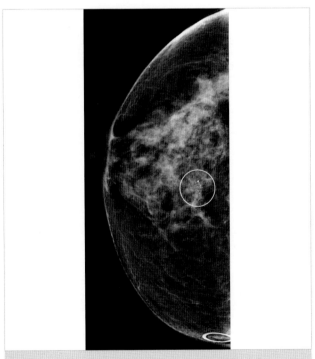

Fig. 42.3 Right craniocaudal (RCC) mammogram with label.

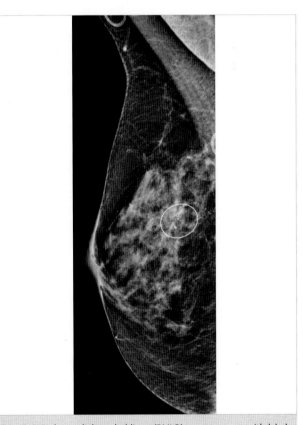

Fig. 42.4 Right mediolateral oblique (RMLO) mammogram with label.

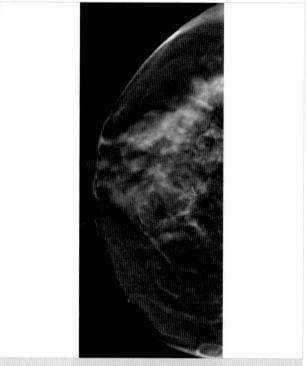

Fig. 42.5 Right craniocaudal digital breast tomosynthesis (RCC DBT), slice 33 of 59.

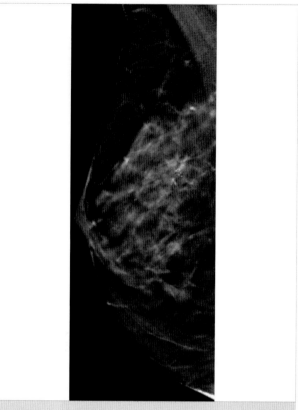

Fig. 42.6 Right mediolateral oblique digital breast tomosynthesis (RMLO DBT), slice 31 of 54.

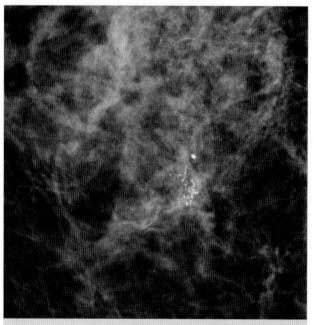

Fig. 42.7 Right craniocaudal (RCC) mammogram spot magnification.

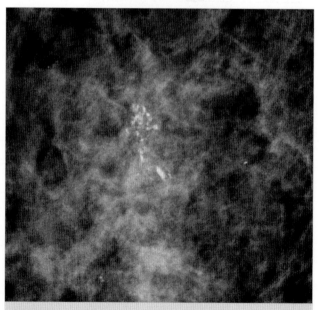

Fig. 42.8 Right mediolateral (RML) mammogram, spot magnification.

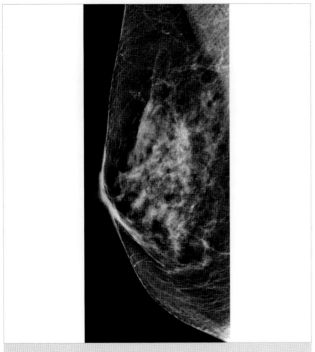

Fig. 42.9 Right mediolateral (RML) mammogram.

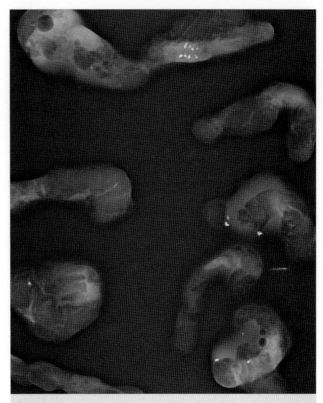

Fig. 42.10 Radiograph of biopsy specimen.

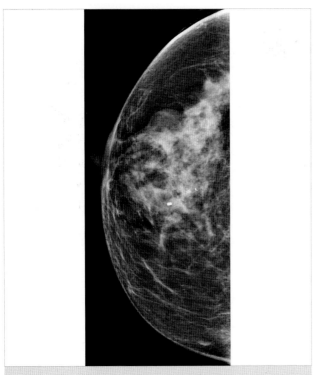

Fig. 42.11 Postbiopsy right craniocaudal (RCC) mammogram.

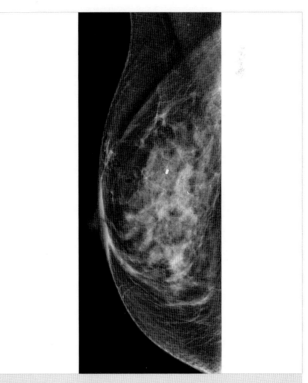

Fig. 42.12 Postbiopsy right mediolateral (RML) mammogram.

43 Amorphous Calcifications

Tanya W. Moseley

43.1 Presentation and Presenting Images

(▶ Fig. 43.1, ▶ Fig. 43.2)

A 58-year-old female presents for routine screening mammography.

43.2 Key Images

(▶ Fig. 43.3, ▶ Fig. 43.4, ▶ Fig. 43.5, ▶ Fig. 43.6)

43.2.1 Breast Tissue Density

The breasts are heterogeneously dense, which may obscure small masses.

43.2.2 Imaging Findings

The imaging of the left breast is normal (*not shown*). A new group of faint calcifications (*circle*) is noted in the upper region of the right breast in the posterior depth, 10 cm from the nipple on the mediolateral oblique (MLO) view (▶ Fig. 43.3). The calcifications are not well seen on the craniocaudal (CC) view (▶ Fig. 43.1). The MLO tomosynthesis movie can be used to localize the calcifications in the CC view. The MLO tomosynthesis movie (▶ Fig. 43.4) localizes the group of calcifications to the lateral portion of the breast, placing them at the 10 to 11 o'clock location, 10 cm from the nipple (▶ Fig. 43.5 and ▶ Fig. 43.6). This localization is helpful for further diagnostic mammographic evaluation.

43.3 BI-RADS Classification and Action

Category 0: Mammography: Incomplete. Need additional imaging evaluation and/or prior mammograms for comparison.

43.4 Diagnostic Images

(▶ Fig. 43.7, ▶ Fig. 43.8, ▶ Fig. 43.9)

43.4.1 Breast Tissue Density

The breasts are heterogeneously dense, which may obscure small masses.

43.5 Imaging Findings

Additional magnification imaging (▶ Fig. 43.7 and ▶ Fig. 43.8) reveals a group of amorphous calcifications. This new finding has a low suspicion of malignancy and underwent stereotactic biopsy. The radiograph of the specimen (▶ Fig. 43.9) from the stereotactic biopsy demonstrates the faint amorphous calcifications (*circles*).

43.6 BI-RADS Classification and Action

Category 4A: Low suspicion for malignancy

43.7 Differential Diagnosis

1. ***Sclerosing adenosis***: Stereotactic biopsy (▶ Fig. 43.7) was performed following a diagnostic evaluation revealing grouped amorphous calcifications. The pathology was consistent with sclerosing adenosis.
2. *Fibrocystic changes*: Fibrocystic changes commonly present as hazy, small, faint calcifications. This diagnosis would be considered concordant if the radiologist felt the calcifications had been adequately sampled.
3. *Ductal carcinoma in situ (DCIS)*: DCIS may present as amorphous calcifications. This would be a concordant biopsy.

43.8 Essential Facts

- With new or increasing calcifications, the next step is diagnostic mammography with magnification views. Magnification views cannot be performed with tomosynthesis.
- Tomosynthesis is helpful in localizing findings, both calcifications and masses, seen on one mammographic view.
- Stereotactic biopsy is recommended for new calcifications with suspicious morphology. Calcifications seen best on tomosynthesis may be biopsied using tomosynthesis-directed stereotactic-guided biopsy.

43.9 Management and DBT Principles

- Spangler and colleagues (2011) found that tomosynthesis was slightly less sensitive than conventional mammography for the detection of calcifications. The authors felt that with improvements in processing algorithms and display, tomosynthesis could potentially improve in the detection of calcifications.
- Kopans and colleagues (2011) found that calcifications can be seen with the same or better clarity on tomosynthesis as on conventional mammography, and tomosynthesis allows for the same and perhaps improved analysis of calcifications.
- Magnification views are performed with conventional mammography; magnification views are not possible with tomosynthesis. Tomosynthesis systems must support both conventional mammography and tomosynthesis.

43.10 Further Reading

[1] Berg WA, Arnoldus CL, Teferra E, Bhargavan M. Biopsy of amorphous breast calcifications: pathologic outcome and yield at stereotactic biopsy. Radiology. 2001; 221(2):495–503

[2] Kopans D, Gavenonis S, Halpern E, Moore R. Calcifications in the breast and digital breast tomosynthesis. Breast J. 2011; 17(6):638–644

[3] Spangler ML, Zuley ML, Sumkin JH, et al. Detection and classification of calcifications on digital breast tomosynthesis and 2D digital mammography: a comparison. AJR Am J Roentgenol. 2011; 196(2):320–324

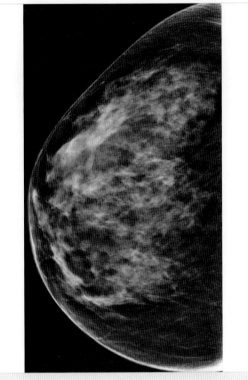

Fig. 43.1 Right craniocaudal (RCC) mammogram.

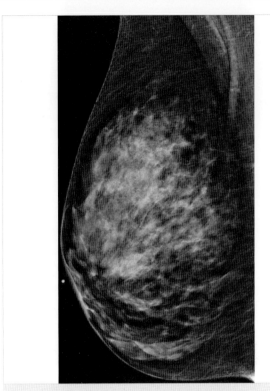

Fig. 43.2 Right mediolateral (RMLO) mammogram.

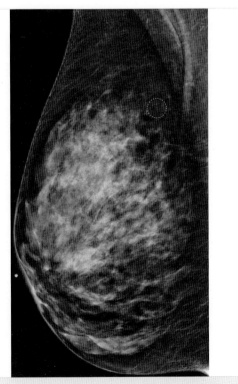

Fig. 43.3 Right mediolateral (RMLO) mammogram with label.

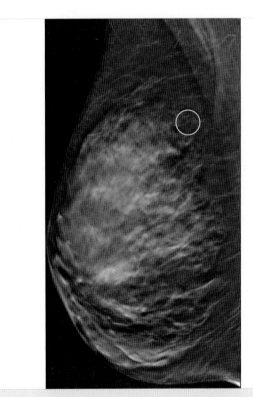

Fig. 43.4 Right mediolateral oblique digital breast tomosynthesis (RMLO DBT), slice 41 of 92, with label.

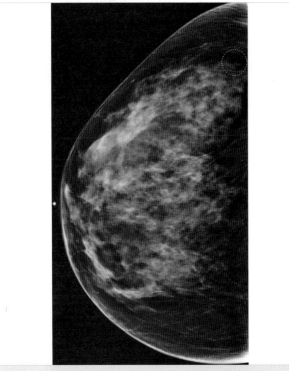

Fig. 43.5 Right craniocaudal (RCC) mammogram with label.

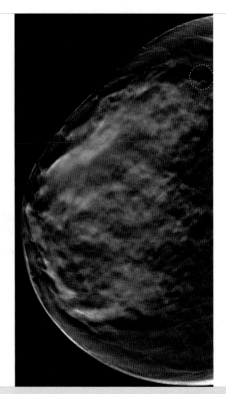

Fig. 43.6 Right craniocaudal digital breast tomosynthesis (RCC DBT), slice 24 of 90, with label.

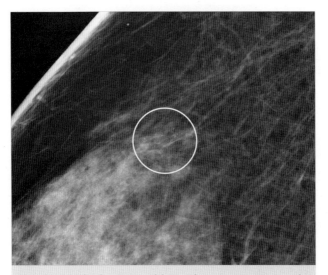

Fig. 43.7 Coned right craniocaudal magnification mammogram with label.

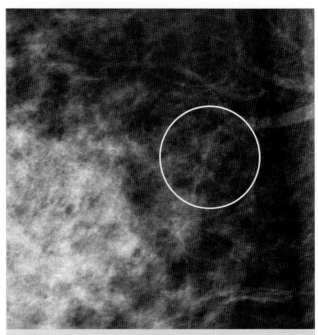

Fig. 43.8 Coned right lateromedial (RLM) magnification mammogram, with label.

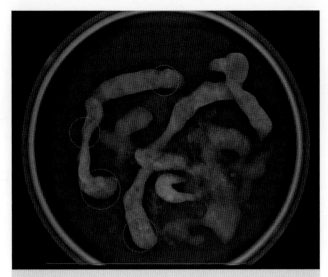

Fig. 43.9 Radiograph of stereotactic samples with label.

44 Developing Asymmetry

Lonie R. Salkowski

44.1 Presentation and Presenting Images

(► Fig. 44.1, ► Fig. 44.2, ► Fig. 44.3, ► Fig. 44.4)

A 70-year-old female presents for screening mammography. Her mother had postmenopausal breast cancer.

44.2 Key Images

(► Fig. 44.5, ► Fig. 44.6)

44.2.1 Breast Tissue Density

The breasts are heterogeneously dense, which may obscure small masses.

44.2.2 Imaging Findings

In the lower inner quadrant of the right breast in the middle depth, there is a focal asymmetry. In comparison to the prior mammograms (► Fig. 44.3 and ► Fig. 44.4), this could also be referred to as a developing asymmetry. The tomosynthesis images help to localize this lesion to the lower inner quadrant and support that this lesion is real and not overlapping fibro-glandular tissue (► Fig. 44.5 and ► Fig. 44.6). This lesion is less apparent on the conventional mammographic mediolateral oblique (MLO) image (► Fig. 44.2) but well seen on the craniocaudal (CC) image (► Fig. 44.1).

44.3 BI-RADS Classification and Action

Category 0: Mammography: Incomplete. Need additional imaging evaluation and/or prior mammograms for comparison.

44.4 Diagnostic Images

(► Fig. 44.7, ► Fig. 44.8, ► Fig. 44.9, ► Fig. 44.10, ► Fig. 44.11, ► Fig. 44.12, ► Fig. 44.13)

44.4.1 Imaging Findings

The diagnostic imaging better defines this focal asymmetry as an 8-mm oval even-density mass with spiculated margins at the 4 o'clock location in the middle depth (► Fig. 44.7 and ► Fig. 44.8). The spot-compression images displace the adjacent tissues with this mass located at the periphery of the breast

tissue. The targeted ultrasound reveals a 7 × 5 × 8 mm oval hypoechoic mass with angular and indistinct margins at the 4 o'clock location, 4 cm from the nipple (► Fig. 44.10 and ► Fig. 44.11). Normal lymph nodes were seen on the axillary ultrasound (*not shown*). This mass was biopsied and the postbiopsy images (► Fig. 44.12 and ► Fig. 44.13) demonstrate the biopsy clip in the appropriate location.

44.5 BI-RADS Classification and Action

Category 4C: High suspicion for malignancy

44.6 Differential Diagnosis

1. ***Breast cancer (invasive ductal carcinoma)***: There are many factors that suggest this mass is highly suspicious for malignancy: it began as a developing asymmetry, the diagnostic imaging confirmed it to be a mass with spiculated margins, and the correlating ultrasound revealed a hypoechoic mass with indistinct and angular margins.
2. *Lymph node*: The location would be atypical for a lymph node. The ultrasound does have a faint hyperechoic central region, which should not be interpreted as a hilum. The other features do not support this as being a lymph node.
3. *Fibroadenoma*: Typically fibroadenomas are hypoechoic oval or gently lobulated masses with circumscribed margins. None of these features are seen with this mass. A biopsy with this diagnosis would be discordant.

44.7 Essential Facts

- Digital breast tomosynthesis (DBT) improves the ability to classify lesions according to BI-RADS.
- DBT is less affected by the surrounding breast tissue density and composition than full-field digital mammography (FFDM).
- Lesions are better seen on the CC view compared to the MLO view on FFDM. On the CC view, the majority of the breast tissue will be located in the subareolar region or upper outer quadrant. On the MLO view, there is considerable overlap of the tissues from the medial and lateral aspects of most of the breast. Thus, it is beneficial to have two mammographic views for optimal interpretation.
- DBT is less impacted by the distribution of tissue because the tomographic technique limits the problems of superimposition of breast tissues.

44.8 Management and Digital Breast Tomosynthesis Principles

- Superimposition of breast tissues will have a greater effect on obscuring a mass with spiculated margins compared to one with a smooth or oval shape.
- DBT can eliminate overlapping tissue effects, enhance local structure separation, and provide localization of an area of interest.
- DBT does improve the recall rate; however, currently there is a doubling of the time that it takes to interpret DBT and FFDM compared to FFDM alone. This may improve as users become more proficient with the technology.

44.9 Further Reading

[1] Andersson I, Ikeda DM, Zackrisson S, et al. Breast tomosynthesis and digital mammography: a comparison of breast cancer visibility and BIRADS classification in a population of cancers with subtle mammographic findings. Eur Radiol. 2008; 18(12):2817–2825

[2] Uematsu T. The emerging role of breast tomosynthesis. Breast Cancer. 2013; 20(3):204–212

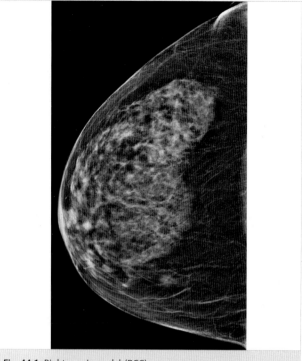

Fig. 44.1 Right craniocaudal (RCC) mammogram.

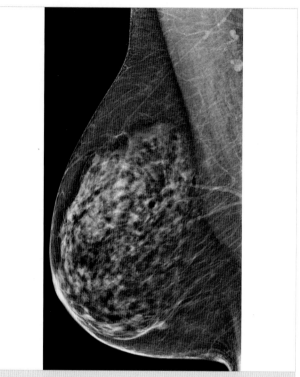

Fig. 44.2 Right mediolateral oblique (RMLO) mammogram.

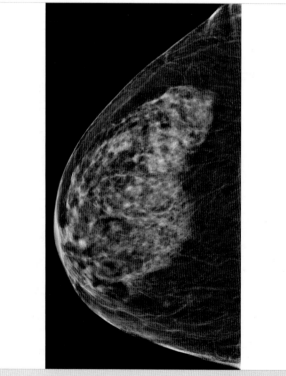

Fig. 44.3 Right craniocaudal (RCC) mammogram 2 years ago.

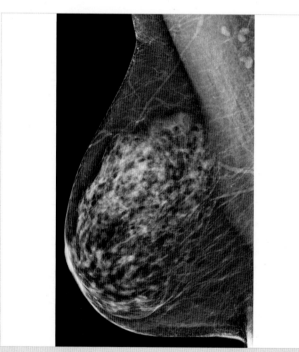

Fig. 44.4 Right mediolateral oblique (RMLO) mammogram 2 years ago.

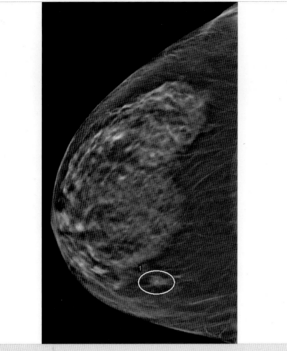

Fig. 44.5 Right craniocaudal digital breast tomosynthesis (RCC DBT), slice 11 of 56, with label.

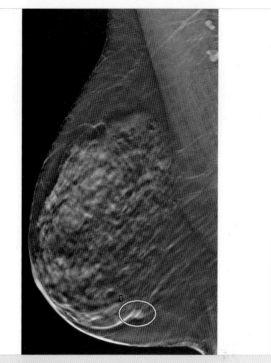

Fig. 44.6 Right mediolateral oblique digital breast tomosynthesis (RMLO DBT), slice 18 of 53, with label.

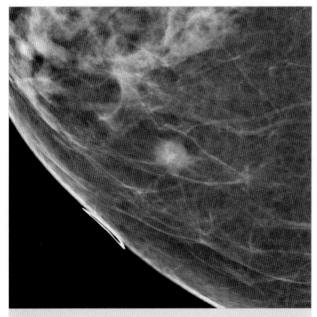

Fig. 44.7 Right craniocaudal (RCC) spot-compression mammogram.

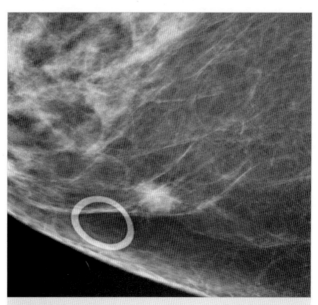

Fig. 44.8 Right mediolateral oblique (RMLO) spot-compression mammogram, with label.

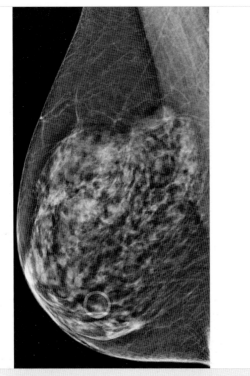

Fig. 44.9 Right mediolateral (RML) mammogram.

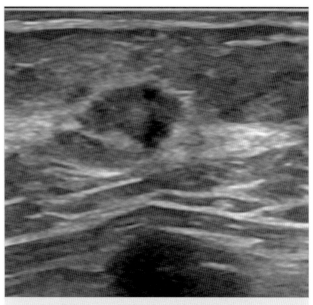

Fig. 44.10 Right breast ultrasound, longitudinal view.

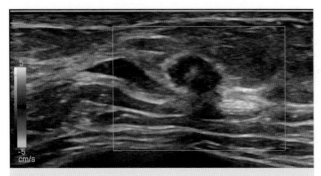

Fig. 44.11 Right breast Doppler ultrasound, transverse view.

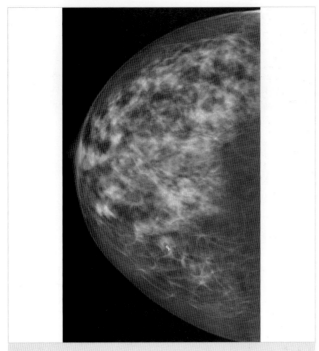

Fig. 44.12 Postbiopsy right craniocaudal (RCC) mammogram.

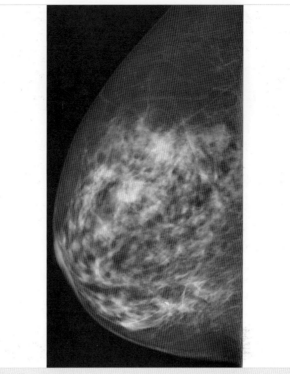

Fig. 44.13 Postbiopsy right mediolateral (RML) mammogram.

45 Focal Asymmetry with Architectural Distortion

Lonie R. Salkowski

45.1 Presentation and Presenting Images

(▶ Fig. 45.1, ▶ Fig. 45.2)

A 68-year-old female presents for screening mammography.

45.2 Key Images

(▶ Fig. 45.3, ▶ Fig. 45.4)

45.2.1 Breast Tissue Density

There are scattered areas of fibroglandular density.

45.2.2 Imaging Findings

In the upper outer quadrant in the posterior depth of the left breast, there is a focal asymmetry (seen on both full-field digital mammography [FFDM] and digital breast tomosynthesis [DBT]) with associated architectural distortion (which is best seen on the DBT). The focal asymmetry is best seen on the mediolateral oblique (MLO) views (▶ Fig. 45.2 and ▶ Fig. 45.4). It is at the very edge of the craniocaudal (CC) views (▶ Fig. 45.1 and ▶ Fig. 45.3), and better seen on the craniocaudal (CC) tomosynthesis image (▶ Fig. 45.3) compared to the conventional CC mammogram (▶ Fig. 45.1). The lateral location of the finding on the MLO DBT slices directs the reader to the corresponding finding in the lateral region on the CC view.

45.3 BI-RADS Classification and Action

Category 0: Mammography: Incomplete. Need additional imaging evaluation and/or prior mammograms for comparison.

45.4 Diagnostic Images

(▶ Fig. 45.5, ▶ Fig. 45.6, ▶ Fig. 45.7, ▶ Fig. 45.8, ▶ Fig. 45.9, ▶ Fig. 45.10, ▶ Fig. 45.11, ▶ Fig. 45.12)

45.4.1 Imaging Findings

The diagnostic imaging demonstrates an 8 × 9 × 8 mm irregular mass with indistinct margins and architectural distortion at the 2 o'clock location in the posterior depth (▶ Fig. 45.5, ▶ Fig. 45.6, ▶ Fig. 45.7, and ▶ Fig. 45.8). Posterior to this mass is a circumscribed oval mass. This is an intramammary lymph node that has been stable for many years (▶ Fig. 45.7 and ▶ Fig. 45.8). The targeted ultrasound demonstrates a lesion that was found with great difficulty. On ultrasound (▶ Fig. 45.9 and ▶ Fig. 45.10), the mass is hypoechoic with indistinct margins and located near the chest wall. It is slightly smaller on ultrasound than on mammography, measuring 7 × 7 × 6 mm. Normal intramammary and low-level axillary lymph nodes were seen (*not shown*). The postprocedure mammograms (▶ Fig. 45.11 and ▶ Fig. 45.12) demonstrate the ribbon biopsy clip 3 mm lateral to the lesion.

45.5 BI-RADS Classification and Action

Category 4B: Moderate suspicion for malignancy

45.6 Differential Diagnosis

1. ***Breast cancer (invasive ductal carcinoma)***: This mass is new and irregular with indistinct margins. Those features alone would raise the suspicion for cancer. The indistinct margins on ultrasound also suggest an invasive process.
2. *Lymph node*: Although there are adjacent lymph nodes, this mass has features that suggest that if it is a lymph node, it will not be a normal lymph node. If an image-guided biopsy resulted in the diagnosis of a metastatic lymph node that would be considered concordant. The next step would involve finding the primary carinoma.
3. *Focal fibrosis*: Focal fibrosis can mimic cancer. An image-guided biopsy of this lesion should yield a histopathologic analysis of this discrete mass If focal fibrosis is the dominant feature of this mass, then this diagnosis is concordant. If a minority of the mass is focal fibrosis, then excision is recommended.

45.7 Essential Facts

- Similar to FFDM, positioning with DBT is extremely important. If the tissue of interest is not appropriately included on the mammogram, no assessment can be made of it.
- Similar to FFDM, the posterior-nipple-line (PNL) depth of the tissue on the CC and MLO views should be within 1 cm on DBT.
- Fat should be posterior to the fibroglandular tissue on both the CC and MLO views. Sometimes an additional exaggerated (XCC) view may be necessary on the screening mammography examination.
- DBT has been shown to improve the specificity and sensitivity in breast cancer screening. The conspicuity of masses and areas of architectural distortion are improved with DBT.
- Taplin and colleagues (2002) observed that that the detection of cancer was highest (84%) when the patients had proper positioning at mammography. This sensitivity falls to 66.3% when positioning is not correct.
- In this case, the DBT images highlighted the finding on the conventional MLO mammogram as being suspicious. The finding is barely included on the conventional CC mammogram. Without DBT, this case might have been among the ones with a missed cancer.

45.8 Management and Digital Breast Tomosynthesis Principles

- Improperly positioned FFDM and DBT can contribute to interval cancers. When the breast tissue is not properly positioned, cancers that were present can go undetected when not imaged.
- Patients should be recalled for repeat imaging when there are technical factors that impede diagnostic interpretation. Some technical factors the can impede diagnosis are patient positioning and motion, radiation exposure (too much or too little) and breast compression (too little).

- Lesions seen only on one view are one cause of missed cancers.
- Posterior lesions are often a cause of missed cancers given that they may only be seen on one view, and not included on the orthogonal view.

45.9 Further Reading

[1] Conant EF. Clinical implementation of digital breast tomosynthesis. Radiol Clin North Am. 2014; 52(3):499–518
[2] Taplin SH, Rutter CM, Finder C, Mandelson MT, Houn F, White E. Screening mammography: clinical image quality and the risk of interval breast cancer. AJR Am J Roentgenol. 2002; 178(4):797–803

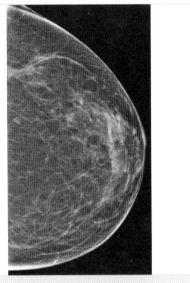

Fig. 45.1 Left craniocaudal (LCC) mammogram.

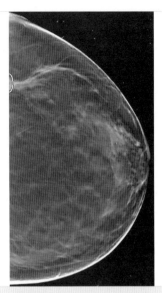

Fig. 45.3 Left craniocaudal digital breast tomosynthesis (LCC DBT), slice 32 of 79.

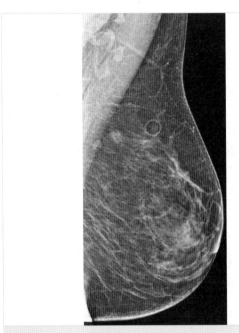

Fig. 45.2 Left mediolateral oblique (LMLO) mammogram.

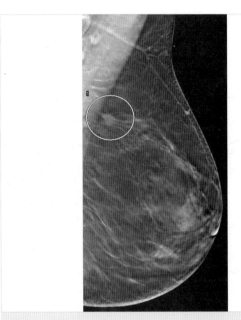

Fig. 45.4 Left mediolateral oblique digital breast tomosynthesis (LMLO DBT), slice 27 of 81, with label.

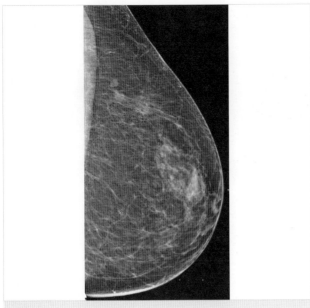

Fig. 45.5 Exaggerated left craniocaudal (LXCC) mammogram.

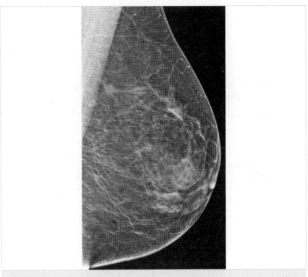

Fig. 45.6 Left mediolateral (LML) mammogram.

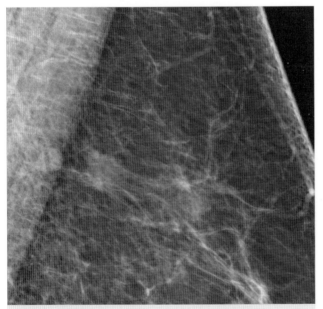

Fig. 45.8 Left mediolateral oblique (LMLO) spot-compression mammogram.

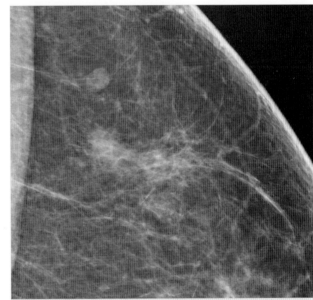

Fig. 45.7 Left craniocaudal (LCC) spot-compression mammogram.

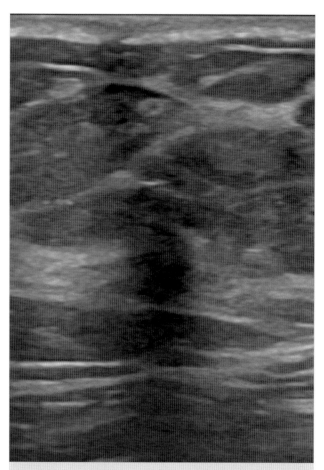

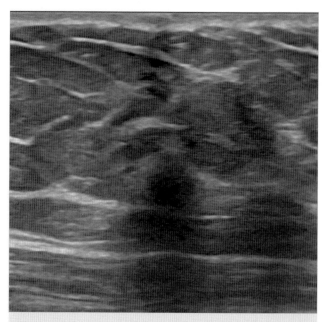

Fig. 45.10 Left breast ultrasound, longitudinal view.

Fig. 45.9 Left breast ultrasound, transverse view.

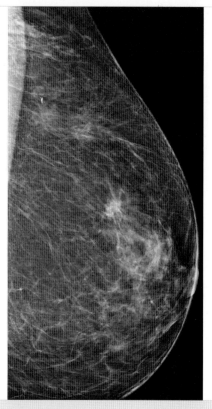

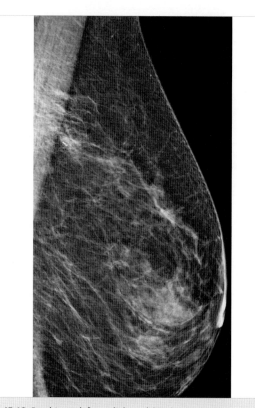

Fig. 45.11 Postbiopsy left craniocaudal (LCC) mammogram.

Fig. 45.12 Postbiopsy left mediolateral (LML) mammogram.

46 Circumscribed Mass on Baseline Mammogram

Lonie R. Salkowski

46.1 Presentation and Presenting Images

(► Fig. 46.1, ► Fig. 46.2)

A 39-year-old female presents for baseline high-risk screening mammography.

46.2 Key Images

(► Fig. 46.3, ► Fig. 46.4)

46.2.1 Breast Tissue Density

The breasts are heterogeneously dense, which may obscure small masses.

46.2.2 Imaging Findings

In the posterior depth of the left breast at the 2 o'clock location, there is an oval circumscribed mass. This is demonstrated on both conventional mammography (► Fig. 46.1 and ► Fig. 46.2) and tomosynthesis (► Fig. 46.3 and ► Fig. 46.4). The location would be classic for a lymph node; however, no defining features are seen to identify this as a lymph node.

46.3 BI-RADS Classification and Action

Category 0: Mammography: Incomplete. Need additional imaging evaluation and/or prior mammograms for comparison.

46.4 Diagnostic Images

(► Fig. 46.5, ► Fig. 46.6, ► Fig. 46.7, ► Fig. 46.8)

46.4.1 Imaging Findings

The diagnostic imaging demonstrates the oval circumscribed mass to be at the 2 o'clock location in the posterior depth (► Fig. 46.5, ► Fig. 46.6, and ► Fig. 46.7). However, these images do not provide any additional information about the nature of the mass. An ultrasound was performed that confirms a 0.9 × 0.5 × 1.0 cm oval hypoechoic mass with a central echogenic hilum located 9 cm from the nipple (► Fig. 46.8). Normal vascularity was seen in the hilum.

46.5 BI-RADS Classification and Action

Category 2: Benign

46.6 Differential Diagnosis

1. **Lymph node**: The location of this mass suggests that a lymph node is a likely diagnosis. However, it does not have the classic features of a fatty hilum on conventional mammography or tomosynthesis. The patient also has no prior imaging for comparison. Additional imaging is warranted. In this case, ultrasound, which demonstrated the mass to be a lymph node, was the most helpful.
2. *Fibroadenoma*: Fibroadenomas can occur anywhere in the breast and are very common in patients this age. Additional imaging is warranted. The ultrasound in this case does not support this diagnosis.
3. *Breast cancer*: Triple-negative cancers have a predilection to occur in the posterior region of the breast and also have a benign appearance. Because the mass is not classic for any specific lesion, additional evaluation is required.

46.7 Essential Facts

- DBT has shown promise in better characterizing benign findings and thus avoiding unnecessary recall mammography.
- Some benign-appearing lesions will only be seen on DBT.
- Recall rates are higher for those with no prior imaging studies than those with prior imaging studies.
- FFDM plus DBT has demonstrated a significant reduction in recall rates in women with a baseline mammogram compared to FFDM alone. There was no associated reduction in sensitivity with the decrease in recall rates.

46.8 Management and Digital Breast Tomosynthesis Principles

- There is a learning curve for reading DBT images before the reader is comfortable and confident.
- Early in the implementation of DBT, there is often a slight increase in recalls owing to readers' readjustment of sensitivity and specificity in reading images from a new modality.
- Although DBT offers the ability to better define lesions and identify them as benign. Care should be taken to ensure that the imaging findings meet all the criteria to dismiss them as benign.

46.9 Further Reading

[1] Roth RG, Maidment AD, Weinstein SP, Roth SO, Conant EF. Digital breast tomosynthesis: lessons learned from early clinical implementation. Radiographics. 2014; 34(4):E89–E102

[2] Sumkin JH, Ganott MA, Chough DM, et al. Recall Rate Reduction with Tomosynthesis During Baseline Screening Examinations: An Assessment From a Prospective Trial. Acad Radiol. 2015; 22(12):1477–1482

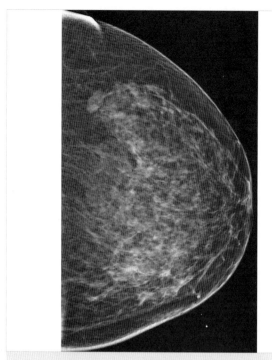

Fig. 46.1 Left craniocaudal (LCC) mammogram.

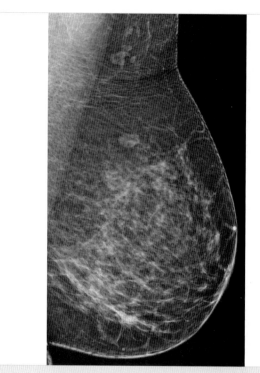

Fig. 46.2 Left mediolateral oblique (LMLO) mammogram.

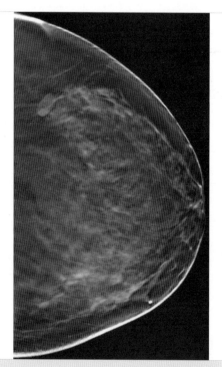

Fig. 46.3 Left craniocaudal digital breast tomosynthesis (LCC DBT), slice 35 of 82.

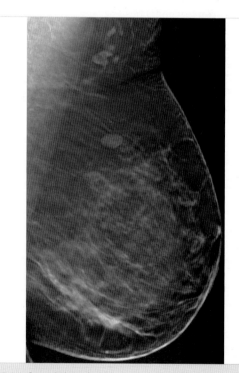

Fig. 46.4 Left mediolateral oblique digital breast tomosynthesis (LMLO DBT), slice 34 of 91.

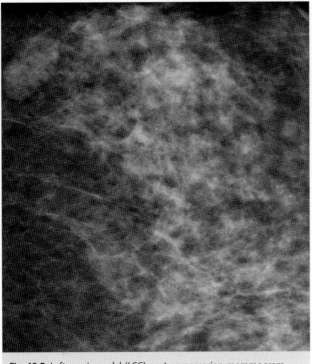

Fig. 46.5 Left craniocaudal (LCC) spot-compression mammogram.

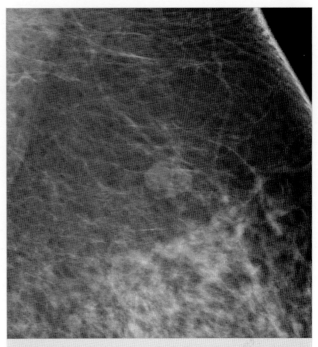

Fig. 46.6 Left mediolateral oblique (LMO) spot-compression mammogram.

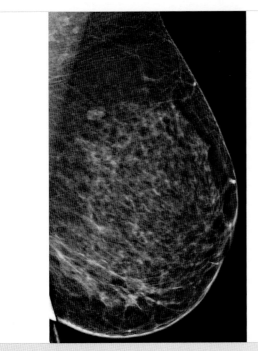

Fig. 46.7 Left mediolateral (LML) mammogram.

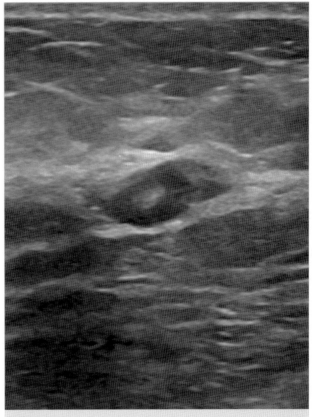

Fig. 46.8 Left breast ultrasound, transverse view.

47 Two Areas of Architectural Distortion

Lonie R. Salkowski

47.1 Presentation and Presenting Images

(► Fig. 47.1, ► Fig. 47.2, ► Fig. 47.3, ► Fig. 47.4)

A 55-year-old female presents for screening mammography.

47.2 Key Images

(► Fig. 47.5, ► Fig. 47.6, ► Fig. 47.7, ► Fig. 47.8)

47.2.1 Breast Tissue Density

There are scattered areas of fibroglandular density.

47.2.2 Imaging Findings

Two areas of possible architectural distortion are seen within the left breast. A more subtle area is present in the upper outer quadrant around the 2 o'clock position and the second area is central to the nipple. These are best seen on the digital breast tomosynthesis (DBT) images (► Fig. 47.5, ► Fig. 47.6, ► Fig. 47.7, and ► Fig. 47.8). The patient had a left breast biopsy 2 years prior, which is marked with a ribbon biopsy clip in the upper inner quadrant. The result of that biopsy was a diagnosis of fibrocystic changes but with findings also suggestive of a radial scar and the usual ductal hyperplasia. The patient elected to observe rather than excise.

47.3 BI-RADS Classification and Action

Category 0: Mammography: Incomplete. Need additional imaging evaluation and/or prior mammograms for comparison.

47.4 Diagnostic Images

(► Fig. 47.9, ► Fig. 47.10, ► Fig. 47.11, ► Fig. 47.12, ► Fig. 47.13, ► Fig. 47.14, ► Fig. 47.15, ► Fig. 47.16, ► Fig. 47.17)

47.4.1 Imaging Findings

The architectural distortion at 2 o'clock did not persist on further diagnostic imaging (*not shown*) and the corresponding ultrasound of the area revealed normal breast tissue (*not shown*). The second area of architectural distortion at 12 o'clock in the middle depth measured approximately 1.9 × 1.3 cm. This area is appreciated on the spot-compression images (► Fig. 47.9, ► Fig. 47.10, and ► Fig. 47.11) and on the lateral view

(► Fig. 47.12). The targeted ultrasound revealed an 1.8 × 0.8 × 0.9 cm irregular hypoechoic mass with indistinct and angular margins at 12 o'clock location, 3 cm from the nipple (► Fig. 47.13 and ► Fig. 47.14). The posterior shadowing present helped to define this mass on ultrasound. Additionally, the axillary ultrasound revealed a lymph node 12 cm from the nipple with mild cortical thickening of 4 mm (► Fig. 47.15). Otherwise all axillary lymph nodes were normal.

47.5 BI-RADS Classification and Action

Category 4C: High suspicion for malignancy

47.6 Differential Diagnosis

1. ***Normal breast tissue and breast cancer (invasive ductal carcinoma with metastatic lymph node)***: More than one lesion can be seen on a screening mammogram. In this case, one was proven to be normal breast tissue and the other cancer.
2. *Radial scar*: The imaging features of a radial scar and carcinoma overlap. It is possible that both lesions could be radial scars since the patient has a history of a prior radial scars. The abnormal lymph node does not support a radial-scar diagnosis.
3. *Summation artifact*: One "lesion" in question did not persist on DBT and likely represents a summation artifact; however, the second lesion is suspicious and warrants tissue sampling.

47.7 Essential Facts

- Architectural distortion accounts for around 6% of imaging detected on screening mammography.
- Architectural distortion accounts for 12 to 45% of missed breast cancers.
- Architectural distortion is better visualized on DBT compared to full-field digital mammography (FFDM).
- In a study by Partyka and colleagues (2014) they found that the cancer detection rate was 21% for architectural distortion lesions seen only on DBT (occult on FFDM).
- Architectural distortion has a positive predictive value of a malignancy of nearly 75%. Thus its presence is highly predictive of cancer.
- Architectural distortion seen at screening is less likely to represent malignancy compared to architectural distortion seen on a diagnostic mammogram.

47.8 Management and Digital Breast Tomosynthesis Principles

- Although architectural distortion is not a very common imaging finding, its detection should warrant complete evaluation due to the high incidence of associated malignancy.
- Architectural distortion seen on DBT that does not persist on FFDM and spot compression images, warrants an ultrasound.
- Architectural distortion without an ultrasound correlate are more likely to represent a radial sclerosing lesion than carcinoma. Larger studies are needed to determine if lesions

falling into this imaging situation can be watched or need to be biopsied.

47.9 Further Reading

[1] Bahl M, Baker JA, Kinsey EN, Ghate SV. Architectural Distortion on Mammography: Correlation With Pathologic Outcomes and Predictors of Malignancy. AJR Am J Roentgenol. 2015; 205(6):1339–1345

[2] Partyka L, Lourenco AP, Mainiero MB. Detection of mammographically occult architectural distortion on digital breast tomosynthesis screening: initial clinical experience. AJR Am J Roentgenol. 2014; 203(1):216–222

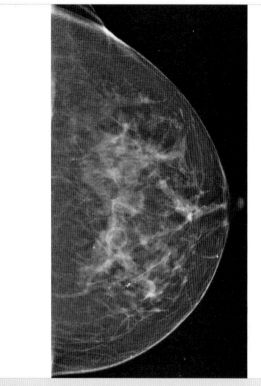

Fig. 47.1 Left craniocaudal (LCC) mammogram.

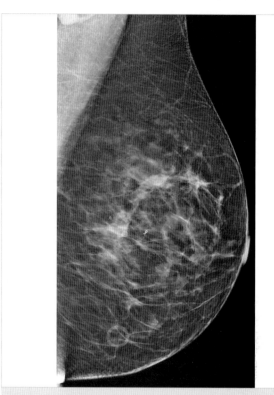

Fig. 47.2 Left mediolateral oblique (LMLO) mammogram.

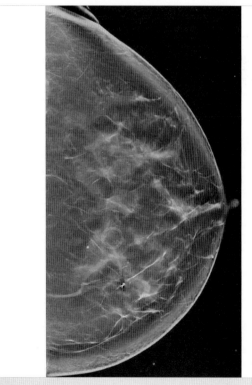

Fig. 47.3 Left craniocaudal (LCC) synthetic mammogram.

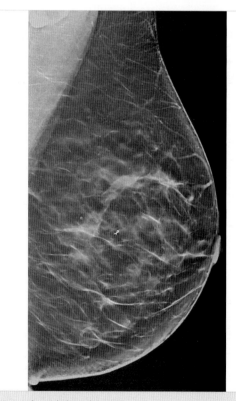

Fig. 47.4 Left mediolateral (LMLO) synthetic mammogram.

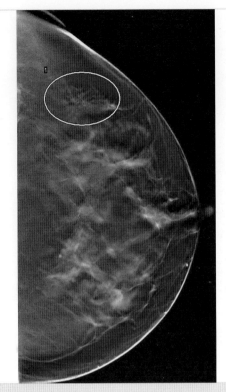

Fig. 47.5 Left craniocaudal digital breast tomosynthesis (LCC DBT), slice 41 of 94, with label.

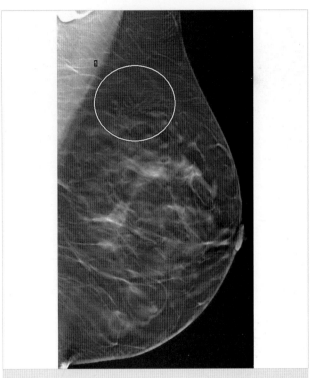

Fig. 47.6 Left mediolateral oblique digital breast tomosynthesis (LMLO DBT), slice 21 of 86, with label.

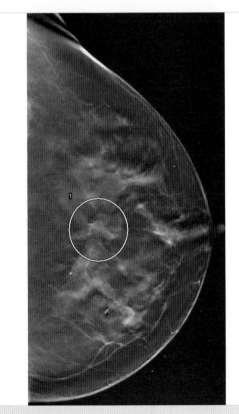

Fig. 47.7 Left craniocaudal digital breast tomosynthesis (LCC DBT), slice 48 of 94, with label.

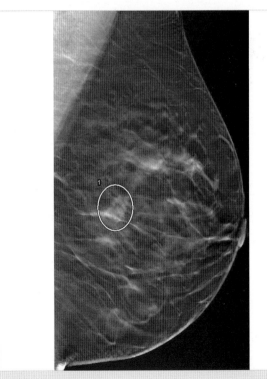

Fig. 47.8 Left mediolateral oblique digital breast tomosynthesis (LMLO DBT), slice 26 of 86, with label.

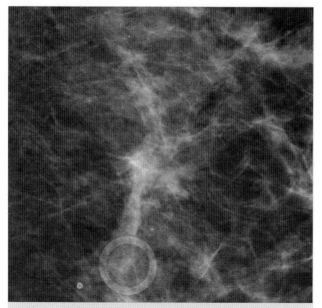

Fig. 47.9 Left craniocaudal (LCC) spot-compression mammogram.

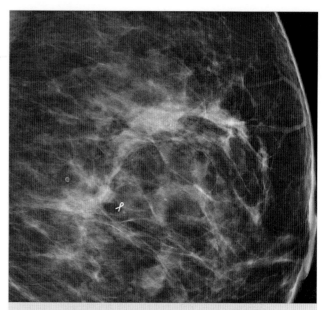

Fig. 47.10 Left mediolateral oblique (LMLO) spot-compression mammogram.

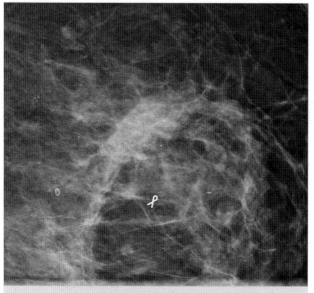

Fig. 47.11 Left mediolateral (LML) spot-compression mammogram.

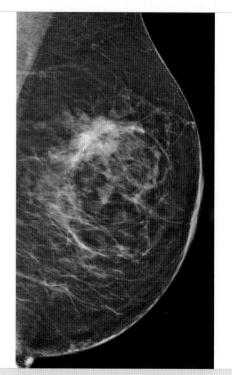

Fig. 47.12 Left mediolateral (LML) mammogram.

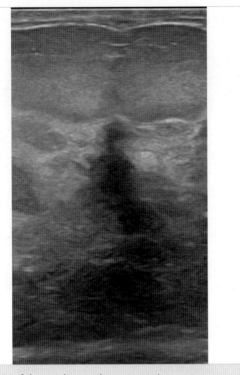

Fig. 47.13 Left breast ultrasound, transverse view.

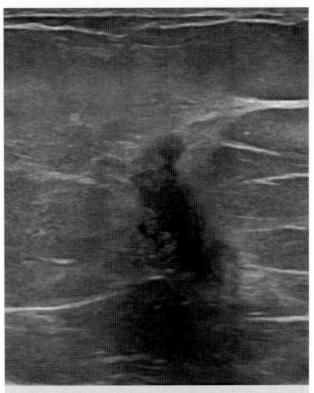

Fig. 47.14 Left breast ultrasound, longitudinal view.

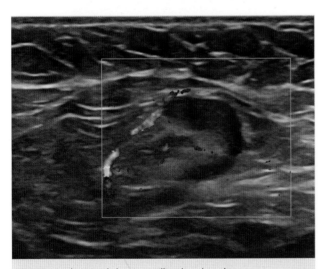

Fig. 47.15 Ultrasound showing axillary lymph node.

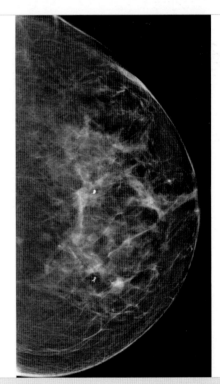

Fig. 47.16 Postbiopsy left craniocaudal (LCC) mammogram.

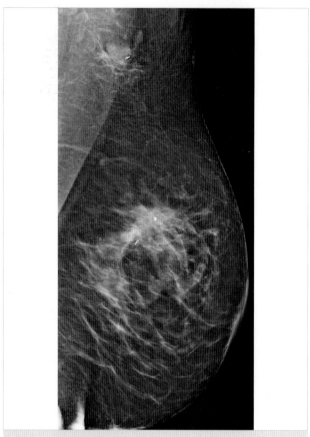

Fig. 47.17 Postbiopsy left mediolateral (LML) mammogram.

48 Architectural Distortion within Dense Breast Tissue

Lonie R. Salkowski

48.1 Presentation and Presenting Images

(▶ Fig. 48.1, ▶ Fig. 48.2, ▶ Fig. 48.3, ▶ Fig. 48.4)

A 50-year-old female with a history of left breast cancer treated 8 years ago presents for screening mammography.

48.2 Key Images

(▶ Fig. 48.5, ▶ Fig. 48.6)

48.2.1 Breast Tissue Density

The breasts are extremely dense, which lowers the sensitivity of mammography.

48.2.2 Imaging Findings

In the upper outer quadrant of the right breast, at the edge of the glandular tissue, there is a possible architectural distortion seen at the 10 o'clock position in the posterior depth. This is only appreciated on the digital breast tomosynthesis (DBT) images (▶ Fig. 48.5 and ▶ Fig. 48.6).

48.3 BI-RADS Classification and Action

Category 0: Mammography: Incomplete. Need additional imaging evaluation and/or prior mammograms for comparison.

48.4 Diagnostic Images

(▶ Fig. 48.7, ▶ Fig. 48.8, ▶ Fig. 48.9, ▶ Fig. 48.10, ▶ Fig. 48.11, ▶ Fig. 48.12, ▶ Fig. 48.13, ▶ Fig. 48.14, ▶ Fig. 48.15, ▶ Fig. 48.16)

48.4.1 Imaging Findings

The diagnostic imaging identifies a 1.1-cm subtle focal asymmetry (▶ Fig. 48.7, ▶ Fig. 48.10 and ▶ Fig. 48.8, ▶ Fig. 48.11) at the edge of the glandular tissue at the 10 o'clock location with the help of the prior screening DBT (▶ Fig. 48.5 and ▶ Fig. 48.6). The targeted ultrasound reveals a 0.6 × 1.0 × 0.9 cm irregular hypoechoic mass with angular and indistinct margins located at 10 o'clock, 10 cm from the nipple (▶ Fig. 48.12 and ▶ Fig. 48.13). There were normal appearing right axillary nodes (*not shown*). The postbiopsy mammogram demonstrates the ribbon biopsy clip is the posterior upper outer quadrant in the expected location (▶ Fig. 48.14 and ▶ Fig. 48.15). Note that the patient does have a coarse calcification in the lateral aspect of the breast (not to be mistaken for the biopsy clip, which is smaller). Due to the patient's prior history and underlying dense breast tissue, she underwent an MR examination. The MR image reveals this solitary enhancing right breast lesion in the upper outer quadrant at the periphery of the glandular tissue (▶ Fig. 48.16).

48.5 BI-RADS Classification and Action

Category 4C: High suspicion for malignancy

48.6 Differential Diagnosis

1. ***Carcinoma (invasive lobular carcinoma [ILC])***: The initial difficulty with this case was detection. The DBT images revealed this lesion and the subsequent imaging, especially the ultrasound in the diagnostic evaluation, confirmed this lesion. This lesion is consistent with carcinoma.
2. *Radial scar*: Typically radial scars do not have a significant mass equivalent on ultrasound. If the diagnosis based on the biopsy of this lesion was a radial scar, to be concordant, the histopathologic size would have to match the imaging size. Otherwise, it would be discordant, and excision of the lesion would be recommended.
3. *Fibroadenoma*: Fibroadenomas have variable features. However, this lesion appears more suspicious, and, thus, a diagnosis of a fibroadenoma on image-guided biopsy would be considered discordant, and excision would be recommended.

48.7 Essential Facts

- ILC accounts for 10 to 15% of invasive breast cancers.
- ILC most frequently manifests mammographically as a mass (44–65% of cases) and secondly as an architectural distortion (10–34% of cases).
- Ray and colleagues (2015) reported that DBT identified 7% of lesions recommended for biopsy that were occult on full-field digital mammography (FFDM). Over half of these mammographically occult lesions were malignant.
- Architectural distortion appears to represent the most common finding seen on DBT that is occult on FFDM.

48.8 Management and Digital Breast Tomosynthesis Principles

- There is a higher false negative rate for ILC (up to 19%) on mammography compared to other invasive breast cancers.
- DBT improves the ability of detecting subtle distortion by reducing the effects of overlapping tissue.

- DBT also allows the dismissal of pseudo–architectural distortion that is created by summation artifacts.
- ILC is the most likely invasive breast cancer to be occult to imaging and physical examination. More studies are needed to see if DBT can have an impact on ILC detection.
- Ray and colleagues' (2015) limited retrospective study suggested that ILC had a higher frequency of detection with DBT, accounting for one-third of their identified cancers.

48.9 Further Reading

[1] Lopez JK, Bassett LW. Invasive lobular carcinoma of the breast: spectrum of mammographic, US, and MR imaging findings. Radiographics. 2009; 29(1): 165–176

[2] Ray KM, Turner E, Sickles EA, Joe BN. Suspicious Findings at Digital Breast Tomosynthesis Occult to Conventional Digital Mammography: Imaging Features and Pathology Findings. Breast J. 2015; 21(5):538–542

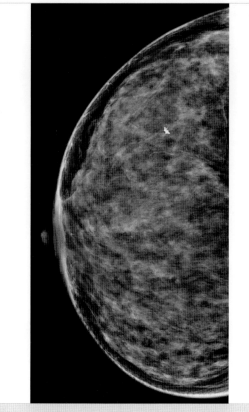

Fig. 48.1 Right craniocaudal (RCC) mammogram.

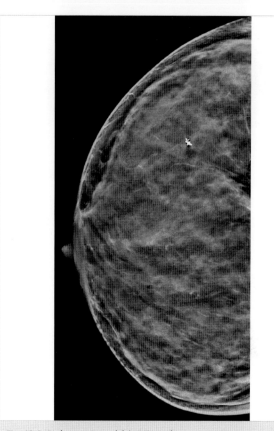

Fig. 48.2 Right craniocaudal (RCC) synthetic mammogram.

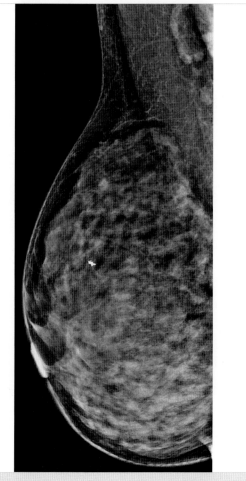

Fig. 48.3 Right mediolateral oblique (RMLO) mammogram.

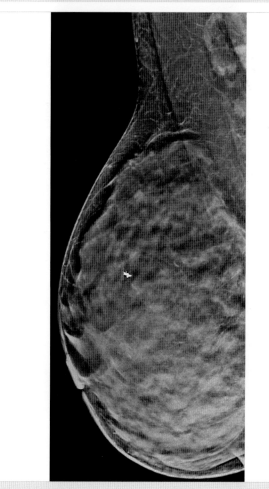

Fig. 48.4 Right mediolateral oblique (RMLO) synthetic mammogram.

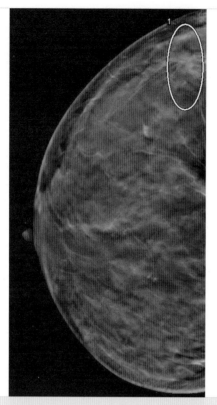

Fig. 48.5 Right craniocaudal digital breast tomosynthesis (RCC DBT), slice 45 of 63, with label.

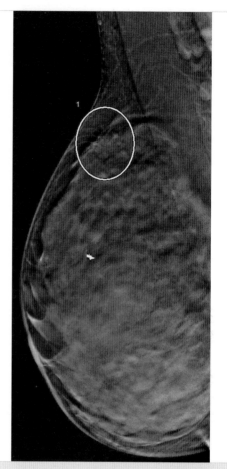

Fig. 48.6 Right mediolateral oblique digital breast tomosynthesis (RMLO DBT), slice 20 of 65, with label.

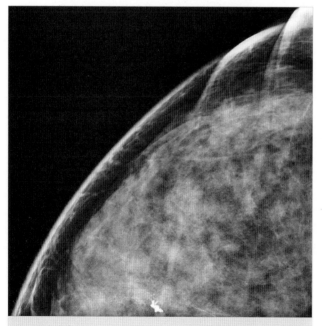

Fig. 48.7 Right craniocaudal (RCC) spot-compression mammogram.

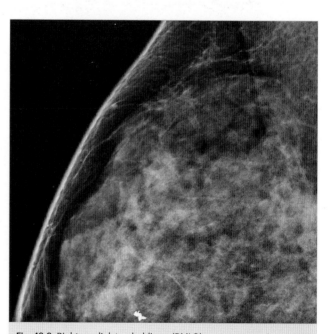

Fig. 48.8 Right mediolateral oblique (RMLO) spot-compression mammogram.

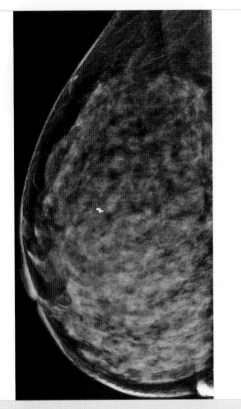

Fig. 48.9 Right mediolateral (RML) mammogram.

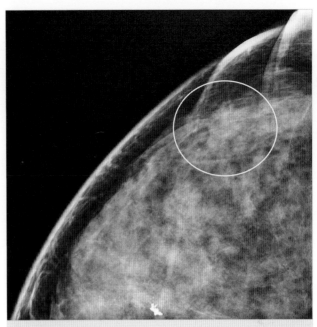

Fig. 48.10 Right craniocaudal (RCC) spot-compression mammogram with label.

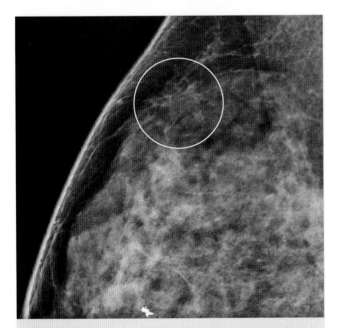

Fig. 48.11 Right mediolateral oblique (RCMLO) spot-compression mammogram with label.

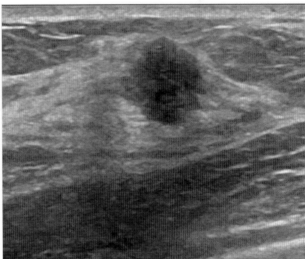

Fig. 48.12 Right breast ultrasound, transverse view.

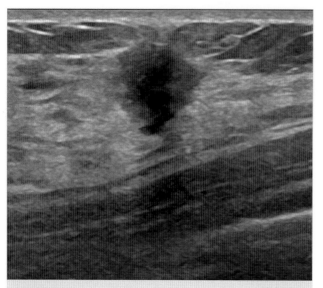

Fig. 48.13 Right breast ultrasound, longitudinal view.

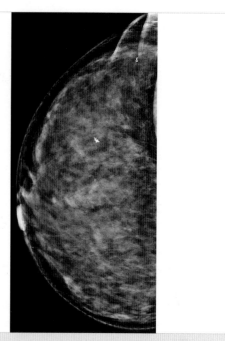

Fig. 48.14 Postbiopsy right craniocaudal (RCC) mammogram.

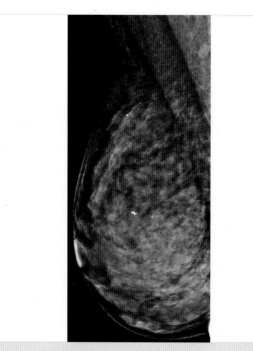

Fig. 48.15 Postbiopsy right mediolateral (RML) mammogram.

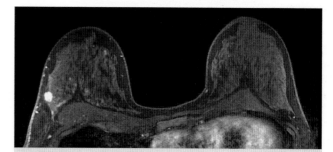

Fig. 48.16 Right breast axial dynamic contrast fat-saturation magnetic resonance (MR) image.

49 Calcifications and Possible Focal Asymmetry

Lonie R. Salkowski

49.1 Presentation and Presenting Images

(▶ Fig. 49.1, ▶ Fig. 49.2, ▶ Fig. 49.3, ▶ Fig. 49.4)

A 81-year-old female presents for screening mammography. She has a personal history of treated bilateral breast cancers. Her most recent breast cancer (ductal carcinoma in situ [DCIS]) was 2 years ago involving the left breast, and was treated with a lumpectomy and radiation therapy.

49.2 Key Images

(▶ Fig. 49.5, ▶ Fig. 49.6, ▶ Fig. 49.7)

49.2.1 Breast Tissue Density

There are scattered areas of fibroglandular density.

49.2.2 Imaging Findings

There is subareolar architectural distortion and retraction, which is marked with a skin line marker that denotes the prior lumpectomy scar. Adjacent to the region, there are grouped linear calcifications (▶ Fig. 49.6 and ▶ Fig. 49.7). In addition, there is a possible focal asymmetry at the 1 o'clock location in the middle depth (▶ Fig. 49.5 and ▶ Fig. 49.6).

49.3 BI-RADS Classification and Action

Category 0: Mammography: Incomplete. Need additional imaging evaluation and/or prior mammograms for comparison.

49.4 Diagnostic Images

(▶ Fig. 49.8, ▶ Fig. 49.9, ▶ Fig. 49.10, ▶ Fig. 49.11, ▶ Fig. 49.12, ▶ Fig. 49.13)

49.4.1 Imaging Findings

The diagnostic imaging resolved the asymmetry (▶ Fig. 49.8 and ▶ Fig. 49.9) in the upper outer quadrant which when compared to prior mammograms appeared to represent a summation artifact. The magnification images further define the 1-cm area of calcifications located at 4 o'clock in the middle depth (▶ Fig. 49.10, ▶ Fig. 49.11, and ▶ Fig. 49.12). These calcifications are fine-linear branching calcifications and are located 1.7 cm inferior to the center of the lumpectomy bed. The other scattered calcifications are stable. A biopsy of these calcifications was performed with calcifications found in several cores (▶ Fig. 49.13).

49.5 BI-RADS Classification and Action

Category 4C: High suspicion for malignancy

49.6 Differential Diagnosis

1. **Summation artifact and DCIS**: The possible asymmetry appeared stable and less worrisome on additional imaging and further comparison to prior imaging studies. The calcifications are in a linear distribution and are suspicious. The biopsy yielded high grade DCIS, which is similar to her prior cancer in this breast.
2. *Fat necrosis*: The calcifications of fat necrosis can mimic those of carcinoma. Typically fat necrosis presents as dystrophic calcifications. These calcifications are suspicious and warrant a biopsy.
3. *Secretory calcifications*: There are no other secretory calcifications in the breast. These calcifications are too fine and branching to be dismissed as benign.

49.7 Essential Facts

- The calcifications in this case would have been detected with or without the digital breast tomosynthesis (DBT) evaluation.
- The detection of microcalcifications on DBT is affected by the detector type, the image acquisition and reconstruction parameters, and blur due to source, detector, or patient motion during acquisition.
- The detection of invasive cancers is increased with the implementation of DBT. The retrospective multi-site study by Friedewald and colleagues (2014) observed a 41% relative increase in the cancer detection rate from 2.9 to 4.1 per 1000. In this same study the detection of DCIS remained unchanged at 1.4 per 1000.
- Early investigation suggests that the synthetic mammogram (reconstructed from the DBT images) performs equally well when compared to the full-field digital mammogram (FFDM). The benefit is in a reduction in patient radiation dose due to performing only DBT and not FFDM and DBT.

49.8 Management and Digital Breast Tomosynthesis Principles

- DBT when included in mammographic screening may add value by increasing the cancer detection rate for invasive cancers, optimizing patient outcomes.
- DBT is well suited to the assessment of asymmetries. Most asymmetry recalls are summation artifacts, which would be effaced by DBT.
- Due to inherent technical factors DBT is less sensitive for the detection of calcifications compared to FFDM.

49.9 Further Reading

[1] Das M, Gifford HC, O'Connor JM, Glick SJ. Evaluation of a variable dose acquisition technique for microcalcification and mass detection in digital breast tomosynthesis. Med Phys. 2009; 36(6):1976–1984
[2] Friedewald SM, Rafferty EA, Rose SL, et al. Breast cancer screening using tomosynthesis in combination with digital mammography. JAMA. 2014; 311 (24):2499–2507
[3] Zuley ML, Guo B, Catullo VJ, et al. Comparison of two-dimensional synthesized mammograms versus original digital mammograms alone and in combination with tomosynthesis images. Radiology. 2014; 271(3):664–671

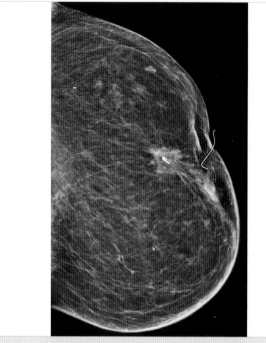

Fig. 49.1 Left craniocaudal (LCC) mammogram.

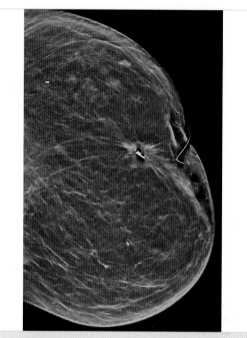

Fig. 49.2 Left craniocaudal (LCC) synthetic mammogram.

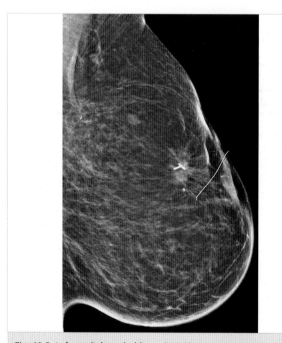

Fig. 49.3 Left mediolateral oblique (LMLO) mammogram.

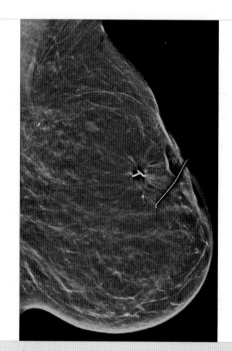

Fig. 49.4 Left mediolateral oblique (LMLO) synthetic mammogram.

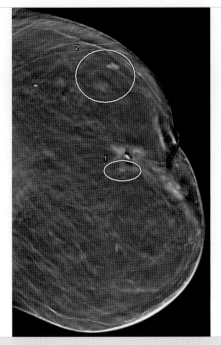

Fig. 49.5 Left craniocaudal digital breast tomosynthesis (LCC DBT), slice 22 of 54, with label.

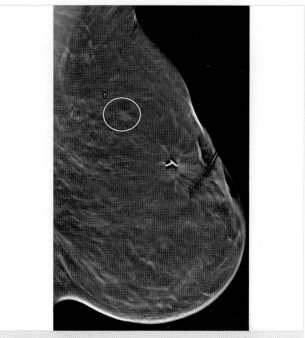

Fig. 49.6 Left mediolateral oblique digital breast tomosynthesis (LMLO DBT), slice 18 of 57, with label.

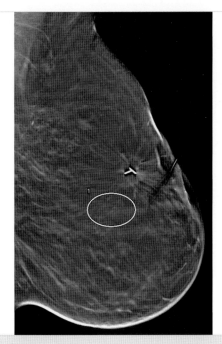

Fig. 49.7 Left mediolateral oblique digital breast tomosynthesis (LMLO DBT), slice 21 of 57, with label.

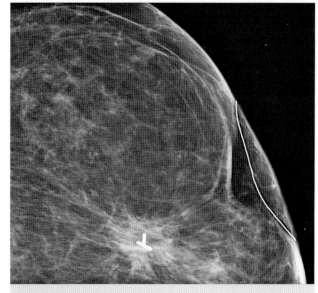

Fig. 49.8 Left craniocaudal (LCC) spot-compression mammogram.

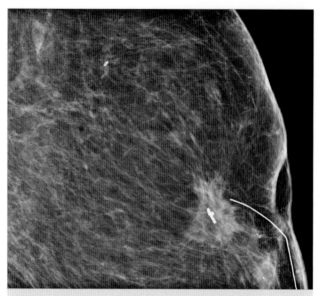

Fig. 49.9 Left mediolateral oblique (LMLO) spot-compression mammogram.

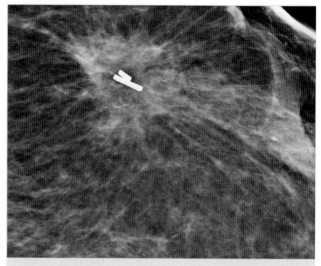

Fig. 49.10 Left craniocaudal (LCC) mammogram, spot magnification.

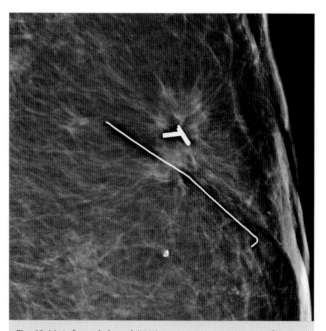

Fig. 49.11 Left mediolateral (LML) mammogram, spot magnification (skin line marker shown).

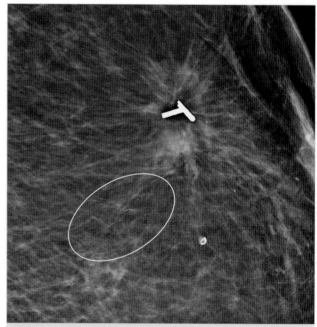

Fig. 49.12 Left mediolateral (LML) mammogram, spot magnification with label.

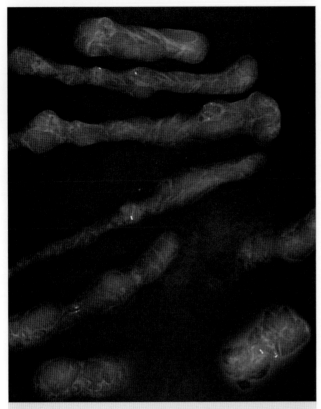

Fig. 49.13 Radiograph of stereotactic biopsy specimens.

50 Developing Asymmetry

Tanya W. Moseley

50.1 Presentation and Presenting Images

(▶ Fig. 50.1, ▶ Fig. 50.2, ▶ Fig. 50.3, ▶ Fig. 50.4, ▶ Fig. 50.5, ▶ Fig. 50.6)

A 72-year-old female presents for routine screening mammography.

50.2 Key Images

(▶ Fig. 50.7, ▶ Fig. 50.8, ▶ Fig. 50.9, ▶ Fig. 50.10, ▶ Fig. 50.11, ▶ Fig. 50.12)

50.2.1 Breast Tissue Density

There are scattered areas of fibroglandular density.

50.2.2 Imaging Findings

The imaging of the right breast is normal (*not shown*). The left breast demonstrates an increasing or developing asymmetry at the 1 to 2 o'clock position in the posterior depth, 8 cm from the nipple (▶ Fig. 50.7 and ▶ Fig. 50.8 and the mammogram comparisons ▶ Fig. 50.9 and ▶ Fig. 50.10). Tomosynthesis confirms the finding and shows it on the left craniocaudal (CC) tomosynthesis movie slice 26 of 62 (▶ Fig. 50.11) and on the left mediolateral oblique (MLO) tomosynthesis movie slice 24 of 69 (▶ Fig. 50.12).

50.3 BI-RADS Classification and Action

Category 0: Mammography: Incomplete. Need additional imaging evaluation and/or prior mammograms for comparison.

50.4 Diagnostic Images

(▶ Fig. 50.13)

50.4.1 Imaging Findings

The ultrasound demonstrated a small group of cysts (*circle*) within a focal asymmetry of fibroglandular tissue, 6.75 cm from the nipple (*dashed line* in ▶ Fig. 50.13). This correlates with the mammographic finding.

50.5 BI-RADS Classification and Action

Category 2: Benign

50.6 Differential Diagnosis

1. **Cysts**: A developing asymmetry has an increased risk for malignancy but may be a benign finding, as in this case. In this situation, this small group of cysts developed in this focal asymmetry of fibroglandular tissue causing this to appear more prominent.
2. *Hematoma*: A developing asymmetry that is due to a hematoma needs to have an appropriate clinical history of trauma or a medical procedure proceeding the development of the finding. This patient had no history of trauma.
3. *Breast cancer*: Developing asymmetries are not common, however are associated with an increased likelihood of malignancy. Imaging should be performed to ensure if the developing asymmetry is benign or malignant. In this case, the ultrasound confirms that the finding is benign.

50.7 Essential Facts

- On mammography, a developing asymmetry is defined as a focal asymmetry that has appeared or increased in size or conspicuity since a previous examination.
- Obtaining a conventional two-dimensional (2D) mammogram and tomosynthesis at the same time allowed direct comparison between the 2D mammogram and the tomosynthesis images. The comparison helped confirm that the finding is a developing asymmetry.
- Developing asymmetries are uncommon. When this finding is identified on screening and diagnostic mammography, the likelihood of malignancy is sufficiently high to justify recall and biopsy. The likelihood of malignancy is 15% at screening mammography and 25% at diagnostic mammography.
- Sonography is useful to confirm or exclude malignancy and to guide biopsy.
- Normal sonographic findings do not exclude malignancy in the case of a developing asymmetry.

50.8 Management and Digital Breast Tomosynthesis Principles

- Tomosynthesis helped to identify and confirm this finding because of its ability to remove the effects of overlapping, obscuring breast tissue.
- Tomosynthesis's ability to unmask lesions increases the number of masses seen on mammography. Not all of these unmasked lesions will be cancer. The morphology of each lesion needs to be assessed.
- With DBT, lesions are unmasked irrespective of the density of the breast tissue.
- When no suspicious findings are seen on ultrasound, tomosynthesis-directed stereotactic biopsy can be performed.

50.9 Further Reading

[1] Leung JW, Sickles EA. Developing asymmetry identified on mammography: correlation with imaging outcome and pathologic findings. AJR Am J Roentgenol. 2007; 188(3):667–675
[2] Sickles EA, D'Orsi CJ, Bassett LW, et al. ACR BI-RADS Mammography. In: ACR BI-RADS Atlas, 5th edition. Reston, VA: American College of Radiology; 2013

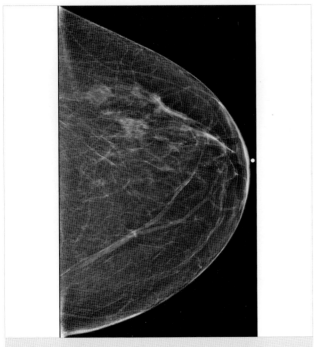

Fig. 50.1 Left craniocaudal (LCC) mammogram.

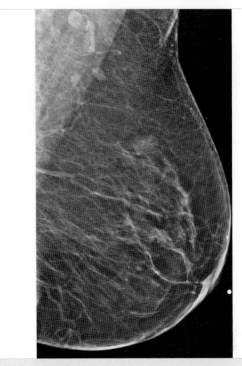

Fig. 50.2 Left mediolateral oblique (LMLO) mammogram.

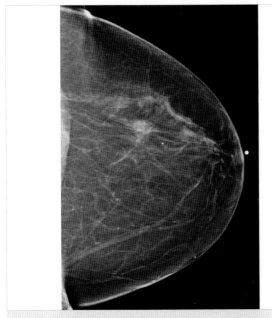

Fig. 50.3 Left craniocaudal (LCC) mammogram comparison.

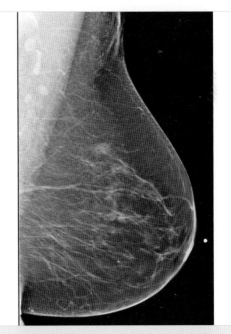

Fig. 50.4 Left mediolateral oblique (LMLO) mammogram comparison.

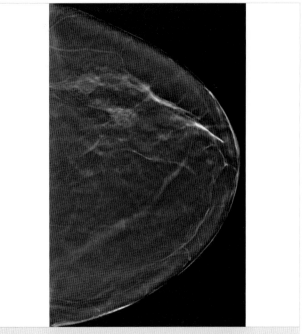

Fig. 50.5 Left craniocaudal digital breast tomosynthesis (LCC DBT), slice 26 of 62.

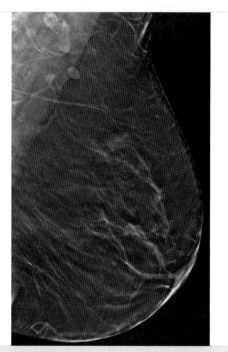

Fig. 50.6 Left mediolateral oblique digital breast tomosynthesis (LMLO DBT), slice 24 of 69.

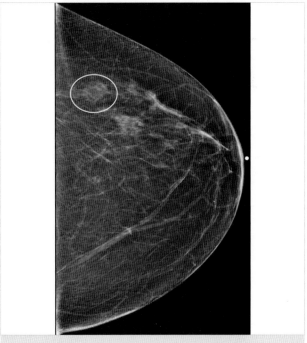

Fig. 50.7 Left craniocaudal (LCC) mammogram with label.

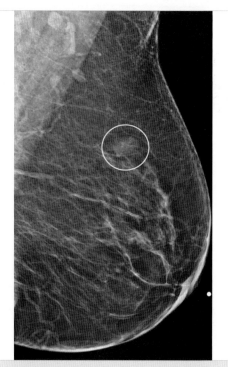

Fig. 50.8 Left mediolateral oblique (LMLO) mammogram with label.

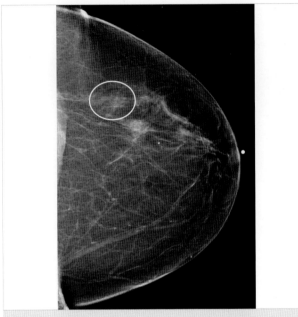

Fig. 50.9 Left craniocaudal (LCC) mammogram comparison with label.

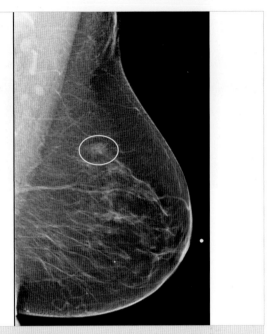

Fig. 50.10 Left mediolateral oblique (LMLO) mammogram comparison with label.

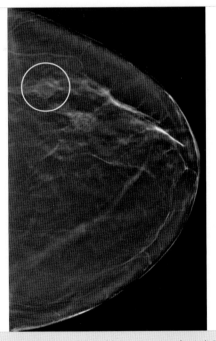

Fig. 50.11 Left craniocaudal digital breast tomosynthesis (LCC DBT), slice 26 of 62 with label.

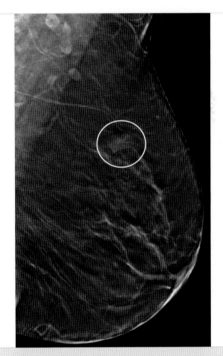

Fig. 50.12 Left mediolateral oblique digital breast tomosynthesis (LMLO DBT), slice 24 of 69 with label.

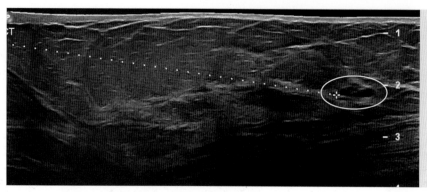

Fig. 50.13 Landscape radial ultrasound at 1 o'clock location.

51 Obscured Mass and Architectural Distortion Findings

Lonie R. Salkowski

51.1 Presentation and Presenting Images

(► Fig. 51.1, ► Fig. 51.2, ► Fig. 51.3, ► Fig. 51.4)

A 74-year-old female presents for screening mammography.

51.2 Key Images

(► Fig. 51.5, ► Fig. 51.6, ► Fig. 51.7, ► Fig. 51.8)

51.2.1 Breast Tissue Density

There are scattered areas of fibroglandular density.

51.2.2 Imaging Findings

There are two lesions identified on the screening mammography examination. At the 11 o'clock location in the posterior depth, there appears to be a mass with a partially convex margin (► Fig. 51.5 and ► Fig. 51.6). Additionally, lateral in the right breast, there is architectural distortion in the middle depth only seen on the craniocaudal (CC) view (► Fig. 51.1). This is better appreciated on the CC synthetic mammogram (► Fig. 51.8) and tomosynthesis images (► Fig. 51.7).

51.3 BI-RADS Classification and Action

Category 0: Mammography: Incomplete. Need additional imaging evaluation and/or prior mammograms for comparison.

51.4 Diagnostic Images

(► Fig. 51.9, ► Fig. 51.10, ► Fig. 51.11, ► Fig. 51.12, ► Fig. 51.13, ► Fig. 51.14, ► Fig. 51.15, ► Fig. 51.16, ► Fig. 51.17)

51.4.1 Imaging Findings

The additional diagnostic imaging confirms the 1.8 × 1.4 cm irregular mass with indistinct calcifications at the 10 o'clock location in the posterior depth (► Fig. 51.9 and ► Fig. 51.10). Ultrasound reveals a corresponding 1.4 × 1.3 × 1.0 cm irregular mass with indistinct and angular margins and posterior acoustic shadowing at the 10 o'clock location, 8 cm from the nipple (► Fig. 51.12). With further review of the initial digital breast tomosynthesis (DBT) images (► Fig. 51.11), the architectural distortion appears to have a correlate on the mediolateral

oblique (MLO) view, at the 9 o'clock location. Ultrasound of this region reveals a 1.2 × 0.8 × 0.7 cm irregular mass with indistinct margins, 5 cm from the nipple (► Fig. 51.13). Similar to the 10 o'clock lesion, this mass also has posterior acoustic shadowing. These lesions occupy the same quadrant of the breast with the 9 o'clock mass anterior and medial to the 10 o'clock mass and separated by 4 cm (► Fig. 51.14). Both lesions were biopsied under ultrasound guidance. The 10 o'clock lesion was marked with a coil biopsy clip and the 9 o'clock lesion was marked with a ribbon clip (► Fig. 51.15 and ► Fig. 51.16). The lesions and their respective biopsy clips can be seen in this lumpectomy specimen (► Fig. 51.17).

51.5 BI-RADS Classification and Action

Category 5: Highly suggestive of malignancy

51.6 Differential Diagnosis

1. *Invasive lobular carcinoma [ILC]*: Both of these lesions were found to be grade 1 ILC. It is important to be aware of the possibility of additional lesions in the breast when an initial lesion is detected.
2. *Invasive ductal carcinoma [IDC]*: The presentation and imaging characteristics of these lesions would be also be consistent with IDC.
3. *Fibrosis*: Fibrosis can mimic carcinoma. To be concordant on image-guided biopsy, the size of the lesion on imaging should closely match the size on histopathology. Both of these lesions are highly suspicious. If there is uncertainty in the radiology–pathology concordance, an excision would be warranted.

51.7 Essential Facts

- The nature of ILC, in its tendency to produce little desmoplastic reaction and its single file growth pattern within the breast tissue, can make it difficult to detect both clinically and by imaging.
- ILC has a variable appearance; it may present as a focal asymmetry, an architectural distortion, a mass, or with no mammographic findings (occult).
- The unmasking benefit of DBT may prove beneficial to the detection of the subtle lesions of ILC. Early studies suggest that there is a higher proportion of ILC detected in the studies the include DBT compared to those that use full-field digital mammography (FFDM) alone.

51.8 Management and Digital Breast Tomosynthesis Principles

- 10 to 30% of breast cancers are missed on conventional mammography.
- The majority of FFDM occult lesions that were identified on DBT were in dense breasts.
- It is important not to rush mammographic interpretation and settle for the first lesion that is detected ("satisfaction of search").

- DBT is very good at detecting architectural distortion. However, not all architectural distortion is cancer. Radial scars and atypical ductal hyperplasia (ADH) are among the frequent sources of false-positive biopsies on DBT.

51.9 Further Reading

[1] Majid AS, de Paredes ES, Doherty RD, Sharma NR, Salvador X. Missed breast carcinoma: pitfalls and pearls. Radiographics. 2003; 23(4):881–895
[2] Ray KM, Turner E, Sickles EA, Joe BN. Suspicious Findings at Digital Breast Tomosynthesis Occult to Conventional Digital Mammography: Imaging Features and Pathology Findings. Breast J. 2015; 21(5):538–542

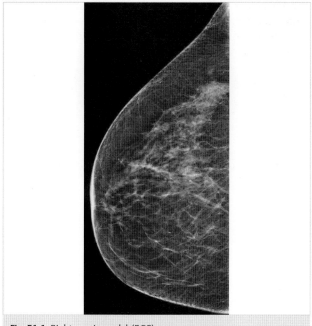

Fig. 51.1 Right craniocaudal (RCC) mammogram.

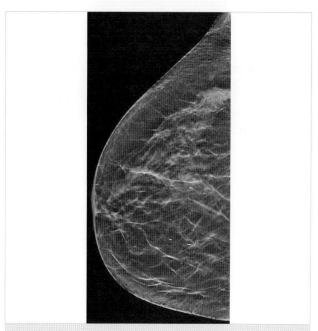

Fig. 51.2 Right craniocaudal (RCC) synthetic mammogram.

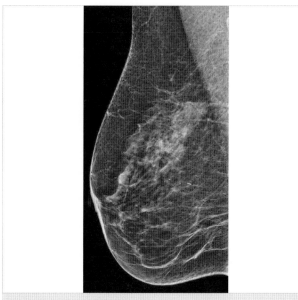

Fig. 51.3 Right mediolateral oblique (RMLO) mammogram.

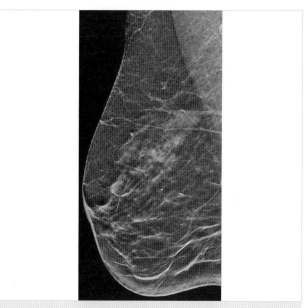

Fig. 51.4 Right mediolateral oblique (RMLO) synthetic mammogram.

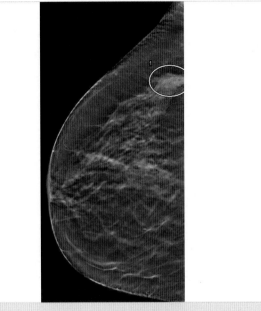

Fig. 51.5 Right craniocaudal digital breast tomosynthesis (RCC DBT), slice 21 of 51, with label.

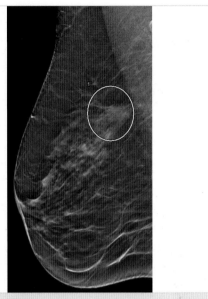

Fig. 51.6 Right mediolateral oblique digital breast tomosynthesis (RMLO DBT), slice 20 of 53, with label.

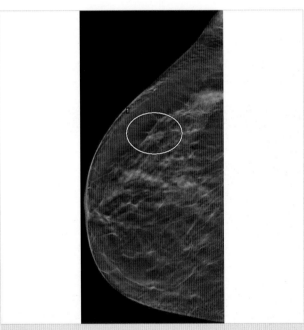

Fig. 51.7 Right craniocaudal digital breast tomosynthesis (RCC DBT), slice 14 of 51, with label.

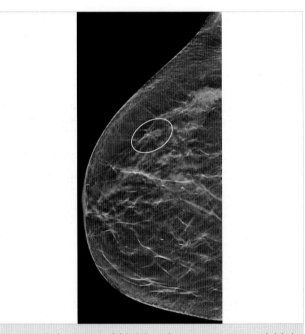

Fig. 51.8 Right craniocaudal (RCC) synthetic mammogram with label.

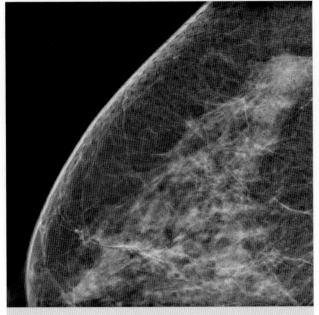

Fig. 51.9 Right craniocaudal (RCC) spot-compression mammogram.

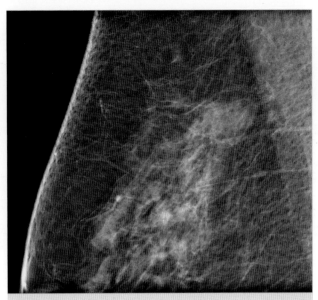

Fig. 51.10 Right mediolateral oblique (RMLO) spot-compression mammogram.

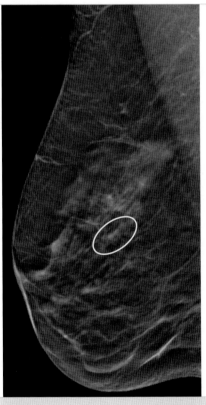

Fig. 51.11 Right mediolateral oblique digital breast tomosynthesis (RMLO DBT), slice 13 of 53 with label.

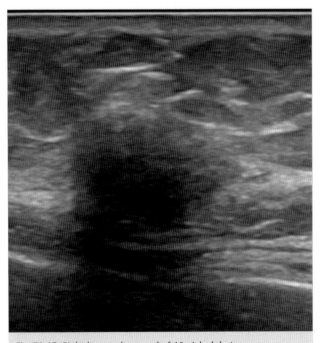

Fig. 51.12 Right breast ultrasound of 10 o'clock lesion.

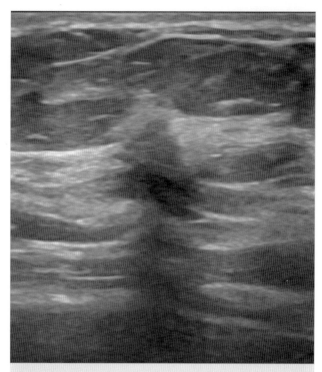

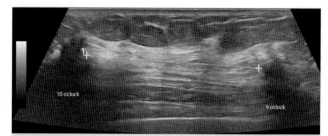

Fig. 51.14 Right breast ultrasound demonstrates 4-cm linear distance between lesions.

Fig. 51.13 Right breast ultrasound of 9 o'clock lesion.

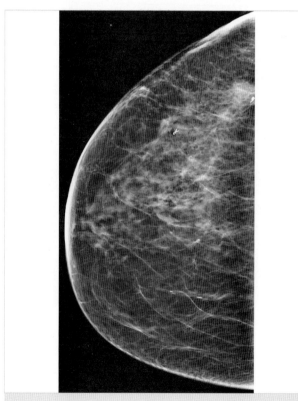

Fig. 51.15 Postbiopsy right craniocaudal (RCC) mammogram.

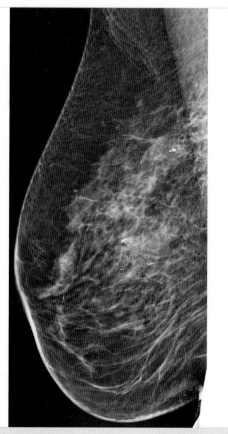

Fig. 51.16 Postbiopsy right mediolateral (RML) mammogram.

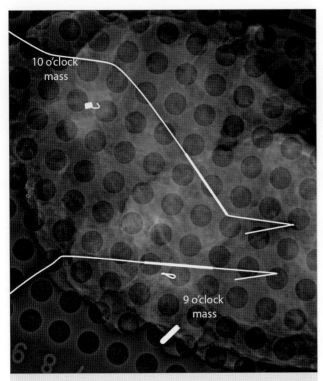

Fig. 51.17 Radiograph of the surgical specimen.

52 Mass After Reduction Mammoplasty

Lonie R. Salkowski

52.1 Presentation and Presenting Images

(► Fig. 52.1, ► Fig. 52.2, ► Fig. 52.3, ► Fig. 52.4)

A 51-year-old female with history of right breast cancer treated with a lumpectomy and more recently a bilateral reduction mammoplasty presents for screening mammography.

52.2 Key Images

(► Fig. 52.5, ► Fig. 52.6, ► Fig. 52.7, ► Fig. 52.8)

52.2.1 Breast Tissue Density

There are scattered areas of fibroglandular density.

52.2.2 Imaging Findings

There are postsurgical changes in the right breast consistent with the patient's lumpectomy, the location of which is marked by the surgical clips at the 9 o'clock location in the posterior depth (► Fig. 52.1 and ► Fig. 52.3). There are bilateral changes due to the bilateral reduction surgery. In the left breast, there is a new mass located at the 7 o'clock location in the middle depth (► Fig. 52.5 and ► Fig. 52.6). This appears to be associated with the skin and is well demonstrated on the digital breast tomosynthesis (DBT) images. Note that it is located on slice 1 of the craniocaudal (CC) tomosynthesis image (► Fig. 52.7 and ► Fig. 52.8). No mention of a skin lesion was noted in the technologist's intake sheet and no skin marker was placed on a skin lesion.

52.3 BI-RADS Classification and Action

Category 0: Mammography: Incomplete. Need additional imaging evaluation and/or prior mammograms for comparison.

52.4 Diagnostic Images

(► Fig. 52.9, ► Fig. 52.10, ► Fig. 52.11)

52.4.1 Imaging Findings

The diagnostic images were taken after a skin marker was placed on the skin lesion (*ring* in ► Fig. 52.9, ► Fig. 52.10, and ► Fig. 52.11). The prior mass seen on the screening mammography and DBT examinations is related to a skin lesion. The patient had a regular follow-up appointment at the breast clinic on the same date as the diagnostic imaging. The clinical notes indicate that this skin lesion is located on the medial aspect of the reduction scar and was likely a "stitch cyst."

52.5 BI-RADS Classification and Action

Category 2: Benign

52.6 Differential Diagnosis

1. **Suture granuloma**: Suture granulomas are benign granulomatous proliferations in response to a retained foreign body (suture material). They are less common with absorbable sutures but may still occur. They can occur anywhere along the suture line.
2. *Epidermal inclusion cyst*: These benign skin lesions can occur anywhere on the hair-bearing areas of the body. They are filled with laminated keratin, and can occur at the site of an obstructed hair follicle or pore and secondary to traumatic implantation of torn epidermis. This would be a reasonable diagnosis for this imaging finding.
3. *Carcinoma*: This is less likely. Carcinoma can occur at suture lines but this tends to be in advanced cancers without clear surgical margins or as a late recurrence of cancer.

52.7 Essential Facts

- Many skin lesions can simulate masses on mammography. Having knowledge and awareness of these skin based lesions is especially helpful to prevent unnecessary patient recalls.
- Many skin lesions have characteristic mammographic and sonographic appearances.
- The most common skin-based lesions are epidermal inclusion cysts and/or sebaceous cysts, moles and keratosis, and surgical scars. Patients with neurofibromatosis can also display skin lesions; however, this is less common.
- It is extremely helpful to have dominant skin lesions marked with skin markers prior to mammographic imaging. Some patients have a large number of skin lesions, and therefore marking all of them can be disruptive to image interpretation.
- When in question, it may require recalling a patient to determine if a lesion close to the skin surface on the mammogram is a skin lesion or a true parenchymal lesion.

52.8 Management and Digital Breast Tomosynthesis Principles

- Tomosynthesis can be used to distinguish lesions that are located in the skin.
- When a "lesion" is seen on the first or last image of a tomosynthesis movie, it is highly likely that this is a skin-based lesion. Making this observation can prevent recalling a patient for additional imaging. In this case, the skin lesion was seen on slice 1 of the CC tomosynthesis movie.

52.9 Further Reading

[1] Kim HS, Cha ES, Kim HH, Yoo JY. Spectrum of sonographic findings in superficial breast masses. J Ultrasound Med. 2005; 24(5):663–680
[2] Rettenbacher T, Macheiner P, Hollerweger A, Gritzmann N, Weismann C, Todoroff B. Suture granulomas: sonography enables a correct preoperative diagnosis. Ultrasound Med Biol. 2001; 27(3):343–350

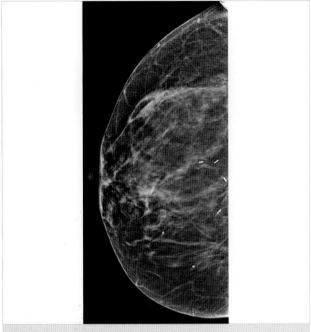

Fig. 52.1 Right craniocaudal (RCC) mammogram.

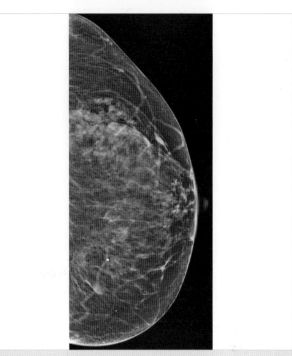

Fig. 52.2 Left craniocaudal (LCC) mammogram.

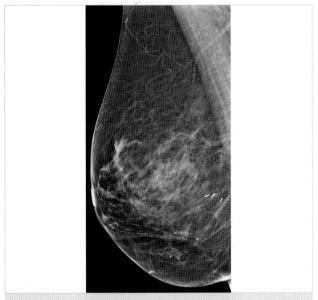

Fig. 52.3 Right mediolateral oblique (RMLO) mammogram.

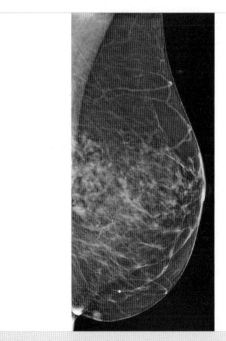

Fig. 52.4 Left mediolateral oblique (LMLO) mammogram.

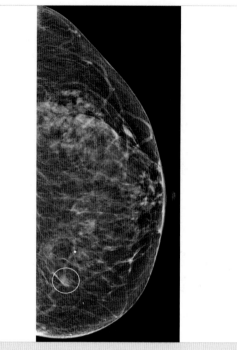

Fig. 52.5 Left craniocaudal (LCC) mammogram with label.

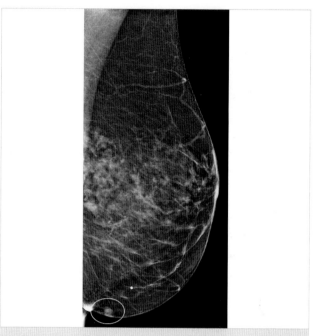

Fig. 52.6 Left mediolateral oblique (LMLO) mammogram with label.

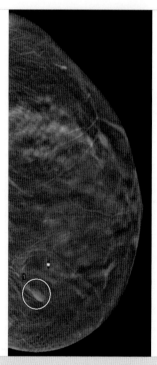

Fig. 52.7 Left craniocaudal digital breast tomosynthesis (LCC DBT), slice 1 of 62 with label.

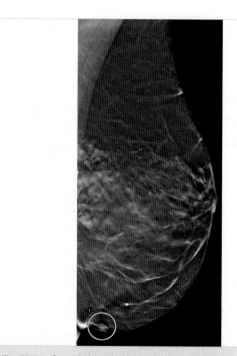

Fig. 52.8 Left mediolateral oblique digital breast tomosynthesis (LMLO DBT), slice 7 of 61 with label.

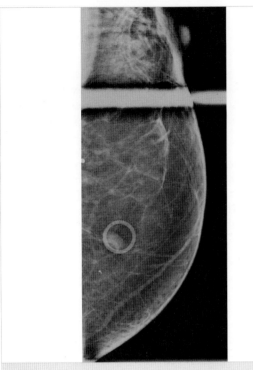

Fig. 52.9 Left craniocaudal (LCC) spot-compression mammogram.

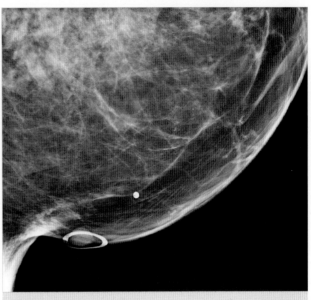

Fig. 52.10 Left mediolateral oblique (LMLO) spot-compression mammogram.

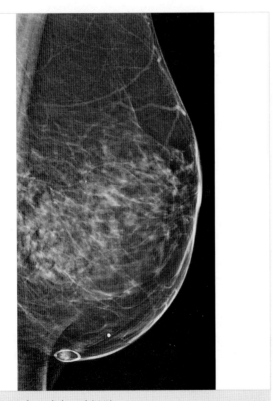

Fig. 52.11 Left mediolateral (LML) mammogram.

53 Architectural Distortion

Lonie R. Salkowski

53.1 Presentation and Presenting Images

(▶ Fig. 53.1, ▶ Fig. 53.2, ▶ Fig. 53.3, ▶ Fig. 53.4)

A 56-year-old female presents for screening mammography.

53.2 Key Images

(▶ Fig. 53.5, ▶ Fig. 53.6)

53.2.1 Breast Tissue Density

The breasts are heterogeneously dense, which may obscure small masses.

53.2.2 Imaging Findings

In the upper outer quadrant of the right breast at the 10 o'clock location in the posterior depth, there is a subtle architectural distortion. It is best seen on the tomosynthesis views (▶ Fig. 53.5 and ▶ Fig. 53.6). Once noted on the tomosynthesis views, the area can be faintly perceived on the conventional digital mammogram.

53.3 BI-RADS Classification and Action

Category 0: Mammography: Incomplete. Need additional imaging evaluation and/or prior mammograms for comparison.

53.4 Diagnostic Images

(▶ Fig. 53.7,▶ Fig. 53.8, ▶ Fig. 53.9, ▶ Fig. 53.10, ▶ Fig. 53.11, ▶ Fig. 53.12, ▶ Fig. 53.13, ▶ Fig. 53.14, ▶ Fig. 53.15, ▶ Fig. 53.16)

53.4.1 Imaging Findings

The diagnostic imaging does not offer much additional information about this area of architectural distortion (▶ Fig. 53.7, ▶ Fig. 53.8, and ▶ Fig. 53.9). The lateral view best identifies this area and suggests that it is about 1 cm in size (▶ Fig. 53.10). The anterior margin of the lesion creates an unnatural angle which makes it perceptible. A targeted ultrasound was performed because the findings seen on tomosynthesis suggested a mass associated with the architectural distortion and the overlying dense breast tissue obscured this finding on the conventional imaging. The ultrasound (▶ Fig. 53.11 and ▶ Fig. 53.12) reveals an irregular 1.5-cm mass with indistinct and angular margins with posterior acoustic shadowing at the 10 o'clock location, 5 cm from the nipple. Normal lymph nodes were seen in the ipsilateral axilla (*not shown*). This breast lesion was biopsied with ultrasound guidance and the postbiopsy mammogram demonstrates the ribbon clip (▶ Fig. 53.13 and ▶ Fig. 53.14) at the site of the initially questioned architectural distortion on the screening examination. A follow-up magnetic resonance (MR) image demonstrates that this is a singular lesion located in the breast with minimal background enhancement (▶ Fig. 53.15). The signal void from the biopsy clip can be seen in the mass on the sagittal MR image (▶ Fig. 53.16).

53.5 BI-RADS Classification and Action

Category 4C: High suspicion for malignancy

53.6 Differential Diagnosis

1. ***Invasive lobular carcinoma [ILC]***: This very subtle lesion was difficult to detect even on DBT. The biopsy revealed a grade 2 ILC. The MR image provides reassurance that there is only one lesion.
2. *Invasive ductal carcinoma [IDC]*: The imaging characteristics are not specific for ILC or IDC. They both would represent concordant results.
3. *Fibroadenoma*: Although this lesion is solid. The other imaging criteria including shape and margin characteristics on imaging should suggest a high suspicion of malignancy. A biopsy result of fibroadenoma would be discordant.

53.7 Essential Facts

- Architectural distortion has a positive predictive value (PPV) of 74.5% on mammography. This study by Bahl and colleagues (2015) did not include digital breast tomosynthesis (DBT). They recognize that DBT may further improve the detection of architectural distortion.
- Early studies have suggested that a diagnostic mammogram could be omitted for DBT findings other than those with calcifications. Brandt and colleagues (2013) found that in 93 to 99% of these cases the two-view screening DBT was adequate for mammographic evaluation.
- Two additional similar studies by Poplack and Hakim found that DBT was equivalent or better to a conventional diagnostic mammogram in 89% and 81% of these cases, respectively.
- In cases with calcifications, DBT has inferior image quality compared to a conventional diagnostic mammogram.

53.8 Management and Digital Breast Tomosynthesis Principles

- Architectural distortion seen on a diagnostic mammogram was more likely to represent a malignancy than that detected on a screening mammogram. It is recognized that some screening findings will eventually be assessed to be benign on diagnostic work-up.
- The implementation of DBT is evolving. Practices may differ from suggested guidelines. More research and experience is needed to determine the optimal imaging protocol.

53.9 Further Reading

[1] Bahl M, Baker JA, Kinsey EN, Ghate SV. Architectural Distortion on Mammography: Correlation With Pathologic Outcomes and Predictors of Malignancy. AJR Am J Roentgenol. 2015; 205(6):1339–1345

[2] Brandt KR, Craig DA, Hoskins TL, et al. Can digital breast tomosynthesis replace conventional diagnostic mammography views for screening recalls without calcifications? A comparison study in a simulated clinical setting. AJR Am J Roentgenol. 2013; 200(2):291–298

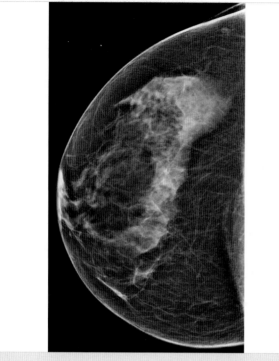

Fig. 53.1 Right craniocaudal (RCC) mammogram.

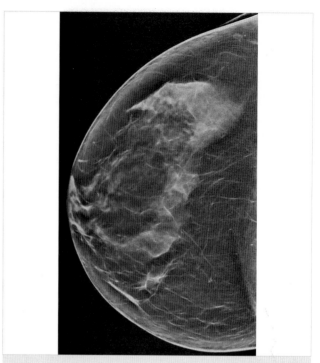

Fig. 53.2 Right craniocaudal (RCC) synthetic mammogram.

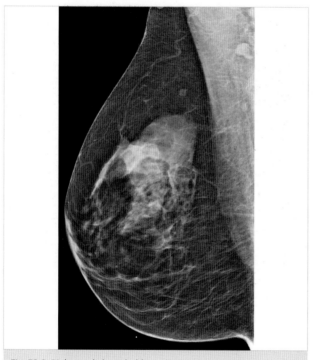

Fig. 53.3 Right mediolateral oblique (RMLO) mammogram.

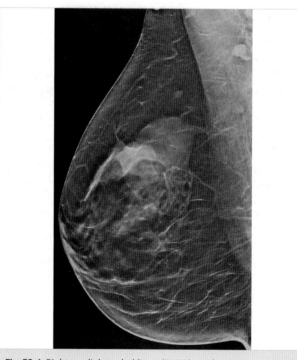

Fig. 53.4 Right mediolateral oblique (RMLO) synthetic mammogram.

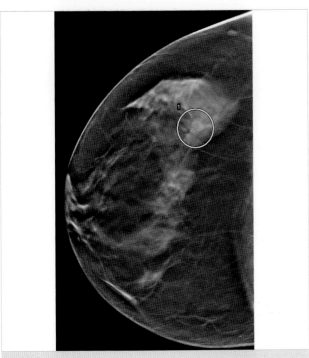

Fig. 53.5 Right craniocaudal digital breast tomosynthesis (RCC DBT), slice 26 of 74, with label.

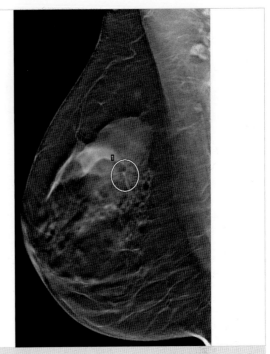

Fig. 53.6 Right mediolateral oblique digital breast tomosynthesis (RMLO DBT), slice 23 of 72, with label.

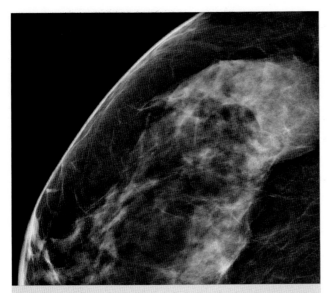

Fig. 53.7 Right craniocaudal (RCC) spot-compression mammogram.

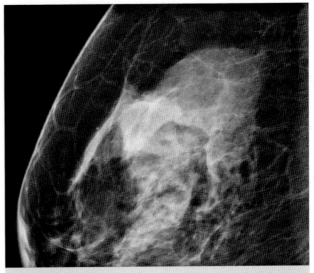

Fig. 53.8 Right mediolateral oblique (RMLO) spot-compression mammogram.

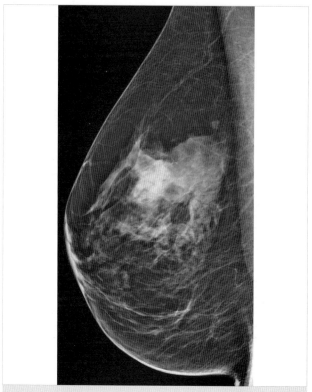

Fig. 53.9 Right mediolateral (RML) mammogram.

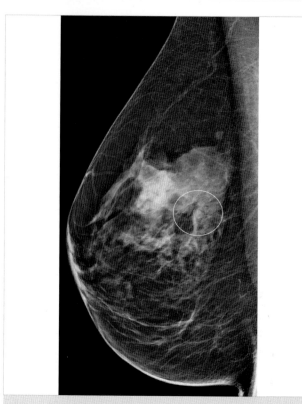

Fig. 53.10 Right mediolateral (RML) mammogram with label.

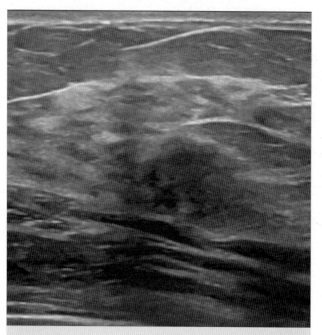

Fig. 53.11 Right breast ultrasound, transverse view.

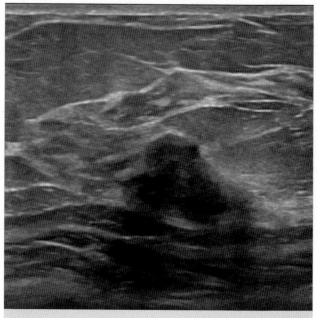

Fig. 53.12 Right breast ultrasound, longitudinal view.

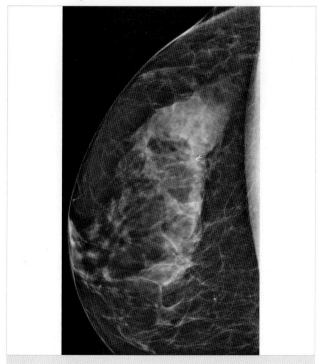

Fig. 53.13 Postbiopsy right craniocaudal (RCC) view.

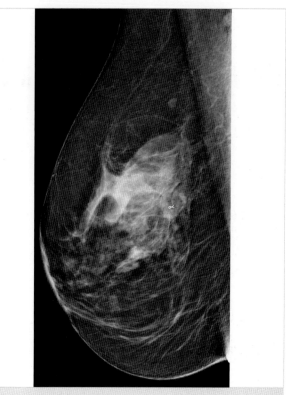

Fig. 53.14 Postbiopsy right mediolateral (RML) view.

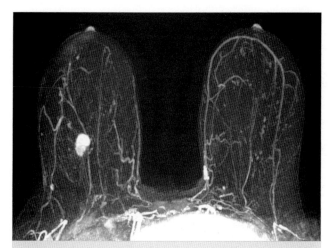

Fig. 53.15 Breast magnetic resonance (MR) maximum-intensity projection (MIP) image.

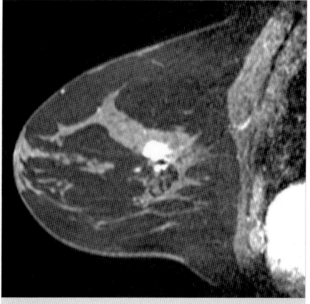

Fig. 53.16 Right breast reconstructed sagittal magnetic resonance (M) image.

54 Obscured Mass

Tanya W. Moseley

54.1 Presentation and Presenting Images

(▶ Fig. 54.1, ▶ Fig. 54.2, ▶ Fig. 54.3, ▶ Fig. 54.4)

A 47-year-old female with a history of an excisional biopsy of a benign left axillary lymph node presents for routine screening mammography.

54.2 Key Images

(▶ Fig. 54.5, ▶ Fig. 54.6, ▶ Fig. 54.7, ▶ Fig. 54.8)

54.2.1 Breast Tissue Density

The breasts are heterogeneously dense, which may obscure small masses.

54.2.2 Imaging Findings

The imaging of the right breast is normal (*not shown*). The left breast demonstrates an obscured mass (*circle* in ▶ Fig. 54.5 and ▶ Fig. 54.6) measuring 7 mm at the 3 o'clock location in the middle depth, 7 cm from the nipple. The left breast tomosynthesis images (▶ Fig. 54.7 and ▶ Fig. 54.8) confirm the findings seen on mammography and that the mass is of low density. Sonography is required to definitively characterize masses. Benign and malignant lesions may present as well-circumscribed masses on tomosynthesis.

54.3 BI-RADS Classification and Action

Category 0: Mammography: Incomplete. Need additional imaging evaluation and/or prior mammograms for comparison.

54.4 Diagnostic Images

(▶ Fig. 54.9)

54.4.1 Imaging Findings

Sonography shows an anechoic well-circumscribed mass with posterior acoustic enhancement at the 3 o'clock location that corresponds directly with the mass seen on the mammogram (▶ Fig. 54.9). Note on the ultrasound that the cyst is located within dense fibroglandular tissue, which can limit the visualization on conventional mammography.

54.5 BI-RADS Classification and Action

Category 2: Benign

54.6 Differential Diagnosis

1. **Cyst**: Cystic and solid masses may have the same appearance on mammography. Sonography can reliably differentiate between cystic and solid masses. This mass is a circumscribed anechoic mass with posterior acoustic enhancement and is consistent with a simple cyst.
2. *Cancer*: High-grade carcinomas and medullary carcinomas can mimic complicated cysts. These carcinomas may be markedly hypoechoic (a nearly anechoic appearance) and rounded.
3. *Fibroadenoma*: Fibroadenomas are oval or gently lobulated masses with parallel orientation and circumscribed margins. The internal echogenicity may range from isoechoic to hypoechoic.

54.7 Essential Facts

- Tomosynthesis can confirm findings seen on conventional mammography and better define the mass and its margins. Tomosynthesis shows that the mass is lower density and well circumscribed.
- The layers of breast tissue are shown separately on tomosynthesis and indeterminate or suspicious lesions seen on conventional mammography may be shown to have a benign appearance on tomosynthesis.
- Radiologists should be careful not to dismiss all benign-appearing tomosynthesis-detected masses as benign.
- If no correlate is seen on sonography, tomosynthesis-directed stereotactic biopsy may be performed.

54.8 Management and Digital Breast Tomosynthesis Principles

- Rafferty and colleagues (2013) found that care must be taken to avoid misclassification of malignancies. It was evident in this study that circumscribed lobular cancers were dismissed as benign.
- Additional studies evaluating circumscribed cancers need to be performed to identify commonalities among these lesions.
- In a letter to the radiology editor (2013), Dr. Kopans described cancers that will be missed with both conventional mammography and tomosynthesis. These cancers arise in fibroglandular tissue, do not have a margin highlighted in fat, do not distort the architecture, and do not produce calcifications.
- Although there are some malignancies that are occult and undetected on all imaging studies, additional studies to evaluate tomosynthesis and missed cancers need to be performed to reduce the numbers of missed and misclassified malignancies.

54.9 Further Reading

[1] Kopans DB. Digital breast tomosynthesis: a better mammogram. Radiology. 2013; 267(3):968–969
[2] Rafferty EA, Park JM, Philpotts LE, et al. Assessing radiologist performance using combined digital mammography and breast tomosynthesis compared with digital mammography alone: results of a multicenter, multireader trial. Radiology. 2013; 266(1):104–113

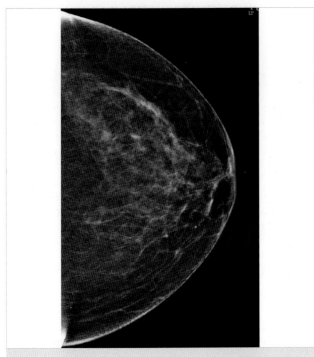

Fig. 54.1 Left craniocaudal (LCC) mammogram.

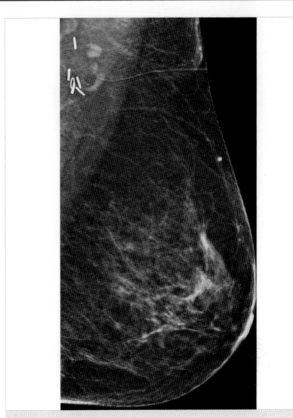

Fig. 54.2 Left mediolateral oblique (LMLO) mammogram.

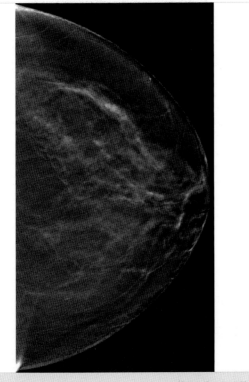

Fig. 54.3 Left craniocaudal digital breast tomosynthesis (LCC DBT), slice 26 of 81.

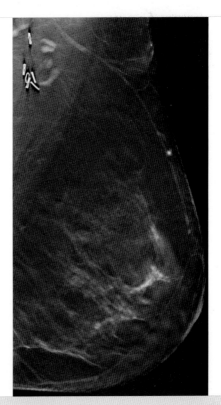

Fig. 54.4 Left mediolateral oblique digital breast tomosynthesis (LMLO DBT), slice 32 of 81.

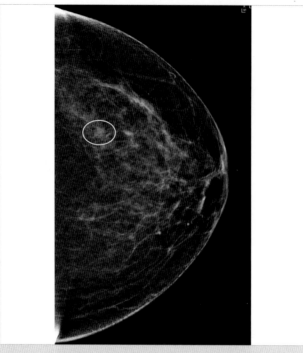

Fig. 54.5 Left craniocaudal (LCC) mammogram with label.

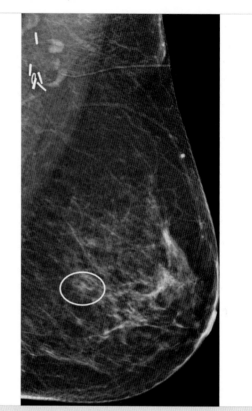

Fig. 54.6 Left mediolateral oblique (LMLO) mammogram with label.

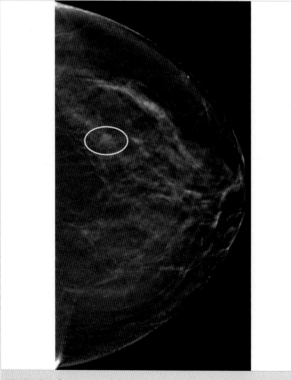

Fig. 54.7 Left craniocaudal digital breast tomosynthesis (LCC DBT), slice 26 of 81 with label.

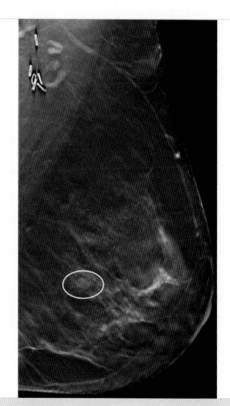

Fig. 54.8 Left mediolateral oblique digital breast tomosynthesis (LMLO DBT), slice 32 of 81 with label.

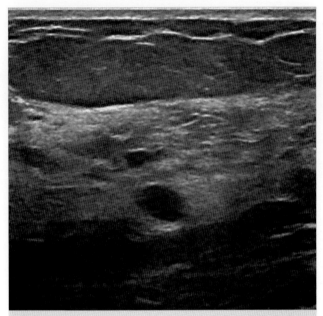

Fig. 54.9 Left breast ultrasound, transverse view of the 3 o'clock mass.

55 Architectural Distortion

Lonie R. Salkowski

55.1 Presentation and Presenting Images

(▶ Fig. 55.1, ▶ Fig. 55.2)

A 71-year-old female presents for screening mammography.

55.2 Key Images

(▶ Fig. 55.3, ▶ Fig. 55.4, ▶ Fig. 55.5, ▶ Fig. 55.6)

55.2.1 Breast Tissue Density

The breasts are heterogeneously dense, which may obscure small masses.

55.2.2 Imaging Findings

In the left breast at the 6 o'clock location in the anterior depth within the dense fibroglandular tissue, there is an area of architectural distortion. It is best seen on the tomosynthesis images (▶ Fig. 55.5 and ▶ Fig. 55.6), but can also be seen on the conventional digital mammograms (▶ Fig. 55.3 and ▶ Fig. 55.4).

55.3 BI-RADS Classification and Action

Category 0: Mammography: Incomplete. Need additional imaging evaluation and/or prior mammograms for comparison.

55.4 Diagnostic Images

(▶ Fig. 55.7, ▶ Fig. 55.8, ▶ Fig. 55.9, ▶ Fig. 55.10, ▶ Fig. 55.11, ▶ Fig. 55.12, ▶ Fig. 55.13, ▶ Fig. 55.14, ▶ Fig. 55.15)

55.4.1 Imaging Findings

The diagnostic imaging nearly suggests that this area of architectural distortion is an artifact (▶ Fig. 55.7 and ▶ Fig. 55.8). However, on the CC spot-compression image (▶ Fig. 55.7 and ▶ Fig. 55.10), there appears to be a persistent finding. A targeted ultrasound was performed revealing a 7 × 7 × 10 mm irregular hypoechoic mass with indistinct margins and posterior acoustic shadowing at the 6 o'clock location, 1 cm from the nipple (▶ Fig. 55.11 and ▶ Fig. 55.12). This mass was biopsied

and the ribbon biopsy clip is placed, as expected, in the location of the architectural distortion that was seen on the tomosynthesis images (▶ Fig. 55.13 and ▶ Fig. 55.14). This mass was eventually excised. The surgical specimen suggests a subtle mass with architectural distortion with the ribbon clip at the center (▶ Fig. 55.15).

55.5 BI-RADS Classification and Action

Category 4C: High suspicion for malignancy

55.6 Differential Diagnosis

1. ***Invasive lobular carcinoma (ILC)***: On image-guided biopsy and excision, this lesion was found to be a grade 1 ILC. This is a concordant diagnosis.
2. *Invasive ductal carcinoma (IDC)*: There is significant overlap in the appearance of IDC and ILC on imaging. IDC would be a concordant diagnosis.
3. *Radial scar*: Radial scars are great mimickers of cancer. This would be concordant if the histopathologic size is similar to the imaging size. There is ongoing controversy about which radial scars need to be excised.

55.7 Essential Facts

- Architectural distortion on mammography can be due to a malignant or a benign lesion.
- Mammography alone often cannot distinguish between the etiology of architectural distortion without additional signs or information.
- Malignancies that present as architectural distortion are typically IDC or ILC; however, ductal carcinoma in situ (DCIS) is also known to present as architectural distortion, but not as frequently.
- Common benign causes of architectural distortion are radial scars, complex sclerosing lesions, and surgical scars (from excisions, lumpectomies, breast reductions, etc.).
- Architectural distortion on screening mammography is less likely to represent malignancy compared to architectural distortion on diagnostic mammography.
- Architectural distortion without a sonographic correlate is less likely to represent a malignancy.

55.8 Management and Digital Breast Tomosynthesis Principles

- The addition of digital breast tomosynthesis (DBT) to full-field digital mammography (FFDM) improves the diagnostic performance of radiologists regardless of their level of experience.
- The addition of DBT to FFDM increases the rate of cancer detection, reducing false-positives.
- The unmasking effects of DBT reduces the underlying anatomical noise in the breast tissue. This is especially noted in dense breast tissue. In this case, the anatomical noise of the breast tissue easily obscures findings. The DBT images helped the reader to determine that the architectural distortion suggested on the craniocaudal (CC) FFDM was likely real and needed further evaluation with a diagnostic mammogram.

55.9 Further Reading

[1] Alakhras MM, Brennan PC, Rickard M, Bourne R, Mello-Thoms C. Effect of radiologists' experience on breast cancer detection and localization using digital breast tomosynthesis. Eur Radiol. 2015; 25(2):402–409

[2] Bahl M, Baker JA, Kinsey EN, Ghate SV. Architectural Distortion on Mammography: Correlation With Pathologic Outcomes and Predictors of Malignancy. AJR Am J Roentgenol. 2015; 205(6):1339–1345

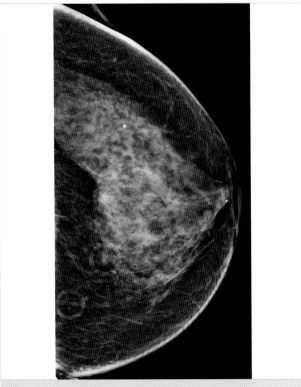

Fig. 55.1 Left craniocaudal (LCC) mammogram.

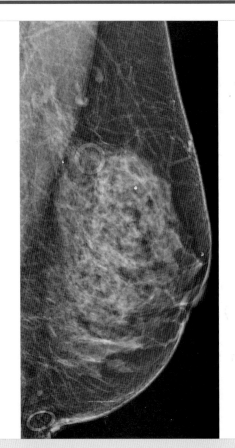

Fig. 55.2 Left mediolateral oblique (LMLO) mammogram.

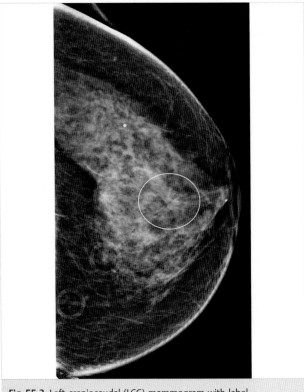

Fig. 55.3 Left craniocaudal (LCC) mammogram with label.

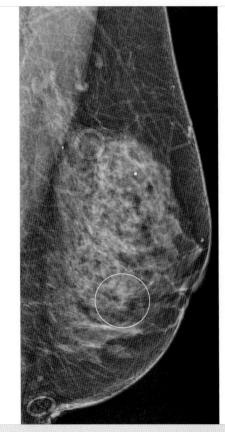

Fig. 55.4 Left mediolateral oblique (LMLO) mammogram with label.

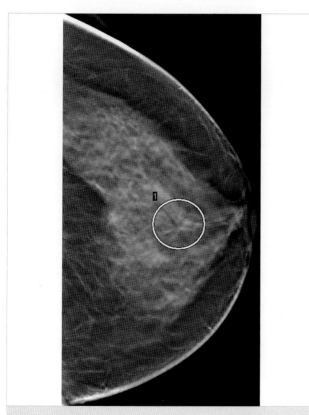

Fig. 55.5 Left craniocaudal digital breast tomosynthesis (LCC DBT), slice 22 of 73, with label.

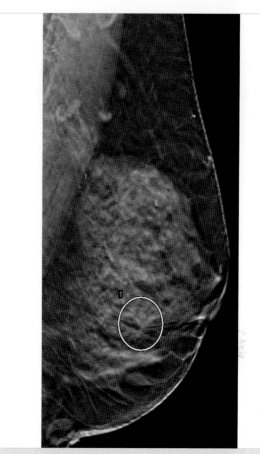

Fig. 55.6 Left mediolateral oblique digital breast tomosynthesis (LMLO DBT), slice 27 of 65, with label.

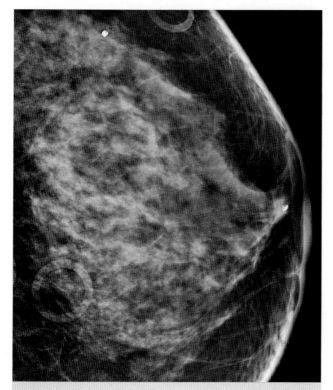

Fig. 55.7 Left craniocaudal (LCC) spot-compression mammogram.

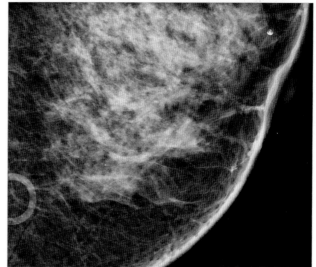

Fig. 55.8 Left mediolateral oblique (LMLO) spot-compression mammogram.

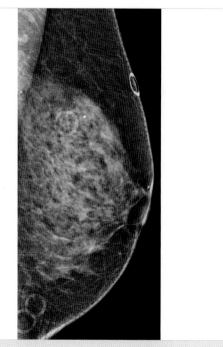

Fig. 55.9 Left mediolateral (LML) mammogram.

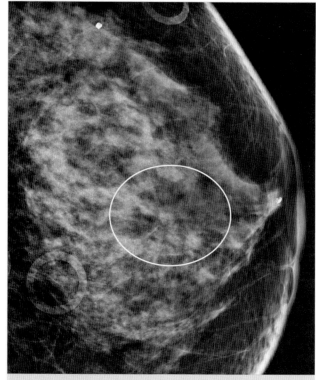

Fig. 55.10 Left craniocaudal (LCC) spot-compression mammogram with label.

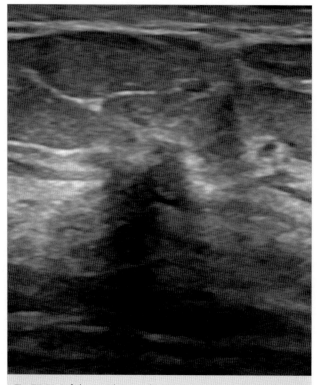

Fig. 55.11 Left breast ultrasound, transverse view.

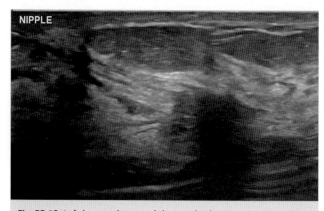

Fig. 55.12 Left breast ultrasound, longitudinal view.

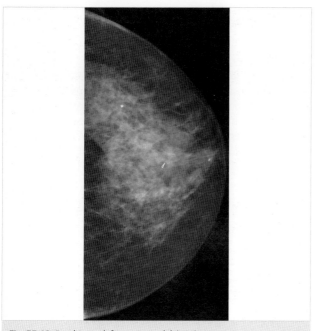

Fig. 55.13 Postbiopsy left craniocaudal (LCC) mammogram.

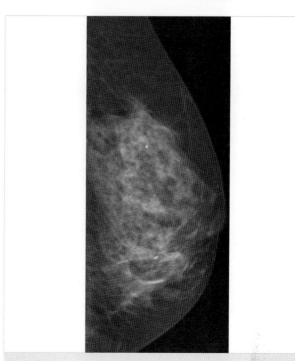

Fig. 55.14 Postbiopsy left mediolateral (LML) mammogram.

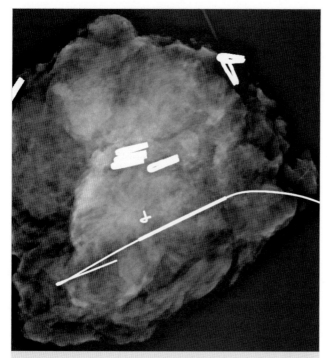

Fig. 55.15 Radiograph of surgical specimen.

56 Linear Calcifications

Lonie R. Salkowski

56.1 Presentation and Presenting Images

(▶ Fig. 56.1, ▶ Fig. 56.2, ▶ Fig. 56.3, ▶ Fig. 56.4)

A 65-year-old female with a history of right breast cancer treated 6 years ago presents for screening mammography.

56.2 Key Images

(▶ Fig. 56.5, ▶ Fig. 56.6, ▶ Fig. 56.7, ▶ Fig. 56.8, ▶ Fig. 56.9, ▶ Fig. 56.10)

56.2.1 Breast Tissue Density

The breasts are heterogeneously dense, which may obscure small masses.

56.2.2 Imaging Findings

There are grouped linear calcifications in the left breast at the 9 o'clock location in the posterior depth (▶ Fig. 56.7 and ▶ Fig. 56.9; DBT images ▶ Fig. 56.5 and ▶ Fig. 56.6). The synthetic mammogams can enhance the appearance of calcifications due to the reconstruction algorithms. In addition, the contrast on the synthetic mammograms is diminished, with the background fibroglandular tissue appearing more flat and thus the calcifications standing out further (▶ Fig. 56.8 and ▶ Fig. 56.10). A single stable coarse calcification is seen in the left breast; otherwise no other calcifications of concern are seen.

56.3 BI-RADS Classification and Action

Category 0: Mammography: Incomplete. Need additional imaging evaluation and/or prior mammograms for comparison.

56.4 Diagnostic Images

(▶ Fig. 56.11, ▶ Fig. 56.12, ▶ Fig. 56.13, ▶ Fig. 56.14, ▶ Fig. 56.15)

56.4.1 Imaging Findings

The diagnostic imaging confirms the segmental fine linear pleomorphic calcifications spanning an area of 0.8 × 3.2 × 0.8 cm at 10 o'clock in the middle depth (▶ Fig. 56.14). The craniocaudal (CC) view tomosynthesis also suggests that there may be an asymmetry associated with the more coarse calcification (▶ Fig. 56.5). This is also suggested on the CC spot magnification image (▶ Fig. 56.14). A correlate is not seen on the mediolateral

oblique (MLO) images likely due to being obscured by the dense overlapping tissue. If further evaluation was required, a spot digital breast tomosynthesis (DBT) could have been performed; however, this area was already assessed as needing a biopsy. The area of segmental calcifications underwent stereotactic biopsy. The specimens from the posterior extent of this area are shown in ▶ Fig. 56.15.

56.5 BI-RADS Classification and Action:

Category 5: Highly suggestive of malignancy

56.6 Differential Diagnosis

1. ***Grade 2 invasive ductal carcinoma (grade 2 IDC) with intermediate grade ductal carcinoma in situ (DCIS)***: Invasive cancers can present as calcifications. On pathologic assessment, the IDC measured 7 mm. In this case, there is a suggestion of an asymmetry on DBT. However, if this asymmetry was not associated with the calcifications, it likely would not have been of interest in recalling the patient.
2. *Ductal carcinoma in situ (DCIS)*: The morphology and linear distribution of these calcifications is highly suspicious for DCIS. This would be a concordant image-guided biopsy result.
3. *Atypical ductal hyperplasia (ADH)*: A biopsy of these calcifications yielding ADH would likely be upgraded to DCIS or IDC.

56.7 Essential Facts

- The calcifications in this case are easily seen on the conventional mammogram. The DBT imaging may have alerted the reader to a possible asymmetry associated with the calcifications. This observation led to performing biopsies at the extent of the calcifications to possibly identify an associated invasive component.
- The diagnosis of an invasive component of a breast cancer will dictate and influence the surgical and oncological treatment.
- Early studies suggest that the synthetic mammogram (a two-dimensional mammogram constructed from DBT images) combined with DBT images is comparable to full-field digital mammography (FFDM) alone or in combination with DBT.

56.8 Management and Digital Breast Tomosynthesis Principles

- The elimination of the routine FFDM during routine mammography, substituting a synthetic mammogram, will decrease the radiation exposure.

- It is estimated that using the synthetic two-dimensional (2D) images has an estimated dose reduction of 45% compared to a FFDM plus DBT.
- There is a significant learning curve for radiologists to add DBT image interpretation to FFDM interpretation. There will be an additional learning curve for the radiologist if and as they convert from the use and interpretation of FFDM to that of synthetic 2D mammograms. Training for this needs to be developed.
- There is not uniform insurance coverage for DBT with FFDM or for synthetic 2D mammograms instead of FFDM. There will be an additional learning curve for the radiologist if they convert from the interpretation of FFDM to synthetic 2D mammograms.

56.9 Further Reading

[1] Skaane P, Bandos AI, Eben EB, et al. Two-view digital breast tomosynthesis screening with synthetically reconstructed projection images: comparison with digital breast tomosynthesis with full-field digital mammographic images. Radiology. 2014; 271(3):655–663

[2] Zuley ML, Guo B, Catullo VJ, et al. Comparison of two-dimensional synthesized mammograms versus original digital mammograms alone and in combination with tomosynthesis images. Radiology. 2014; 271(3):664–671

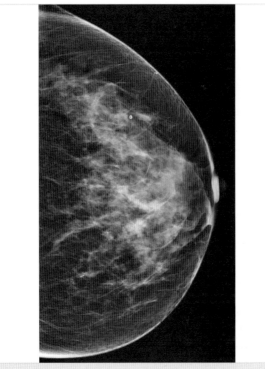

Fig. 56.1 Left craniocaudal (LCC) mammogram.

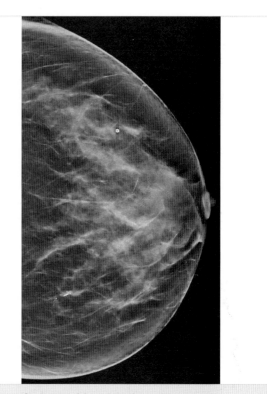

Fig. 56.2 Left craniocaudal (LCC) synthetic mammogram.

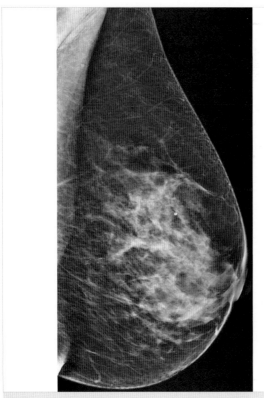

Fig. 56.3 Left mediolateral oblique (LMLO) mammogram.

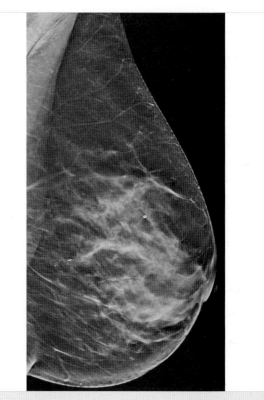

Fig. 56.4 Left mediolateral oblique (LMLO) synthetic mammogram.

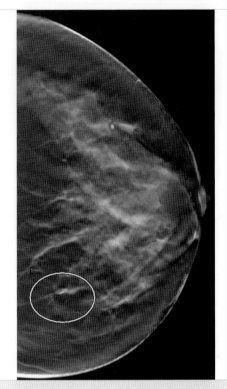

Fig. 56.5 Left craniocaudal digital breast tomosynthesis (LCC DBT), slice 33 of 66, with label.

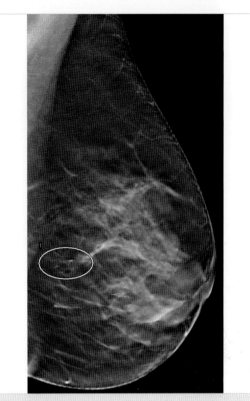

Fig. 56.6 Left mediolateral oblique digital breast tomosynthesis (LMLO DBT), slice 37 of 65, with label.

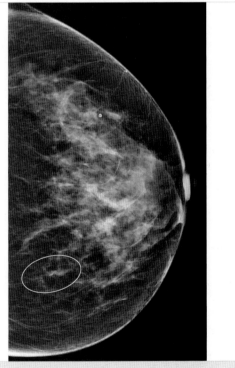

Fig. 56.7 Left craniocaudal (LCC) mammogram with label.

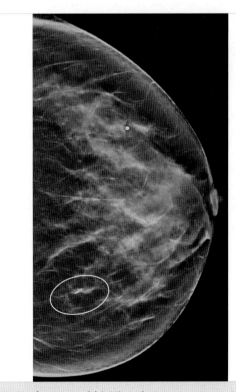

Fig. 56.8 Left craniocaudal (LCC) synthetic mammogram with label.

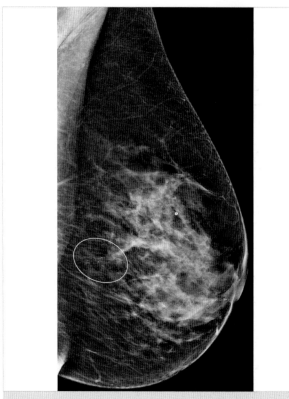

Fig. 56.9 Left mediolateral oblique (LMLO) mammogram with label.

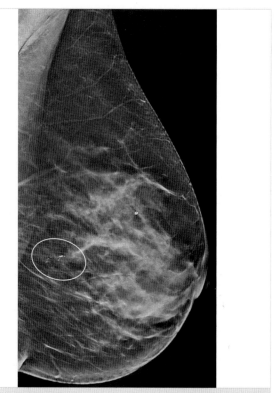

Fig. 56.10 Left mediolateral oblique (LMLO) synthetic mammogram with label.

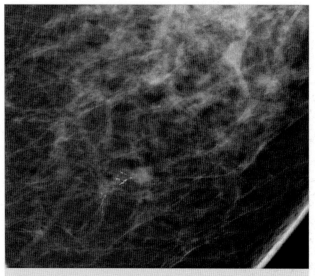

Fig. 56.11 Left craniocaudal (LCC) mammogram, spot magnification.

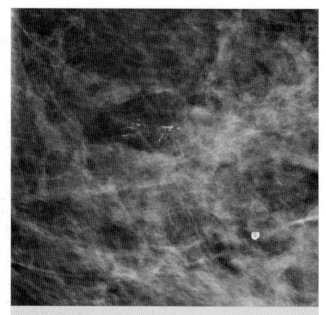

Fig. 56.12 Left mediolateral oblique (LML) mammogram, spot magnification.

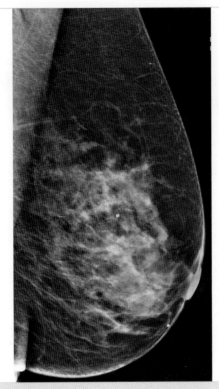

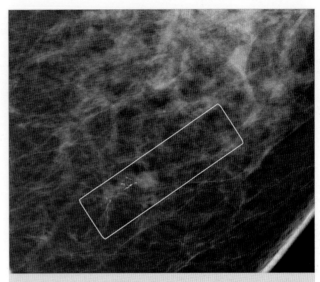

Fig. 56.14 Left craniocaudal (LCC) mammogram, spot magnification with label.

Fig. 56.13 Left mediolateral (LML) mammogram.

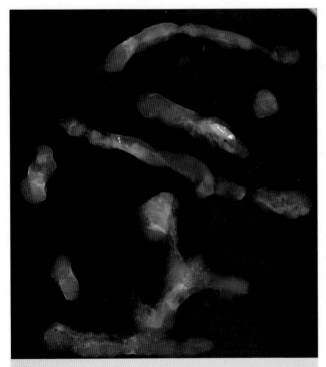

Fig. 56.15 Radiograph of core needle biopsy specimens.

57 Developing Asymmetry

Lonie R. Salkowski

57.1 Presentation and Presenting Images

(▶ Fig. 57.1, ▶ Fig. 57.2)

A 70-year-old female presents for screening mammography. She has a history of left breast cancer treated 2 years ago with a lumpectomy but not radiation therapy, which she declined.

57.2 Key Images

(▶ Fig. 57.3, ▶ Fig. 57.4, ▶ Fig. 57.5)

57.2.1 Breast Tissue Density

The breasts are almost entirely fatty.

57.2.2 Imaging Findings

There are postsurgical changes in the upper outer quadrant consistent with the patient's prior lumpectomy for DCIS 2 years ago. The skin incision is marked with a wire marker. On the conventional craniocaudal (CC) mammogram, there is an asymmetry that is just lateral to the prior lumpectomy site (▶ Fig. 57.3). The corresponding tomosynthesis images demonstrate a focal asymmetry at the 2 o'clock location in the middle depth (▶ Fig. 57.4 and ▶ Fig. 57.5). The asymmetry was obscured by the overlapping tissue on the conventional mediolateral oblique (MLO) mammogram (▶ Fig. 57.2).

57.3 BI-RADS Classification and Action

Category 0: Mammography: Incomplete. Need additional imaging evaluation and/or prior mammograms for comparison.

57.4 Diagnostic Images

(▶ Fig. 57.6, ▶ Fig. 57.7, ▶ Fig. 57.8, ▶ Fig. 57.9, ▶ Fig. 57.10, ▶ Fig. 57.11, ▶ Fig. 57.12, ▶ Fig. 57.13, ▶ Fig. 57.14)

57.4.1 Imaging Findings

The diagnostic imaging further delineates the developing asymmetry on the both the CC and MLO spot-compression images (▶ Fig. 57.6, ▶ Fig. 57.9 and ▶ Fig. 57.7, ▶ Fig. 57.10) to be at the 2 o'clock location, 6 cm from the nipple. The targeted ultrasound demonstrates the 4-mm hypoechoic mass with indistinct margins at the 2 o'clock location, 6 cm from the nipple (▶ Fig. 57.11 and ▶ Fig. 57.12). This mass is at the medial edge of the patient's incision scar from the prior lumpectomy. The mass was biopsied with ultrasound guidance and the ribbon clip, placed at biopsy, is found at the location of the mass seen on tomosynthesis (*arrow* in ▶ Fig. 57.13 and ▶ Fig. 57.14).

57.5 BI-RADS Classification and Action

Category 4B: Moderate suspicion for malignancy

57.6 Differential Diagnosis

1. **Ductal carcinoma in situ (DCIS)**: DCIS is more common to present as calcifications. It can also present as a focal asymmetry, a mass, or an architectural distortion. This patient had prior DCIS treated with lumpectomy and without radiation therapy. This lesion is in the local vicinity of her prior cancer treated 2 years ago and likely represents local treatment failure.
2. *Invasive cancer*: Invasive cancers can present in the same areas as DCIS. A biopsy yielding invasive cancer would be concordant and similarly would represent local treatment failure.
3. *Fat necrosis*: Fat necrosis can resemble tumor recurrence. It can appear as a focal asymmetry, a mass, or dystrophic calcifications. When the imaging findings are not characteristic, biopsy is often necessary to differentiate fat necrosis from carcinoma.

57.7 Essential Facts

- Local treatment failure is likely to occur at or near the site of the original cancer and appear within the first 5 to 7 years after treatment.
- Local recurrence can be in situ or invasive cancer.
- Fat necrosis can occur around a surgical site and resemble a tumor. It typically occurs approximately 2 years after treatment.
- Mammographic detection of small cancers at screening allows for the decision for breast-conserving therapy.
- Not all patients have the same breast-conserving therapy. It is important to know the patient's surgical outcome (surgical margin status) and whether they had radiation, chemotherapy, or hormonal therapy. These factors can influence local recurrence.
- As patients undergo breast-conserving therapy, it is important to be aware of the normal treatment changes that can occur in the breast over time, and those that are abnormal and need further evaluation.

57.8 Management and Digital Breast Tomosynthesis Principles

- Initial reports suggest that the interpretation time for digital breast tomosynthesis (DBT) with FFDM is roughly double that of full-field digital mammography (FFDM) alone. This is an important consideration if an entire screening practice is converted from FFDM alone to FFDM plus DBT. Additional time will need to be allocated for interpretation.

- It is uncertain if the interpretation time persists or decreases over time with experience.
- Many of the initial studies in DBT were simulations with inflated numbers of cancers, thus the results may not extrapolate to the real world. This should be taken into consideration when evaluating sensitivity and specificity, which in these experimental situations may be overstated.
- Prevalent detection bias occurs when a new technology or test is introduced into a population. This can lead to increased cancer detection rates and outcomes when first introduced that are not observed in subsequent years.

57.9 Further Reading

[1] Conant EF. Clinical implementation of digital breast tomosynthesis. Radiol Clin North Am. 2014; 52(3):499–518

[2] Dershaw DD. Breast imaging and the conservative treatment of breast cancer. Radiol Clin North Am. 2002; 40(3):501–516

[3] Helvie MA. Digital mammography imaging: breast tomosynthesis and advanced applications. Radiol Clin North Am. 2010; 48(5):917–929

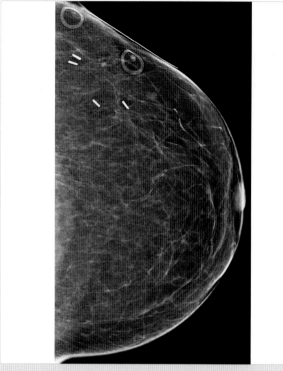

Fig. 57.1 Left craniocaudal (LCC) mammogram.

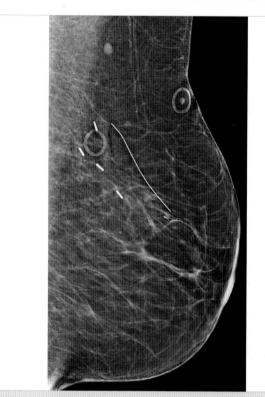

Fig. 57.2 Left mediolateral oblique (LMLO) mammogram.

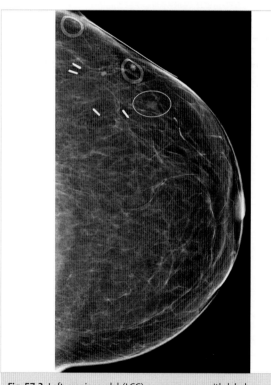

Fig. 57.3 Left craniocaudal (LCC) mammogram with label.

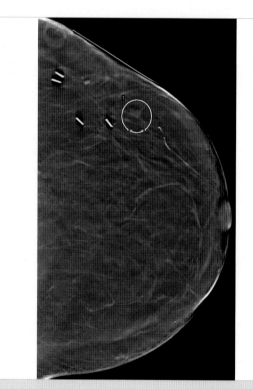

Fig. 57.4 Left craniocaudal digital breast tomosynthesis (LCC DBT), slice 17 of 56, with label.

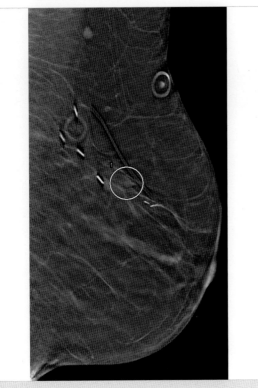

Fig. 57.5 Left mediolateral oblique digital breast tomosynthesis (LMLO DBT), slice 10 of 54, with label.

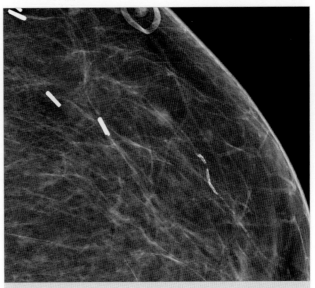

Fig. 57.6 Left craniocaudal (LCC) spot-compression mammogram.

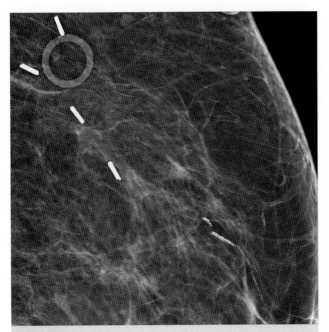

Fig. 57.7 Left mediolateral oblique (LMLO) spot-compression mammogram.

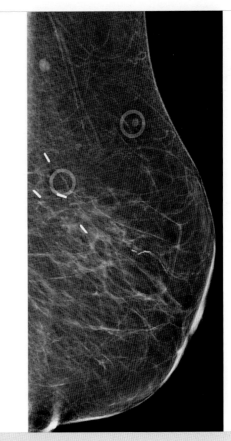

Fig. 57.8 Left mediolateral (LML) mammogram.

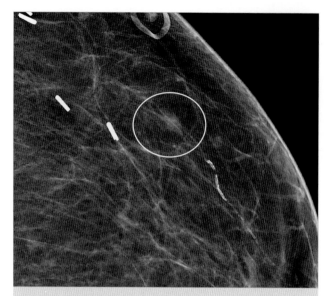

Fig. 57.9 Left craniocaudal (LCC) spot-compression mammogram with label.

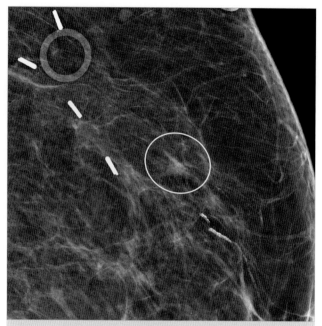

Fig. 57.10 Left mediolateral oblique (LMLO) spot-compression mammogram with label.

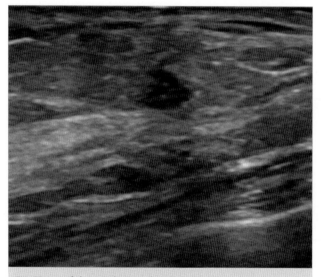

Fig. 57.11 Left breast ultrasound, transverse view

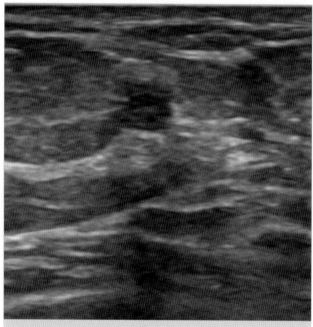

Fig. 57.12 Left breast ultrasound, longitudinal view.

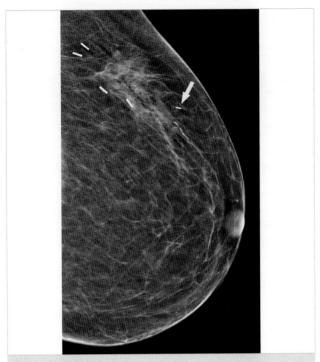

Fig. 57.13 Postbiopsy left craniocaudal (LCC) mammogram with label.

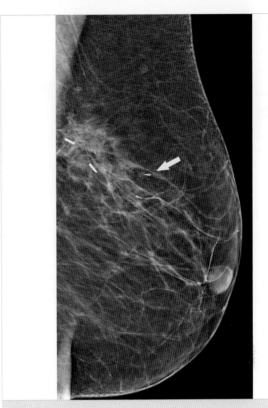

Fig. 57.14 Postbiopsy left mediolateral (LML) mammogram with label.

58 Enlarging Mass

Tanya W. Moseley

58.1 Presentation and Presenting Images

(▶ Fig. 58.1, ▶ Fig. 58.2, ▶ Fig. 58.3, ▶ Fig. 58.4, ▶ Fig. 58.5)

A 49-year-old female with elevated lifetime risk for breast cancer (20%) presents for routine screening mammography.

58.2 Key Images

(▶ Fig. 58.6, ▶ Fig. 58.7, ▶ Fig. 58.8, ▶ Fig. 58.9, ▶ Fig. 58.10)

58.2.1 Breast Tissue Density

The breasts are heterogeneously dense, which may obscure small masses.

58.2.2 Imaging Findings

The imaging of the right breast is normal (*not shown*). The left breast demonstrates a 3-cm mass (*circle*) in the upper outer quadrant of the left breast in the posterior depth, 5.5 cm from the nipple (▶ Fig. 58.6 and ▶ Fig. 58.7). The mass has increased in size since the prior mammogram (▶ Fig. 58.8 and ▶ Fig. 58.9). The mass is best seen on the left craniocaudal (CC) tomosynthesis slice 36 of 85 (▶ Fig. 58.10). It is not well seen on the left conventional mediolateral oblique (MLO) mammogram (▶ Fig. 58.7) or the MLO tomosynthesis movie.

58.3 BI-RADS Classification and Action

Category 0: Mammography: Incomplete. Need additional imaging evaluation and/or prior mammograms for comparison.

58.4 Diagnostic Images

(▶ Fig. 58.11)

58.4.1 Imaging Findings

Ultrasound was performed and demonstrated a circumscribed anechoic mass with posterior acoustic enhancement located at 3 o'clock (▶ Fig. 58.11). The distance to the mass is 5.5 cm (*dotted line*). The ultrasound evaluation is consistent with a cyst.

58.5 BI-RADS Classification and Action

Category 2: Benign

58.6 Differential Diagnosis

1. **Cyst**: Cystic and solid masses may have similar appearances on mammography. Sonography reliably differentiates cystic and solid masses. This circumscribed anechoic mass with posterior acoustic enhancement is consistent with a simple cyst.
2. *Fibroadenoma*: Fibroadenomas are oval masses with parallel orientation. Gentle lobulations (typically fewer than 4) may be present but the margins should be circumscribed. The internal echogenicity may range from isoechoic to hypoechoic.
3. *Cancer*: High-grade carcinomas and medullary carcinomas can be markedly hypoechoic and rounded in shape, mimicking complicated cysts.

58.7 Essential Facts

- A mass that enlarges over time may be benign or malignant. Benign versus malignant findings may be difficult to distinguish on conventional mammography. Tomosynthesis is helpful to further characterize masses. Sonography is used to determine the cystic or solid nature of a mass.
- Cysts result from distension of the terminal duct lobular units (TDLU) due to progressive filling with fluid.
- Cysts may be classified as simple, complicated, and complex.
  - Simple cysts are anechoic, well-circumscribed masses with posterior acoustic enhancement and subtle acoustic edge shadows.
  - Complicated cysts are not purely anechoic. These cysts contain diffuse low level echoes. Needle biopsy should be performed if this diagnosis cannot be confidently made.
  - Complex cysts may indicate the presence of malignancy or infection. Complex cysts have solid and cystic components.

58.8 Management and Digital Breast Tomosynthesis Principles

- With mammography, a two-dimensional picture (mammogram) is taken of the three-dimensional breast. The third dimension, breast thickness, is projected in a single plane. Overlapping breast tissue limits interpretation in mammography, particularly in women with denser breast parenchyma.
- The breast is positioned the same way in tomosynthesis as it is in conventional mammography. The X-ray tube moves in an arc around the breast while images are taken. This data is processed in a sequential slice format from side to side or top to bottom and viewed as a movie, thus allowing for the breast tissue to be viewed as a three-dimensional (3D) object,
- These 3D images of tomosynthesis eliminate the overlapping breast tissue and often make lesions more conspicuous.

58.9 Further Reading

[1] Masciadri N, Ferranti C. Benign breast lesions: Ultrasound. J Ultrasound. 2011; 14(2):55–65
[2] Rahbar G, Sie AC, Hansen GC, et al. Benign versus malignant solid breast masses: US differentiation. Radiology. 1999; 213(3):889–894

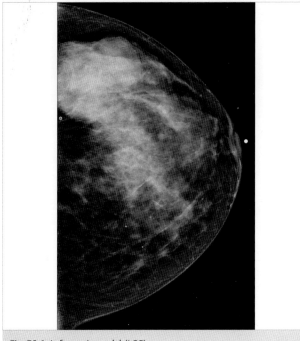

Fig. 58.1 Left craniocaudal (LCC) mammogram.

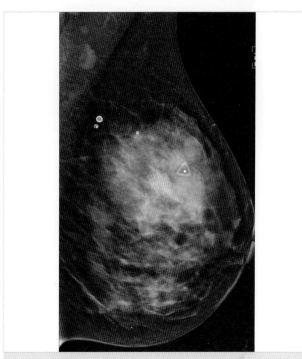

Fig. 58.2 Left mediolateral oblique (LMLO) mammogram.

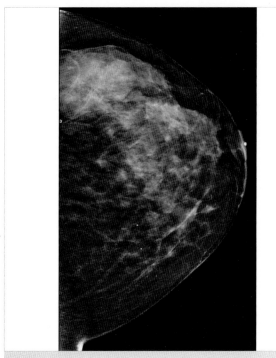

Fig. 58.3 Left craniocaudal (LCC) mammogram comparison.

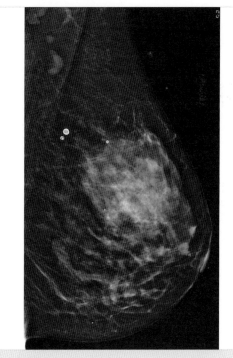

Fig. 58.4 Left mediolateral oblique (LMLO) mammogram comparison.

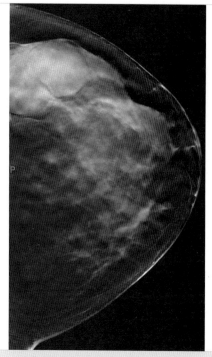

Fig. 58.5 Left craniocaudal digital breast tomosynthesis (LCC DBT), slice 36 o f 85.

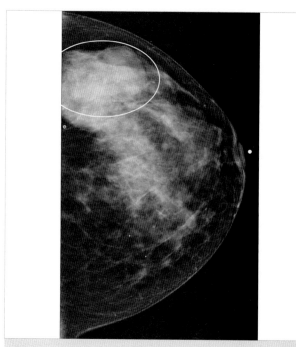

Fig. 58.6 Left craniocaudal (LCC) mammogram with label.

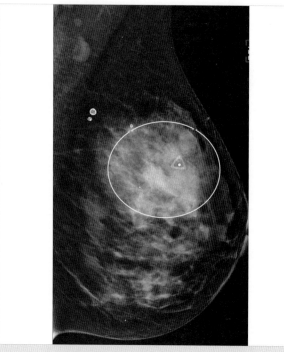

Fig. 58.7 Left mediolateral oblique (LMLO) mammogram with label.

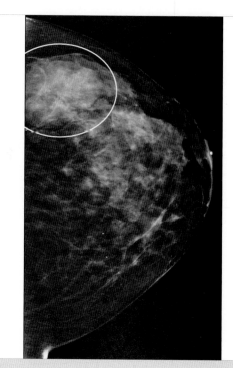

Fig. 58.8 Left craniocaudal (LCC) mammogram comparison with label.

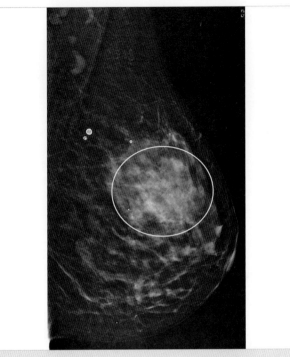

Fig. 58.9 Left mediolateral oblique (LMLO) mammogram comparison with label.

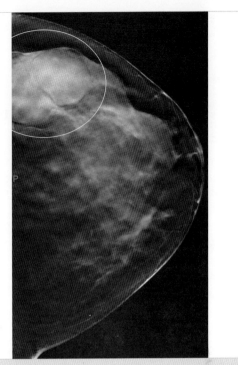

Fig. 58.10 Left craniocaudal digital breast tomosynthesis (LCC DBT), slice 36 of 85 with label.

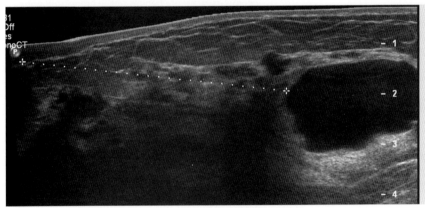

Fig. 58.11 Left breast ultrasound.

59 Developing Asymmetry in a Patient with Treated Breast Cancer

Lonie R. Salkowski

59.1 Presentation and Presenting Images

(▶ Fig. 59.1, ▶ Fig. 59.2)

A 39-year-old female treated for left breast cancer with a lumpectomy, chemotherapy, and radiation therapy more than 10 years ago presents for screening mammography.

59.2 Key Images

(▶ Fig. 59.3, ▶ Fig. 59.4)

59.2.1 Breast Tissue Density

There are scattered areas of fibroglandular density.

59.2.2 Imaging Findings

In the upper outer quadrant of the left breast, there are significant postsurgical changes that can be very distracting when reviewing a mammogram and looking for any changes (▶ Fig. 59.1 and ▶ Fig. 59.2). On first glance, the mammograms appear very similar to prior exams. However, the digital breast tomosynthesis (DBT) images suggest a developing asymmetry (*comparisons not shown*) adjacent to the postsurgical changes at the 3 o'clock location in the posterior depth (▶ Fig. 59.3 and ▶ Fig. 59.4).

59.3 BI-RADS Classification and Action

Category 0: Mammography: Incomplete. Need additional imaging evaluation and/or prior mammograms for comparison.

59.4 Diagnostic Images

(▶ Fig. 59.5, ▶ Fig. 59.6, ▶ Fig. 59.7, ▶ Fig. 59.8, ▶ Fig. 59.9, ▶ Fig. 59.10, ▶ Fig. 59.11)

59.4.1 Imaging Findings

The diagnostic imaging confirms the presence of an irregular mass with indistinct margins at the 3 o'clock location in the posterior depth (▶ Fig. 59.5, ▶ Fig. 59.6, and ▶ Fig. 59.7). The accompanying ultrasound examination demonstrates a 1.2 × 1.3 × 1.2 cm irregular mass with angular and indistinct margins located at 3 o'clock, 7 cm from the nipple (▶ Fig. 59.8 and ▶ Fig. 59.9). The mass has posterior acoustic shadowing. This mass was biopsied with ultrasound guidance, and the ribbon marker placed at the completion of the biopsy is located in the developing asymmetry, originally seen on the screening mammogram (▶ Fig. 59.10 and ▶ Fig. 59.11).

59.5 BI-RADS Classification and Action

Category 4C: High suspicion for malignancy

59.6 Differential Diagnosis

1. ***Recurrent invasive ductal carcinoma***: The patient had cancer of the left breast many years ago, receiving a lumpectomy, radiation and chemotherapy. New masses or developing asymmetries near or at a surgical sight always raises concern for recurrent breast cancer.
2. *Scar tissue*: Post-treatment changes of the breast following surgery and radiation continue to evolve over time. A developing mass or calcifications in the treated breast need to be evaluated prior to dismissing it as post-treatment changes.
3. *Fat necrosis*: Fat necrosis can have many forms, from calcifications to spiculated masses. Similar to scars, developing changes need to evaluated prior to dismissing as part of the spectrum of fat necrosis changes.

59.7 Essential Facts

- Breast-conserving therapy (BCT) is widely used for treating localized cancer. It is important to recognize the mammographic changes that occur in a conservatively treated breast.
- Local recurrence after BCT is approximately 1 to 2% per year. Based on this estimate, a patient who has a mammogram 10 years after her initial cancer, has a 10 to 20% chance of recurrence at 10 years.
- DBT allows the ability to scroll through image sets thus revealing findings that may have been obscured by background noise.
- Lesions seen better on DBT can be more accurately assessed using the BIRADS classification.

59.8 Management and Digital Breast Tomosynthesis Principles

- Any new or developing suspicious mammographic finding warrants evaluation regardless of how its appearance compares to the original cancer.
- Factors that affect the detection of cancer lesions on mammography are technique sensitivity, distracting lesions, tumor growth rate, tumor growth pattern, and the background upon which the tumor is displayed.

- The mammographic appearance of a recurrence does not always correlate with the appearance of the initial breast cancer.

59.9 Further Reading

[1] Andersson I, Ikeda DM, Zackrisson S, et al. Breast tomosynthesis and digital mammography: a comparison of breast cancer visibility and BIRADS classification in a population of cancers with subtle mammographic findings. Eur Radiol. 2008; 18(12):2817–2825

[2] Weinstein SP, Orel SG, Pinnamaneni N, et al. Mammographic appearance of recurrent breast cancer after breast conservation therapy. Acad Radiol. 2008; 15(2):240–244

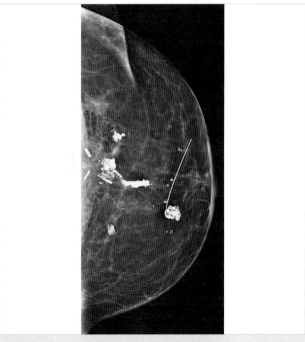

Fig. 59.1 Left craniocaudal (LCC) mammogram.

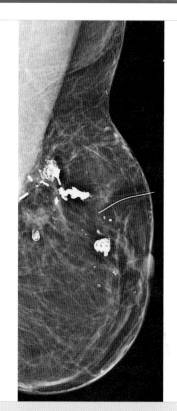

Fig. 59.2 Left mediolateral oblique (LMLO) mammogram.

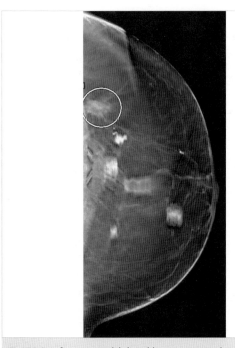

Fig. 59.3 Left craniocaudal digital breast tomosynthesis (LCC DBT), slice 26 of 87, with label.

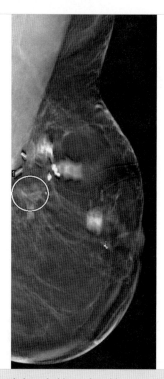

Fig. 59.4 Left mediolateral oblique digital breast tomosynthesis (LMLO DBT), slice 27 of 80, with label.

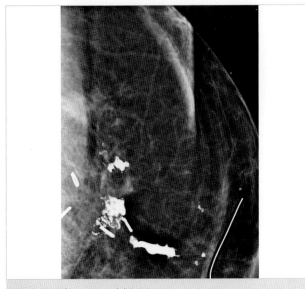

Fig. 59.5 Left craniocaudal (LCC) spot-compression mammogram.

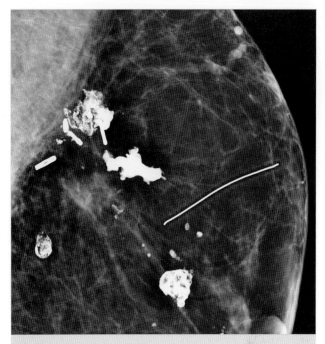

Fig. 59.6 Left mediolateral oblique (LMLO) spot-compression mammogram.

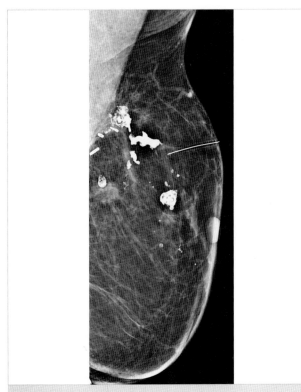

Fig. 59.7 Left mediolateral (LML) mammogram.

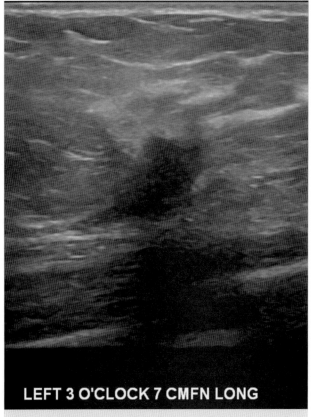

LEFT 3 O'CLOCK 7 CMFN LONG

Fig. 59.8 Left breast ultrasound, longitudinal view.

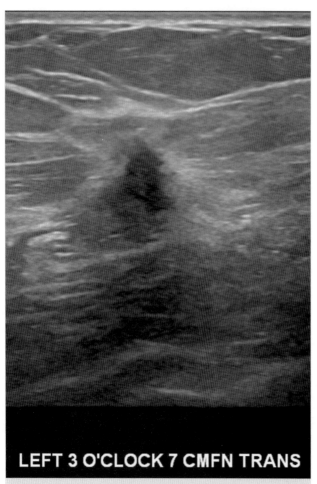

LEFT 3 O'CLOCK 7 CMFN TRANS

Fig. 59.9 Left breast ultrasound, transverse view.

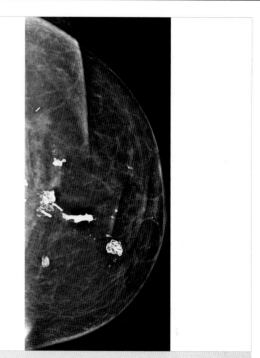

Fig. 59.10 Postbiopsy left craniocaudal (LCC) mammogram.

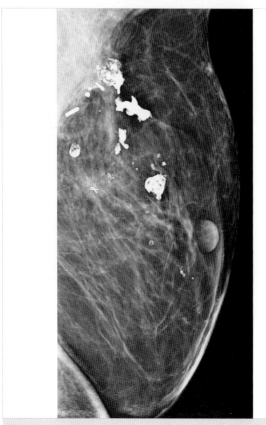

Fig. 59.11 Postbiopsy left mediolateral (LML) mammogram.

Part IV

**Cases with Screening and
Diagnostic Tomosynthesis
Evaluations**

IV

60 Circumscribed Mass

Tanya W. Moseley

60.1 Presentation and Presenting Images

(► Fig. 60.1, ► Fig. 60.2, ► Fig. 60.3, ► Fig. 60.4, ► Fig. 60.5, ► Fig. 60.6)

A 42-year-old female with right breast cancer treated with a mastectomy presents for screening mammography.

60.2 Key Images

(► Fig. 60.7, ► Fig. 60.8, ► Fig. 60.9, ► Fig. 60.10, ► Fig. 60.11)

60.2.1 Breast Tissue Density

The breasts are heterogeneously dense, which may obscure small masses.

60.2.2 Imaging Findings

The right breast is surgically absent. The left breast demonstrates an oval mass with obscured margins (*circle*) in the lower inner quadrant at the 7 o'clock location in the anterior depth, 3 cm from the nipple (► Fig. 60.7, ► Fig. 60.8, ► Fig. 60.9, ► Fig. 60.10, and ► Fig. 60.11). There are two postbiopsy clips in the left breast that denote the sites of prior benign biopsies. The bar-shaped clip marks a prior magnetic resonance (MR) biopsy of a fibroadenomatoid change, stromal fibrosis, and findings suggestive of intraductal papilloma. The baby-diaper–shaped clip marks a prior ultrasound biopsy of a fibroadenoma.

60.3 BI-RADS Classification and Action

Category 0: Incomplete. Need additional imaging evaluation and/or prior mammograms for comparison.

60.4 Diagnostic Images

(► Fig. 60.12, ► Fig. 60.13, ► Fig. 60.14, ► Fig. 60.15)

60.4.1 Imaging Findings

Spot-compression digital breast tomosynthesis (DBT) movies were done to further evaluate the obscured mass in the left breast. Slices from these movies confirm the mammographic suspicion of a mass and show the mass's margins to be circumscribed (► Fig. 60.12 and ► Fig. 60.13). A targeted ultrasound reveals an oval hypoechoic mass with circumscribed margins at the 6 o'clock location (► Fig. 60.14 and ► Fig. 60.15). This mass underwent ultrasound-guided biopsy.

60.4.2 BI-RADS Classification and Action

Category 4A: Low suspicion for malignancy

60.5 Differential Diagnosis

1. *Fibroadenoma*: Fibroadenomas may range from isoechoic to hypoechoic with variable posterior acoustic enhancement. Fibroadenomas do not have a true capsule; the thin echogenic capsule seen on sonography is a pseudocapsule caused by the compression of adjacent tissue. The vascularity of solid masses does not help distinguish a cancer from a fibroadenoma.
2. *Complicated cyst*: Complicated cysts may have sonographic features similar to fibroadenomas.
3. *Ductal carcinoma in situ (DCIS)*: DCIS typically presents as a group of calcifications varying in size, density, and form. A mass lesion is an uncommon presentation for DCIS.

60.6 Essential Facts

- Fibroadenomas are solid, benign fibroepithelial breast masses that occur most often in young women.
- Benign-appearing masses should not be dismissed as benign. Sonography is required to definitively characterize masses. Benign and malignant entities may present as benign-appearing or well-circumscribed masses on tomosynthesis.
- In this case, specifically, this patient is at an increased risk of developing a malignancy given her personal history of breast cancer.
- The mass is better seen on tomosynthesis than on conventional mammography. Digital breast tomosynthesis (DBT) is excellent at localizing masses, which is helpful to guide the sonographic evaluation.
- If the finding was not seen on sonography, it could have been biopsied under the guidance of tomosynthesis.

60.7 Management and Digital Breast Tomosynthesis Principles

- Tomosynthesis systems are highly flexible and support screening mammography, diagnostic mammography, stereotactic biopsies, and tomosynthesis all with one machine.
- The anatomical structures of the breast inherently can obscure findings due to overlapping tissue. DBT overcomes the limitations of overlapping tissue.
- The DBT system moves in an arc over the breast generating low-dose images. The data is compiled into a three-dimensional (3D) volume set, which may be viewed as a single slices or a cine movie. This allows for better detection and analysis of breast lesions over conventional imaging.
- Only findings within an imaged section appear sharp, whereas those above or below appear out of focus.

60.8 Further Reading

[1] Enhancing imaging capabilities with breast tomosynthesis. Siemens white paper. Accessed 12/25/2015. Available at: http://www.healthcare.siemens.com/siemens_hwem-hwem_ssxa_websites-context-root/wcm/idc/groups/public/@global/@imaging/@mammo/documents/download/mdaw/mtuy/~edisp/enhancing_imaging_capabilities_with_breast_tomosynthesis-00078508.pdf

[2] Smith A. Fundamentals of breast tomosynthesis. Improving the performance of mammography. Hologic white paper. Accessed 12/25/2015. Available at: http://www.hologic.com/sites/default/files/Fundamentals%20of%20Breast%20Tomosynthesis_WP-00007.pdf

[3] Souchay H, Carton A-K, lordache R. Boosting dose efficiency with digital breast tomosynthesis. GE white paper. Accessed 12/25/2015. Available at: https://www.google.co.in/url?sa=t&rct=j&q=&esrc=s&source=web&cd=1&cad=rja&uact=8&ved=0ahUKEwjA-NnigePMAhWKNI8KHRh6AP8QFggh-MAA&url=http%3A%2F%2Fwww3.gehealthcare.com.br%2F~%2Fmedia%2Fdownloads%2Fbr%2Fsenoclaire_dose_white_paper_-_doc1403841.pdf%3FParent%3D%257B10196544-07D9-4A31-95BB-DD2D94F05C16%257D&usg=AFQjCNEZqb51t7uNyS1TGyT2S_kzhrHkJA&bvm=bv.122129774,d.c2I

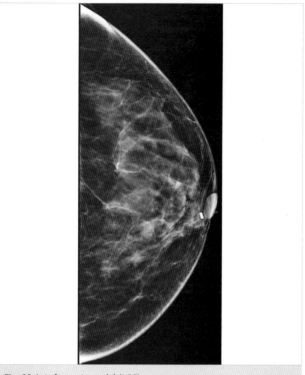

Fig. 60.1 Left craniocaudal (LCC) mammogram.

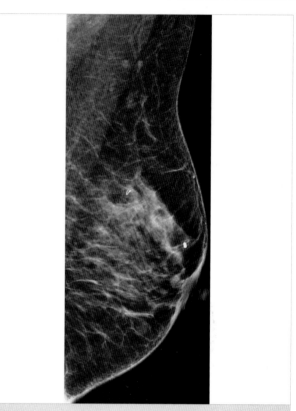

Fig. 60.2 Left mediolateral oblique (LMLO) mammogram.

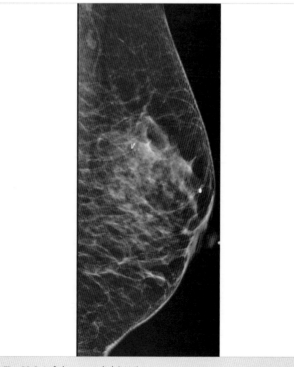

Fig. 60.3 Left lateromedial (LLM) mammogram.

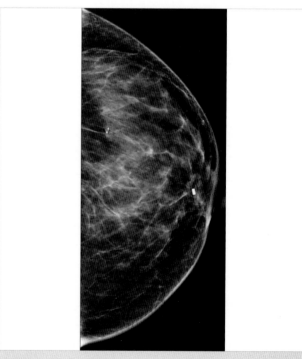

Fig. 60.4 Left craniocaudal (LCC) mammogram comparison.

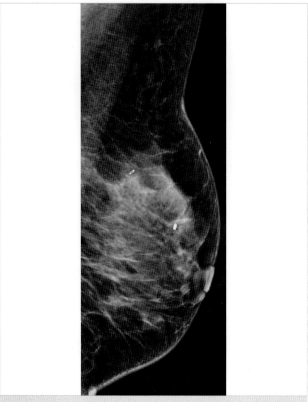

Fig. 60.5 Left mediolateral oblique (LMLO) mammogram comparison.

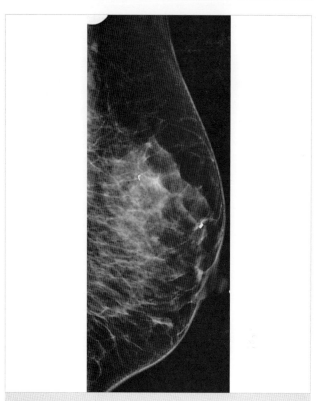

Fig. 60.6 Left lateromedial (LLM) mammogram comparison.

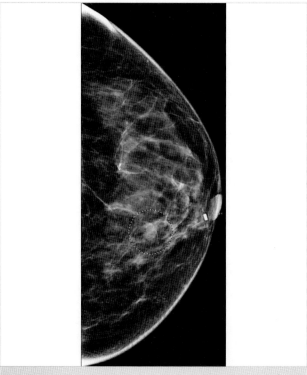

Fig. 60.7 Left craniocaudal (LCC) mammogram with label.

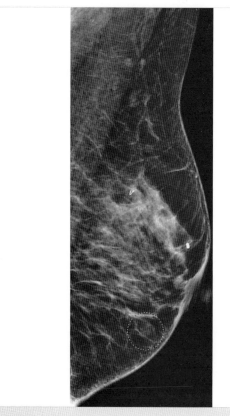

Fig. 60.8 Left mediolateral oblique (LMLO) mammogram with label.

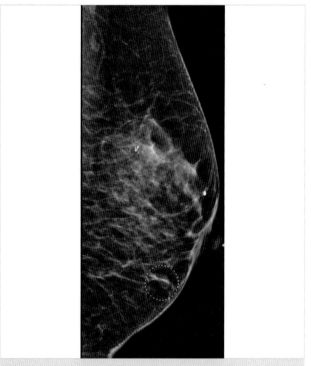

Fig. 60.9 Left lateromedial (LLM) mammogram with label.

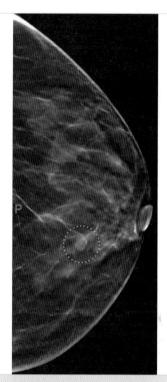

Fig. 60.10 Left craniocaudal digital breast tomosynthesis (LCC DBT), slice 11 of 55 with label.

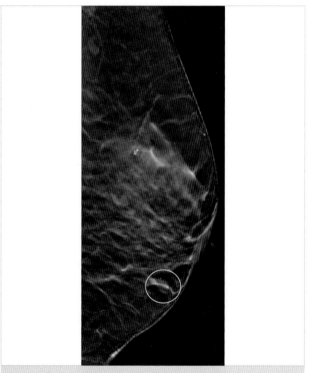

Fig. 60.11 Left lateromedial digital breast tomosynthesis (LLM DBT), slice 26 of 47 with label.

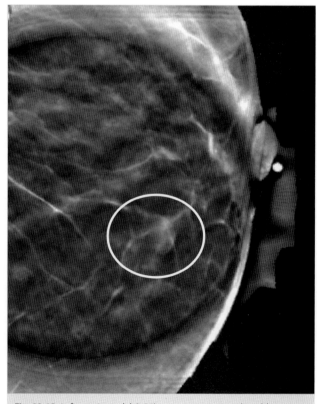

Fig. 60.12 Left craniocaudal (LCC) spot-compression digital breast tomosynthesis (DBT), slice 8 of 40, with label.

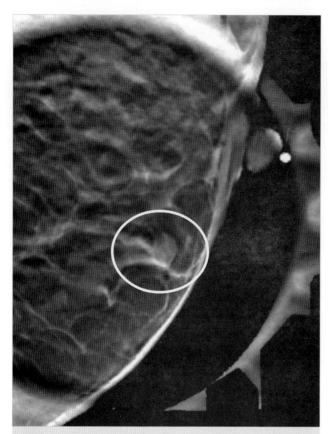

Fig. 60.13 Left lateromedial (LLM) spot-compression digital breast tomosynthesis (DBT), slice 17 of 34, with label.

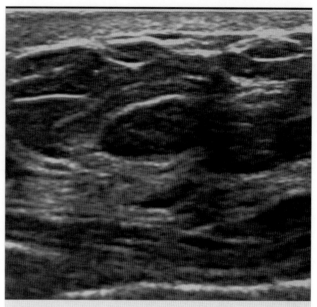

Fig. 60.14 Left breast ultrasound, longitudinal view.

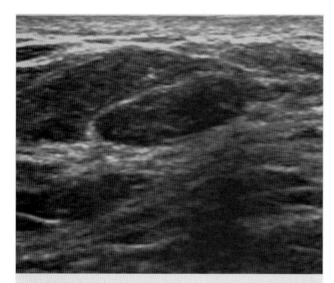

Fig. 60.15 Left breast ultrasound, transverse view.

61 Developing Asymmetry

Lonie R. Salkowski

61.1 Presentation and Presenting Images

(▶ Fig. 61.1, ▶ Fig. 61.2)

A 65-year-old female with a history of right breast cancer treated 4 years ago presents for asymptomatic screening mammography.

61.2 Key Images

(▶ Fig. 61.3, ▶ Fig. 61.4)

61.2.1 Breast Tissue Density

There are scattered areas of fibroglandular density.

61.2.2 Imaging Findings

In the upper outer quadrant of the left breast there is a small area of architectural distortion at the 1 o'clock location in the posterior depth (▶ Fig. 61.3 and ▶ Fig. 61.4). It is best seen on the tomosynthesis images; however, it can be seen retrospectively on the conventional digital mammogram.

61.3 BI-RADS Classification and Action

Category 0: Mammography: Incomplete. Need additional imaging evaluation and/or prior mammograms for comparison.

61.4 Diagnostic Imaging

(▶ Fig. 61.5, ▶ Fig. 61.6, ▶ Fig. 61.7, ▶ Fig. 61.8, ▶ Fig. 61.9, ▶ Fig. 61.10, ▶ Fig. 61.11, ▶ Fig. 61.12)

61.4.1 Imaging Findings

Sometimes small areas of architectural distortion can resolve with additional imaging. In this diagnostic evaluation, spot-compression digital breast tomosynthesis (DBT) combination views were obtained in the craniocaudal (CC) (▶ Fig. 61.5 and ▶ Fig. 61.7) and mediolateral (ML) projections (▶ Fig. 61.9 and ▶ Fig. 61.11). The imaging confirms a 6-mm irregular mass with indistinct and spiculated margins at the 1 o'clock location 14 cm from the nipple. A targeted ultrasound reveals a 3 × 6 × 4 mm hypoechoic mass with posterior acoustic

shadowing (▶ Fig. 61.12). The axillary lymph nodes were normal (*not shown*).

61.5 BI-RADS Classification and Action

Category 4B: Moderate suspicion for malignancy

61.6 Differential Diagnosis

1. ***Invasive cancer***: Although this lesion is small, it has suspicious features and the biopsy revealed invasive tubulolobular carcinoma.
2. *Fibromatosis*: Fibromatosis is not very common (0.2% of all breast tumors). These lesions present as small spiculated lesions near the chest wall and often mimic breast cancer on imaging.
3. *Radial scar*: Radial scars can mimic breast cancers and would be consistent with the presentation of this lesion.

61.7 Essential Facts

- Tubulolobular carcinoma is a subtype of mammary carcinoma with an incidence of 0.9%.
- Currently tubulolobular carcinoma is thought to be a variant of a well-differentiated ductal carcinoma with a lobular growth pattern.
- There is an excellent prognosis for patients with tubulolobular carcinoma with an over 90% 10-year survival rate.
- Most tubulolobular carcinoma lesions are less than 2 cm in size, and they are often found on screening mammography.
- Most common mammographic presentation of tubulolobular carcinoma is a mass without calcifications, of irregular shape, and with spiculated or indistinct margins.
- The typical sonographic appearance of a tubulolobular carcinoma lesion is a hypoechoic, mass with spiculated or microlobulated margins, and with posterior acoustic shadowing in about half the cases.

61.8 Management and Digital Breast Tomosynthesis Principles

- This lesion is very small and is in the midst of the anatomical noise of the underlying breast tissue. Spot-compression digital breast tomosynthesis (DBT) could help localize this finding and further help to characterize this small lesion. It would reveal the spiculated nature of the lesion, which is not fully appreciated on conventional diagnostic imaging.

- Early studies suggest that DBT with full-field digital mammography (FFDM) appears to be better than FFDM and additional diagnostic imaging in over half of the assessments. DBT had better margin assessment than diagnostic imaging for noncalcified lesions.
- DBT may be able to replace conventional diagnostic mammography for noncalcified lesions recalled from screening. Some studies suggest that these noncalcified lesions on screening DBT could bypass diagnostic mammography and proceed to ultrasound examination. Larger studies are needed

to determine the optimal imaging protocol for attaining diagnostic information while minimizing patient radiation dose.

61.9 Further Reading

[1] Brandt KR, Craig DA, Hoskins TL, et al. Can digital breast tomosynthesis replace conventional diagnostic mammography views for screening recalls without calcifications? A comparison study in a simulated clinical setting. AJR Am J Roentgenol. 2013; 200(2):291–298

[2] Günhan-Bilgen I, Oktay A. Tubulolobular carcinoma of the breast: clinical, mammographic and sonographic findings. Eur J Radiol. 2006; 60(3):418–424

[3] Hakim CM, Catullo VJ, Chough DM, et al. Effect of the Availability of Prior Full-Field Digital Mammography and Digital Breast Tomosynthesis Images on the Interpretation of Mammograms. Radiology. 2015; 276(1):65–72

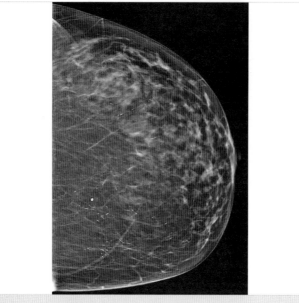

Fig. 61.1 Left craniocaudal (LCC) mammogram.

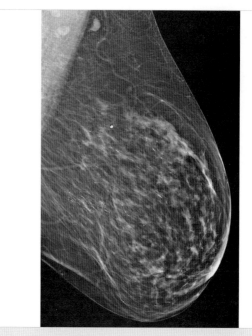

Fig. 61.2 Left mediolateral oblique (LMLO) mammogram.

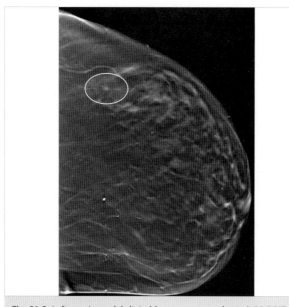

Fig. 61.3 Left craniocaudal digital breast tomosynthesis (LCC DBT), slice 41 of 79, with label.

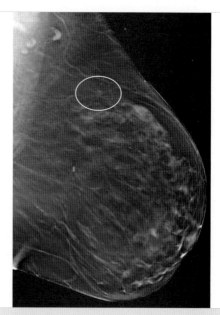

Fig. 61.4 Left mediolateral oblique digital breast tomosynthesis (LMLO DBT), slice 42 of 87, with label.

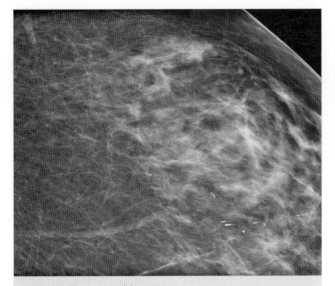

Fig. 61.5 Left craniocaudal (LCC) spot-compression mammogram.

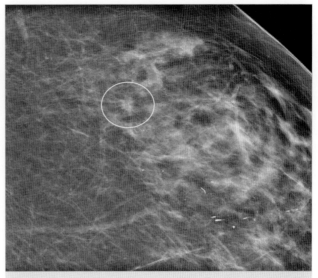

Fig. 61.6 Left craniocaudal (LCC) spot-compression mammogram with label.

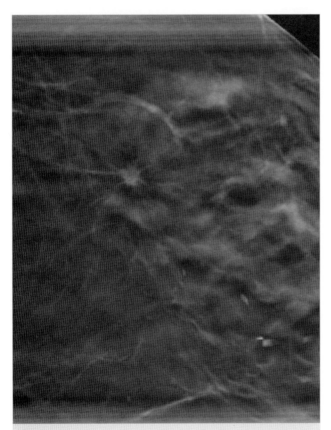

Fig. 61.7 Left craniocaudal (LCC) spot-compression digital breast tomosynthesis (DBT), slice 33 of 60.

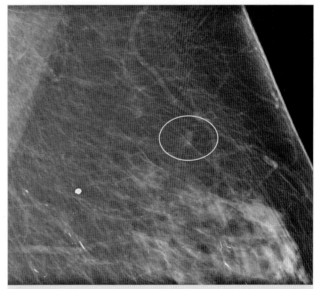

Fig. 61.8 Left mediolateral oblique (LMLO) spot-compression mammogram with label.

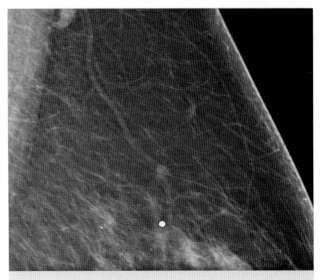

Fig. 61.9 Left mediolateral (LML) spot-compression mammogram.

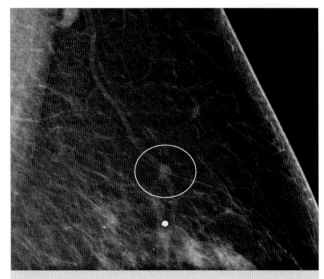

Fig. 61.10 Left mediolateral (LML) spot-compression mammogram with label.

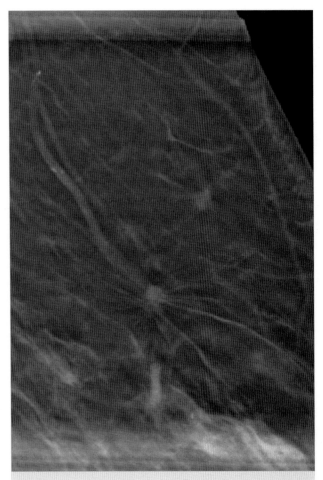

Fig. 61.11 Left mediolateral digital breast tomosynthesis (LML DBT), slice 22 of 70.

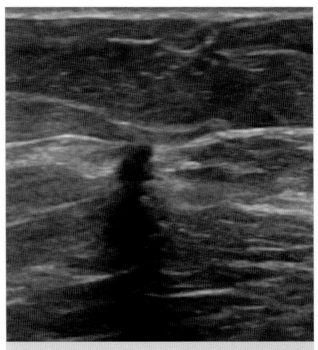

Fig. 61.12 Left breast ultrasound, transverse view.

Part V

Cases with Diagnostic Tomosynthesis Evaluation Recalled from Conventional Screening Mammogram

V

62 Possible Focal Asymmetry

Lonie R. Salkowski

62.1 Presentation and Presenting Images

(▶ Fig. 62.1, ▶ Fig. 62.2)
A 42-year-old female presents for screening mammography.

62.2 Key Images

(▶ Fig. 62.3, ▶ Fig. 62.4)

62.2.1 Breast Tissue Density

The breasts are heterogeneously dense, which may obscure small masses.

62.2.2 Imaging Findings

The patient had a conventional digital screening mammogram. In the lower inner quadrant of the left breast, there is a possible focal asymmetry (▶ Fig. 62.3 and ▶ Fig. 62.4).

62.3 BI-RADS Classification and Action

Category 0: Mammography: Incomplete. Need additional imaging evaluation and/or prior mammograms for comparison.

62.4 Diagnostic Images

(▶ Fig. 62.5, ▶ Fig. 62.6, ▶ Fig. 62.7)

62.4.1 Imaging Findings

The diagnostic imaging demonstrates a possible persistent asymmetry on the craniocaudal (CC) spot-compression mammogram (▶ Fig. 62.5). The mediolateral oblique (MLO) spot-compression (▶ Fig. 62.6) and medioateral (ML) mammograms (▶ Fig. 62.7) are less suggestive of a true asymmetry. The corresponding CC and MLO digital breast tomosynthesis (DBT) movies demonstrate that the focal asymmetry seen on screening mammography is a summation artifact created by overlapping tissues in the same imaging plane.

62.5 BI-RADS Classification and Action

Category 1: Negative

62.6 Differential Diagnosis

1. **Summation artifact (superimposition of breast tissue)**: The DBT movies obtained at the diagnostic evaluation best demonstrated that this asymmetry is created by overlapping tissue.
2. *Radial scar*: Subtle asymmetries can represent a radial scar. The DBT images did not support any underlying architectural distortion or other suspicious findings.
3. *Carcinoma*: Carcinomas can initially present as subtle findings, especially lobular carcinoma. It is reassuring that the DBT images revealed overlapping tissue.

62.7 Essential Facts

- Many screening mammograms are recalled for summation artifacts.
- DBT is designed to reduce the summation effects of overlapping tissues and improve lesion conspicuity.
- DBT makes suspicious findings more apparent and helps the reader to recognize normal structures more clearly.
- In DBT the reconstruction of the three-dimensional breast image into slices helps to uncover those areas of overlapping tissue.

62.8 Management and Digital Breast Tomosynthesis Principles

- DBT has demonstrated a reduction in recall rate from 7 to 15% in clinical studies.
- Improvements in sensitivity and specificity are seen on DBT irrespective of breast tissue density.
- DBT is approved for screening and diagnostic mammography imaging. The role in breast imaging is evolving.
- Drawbacks to DBT are the increased radiation for combination exams (FFDM and DBT) and the increased time for reading a study (reported as twice the time).
- DBT produces extremely large data files that require extra PACS (picture archiving and communication system) storage capacity.

62.9 Further Reading

[1] Brandt KR, Craig DA, Hoskins TL, et al. Can digital breast tomosynthesis replace conventional diagnostic mammography views for screening recalls without calcifications? A comparison study in a simulated clinical setting. AJR Am J Roentgenol. 2013; 200(2):291–298

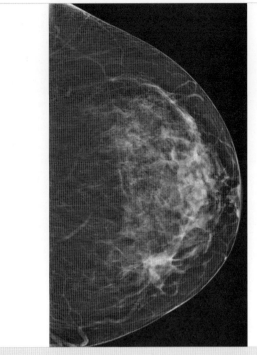

Fig. 62.1 Left craniocaudal (LCC) mammogram.

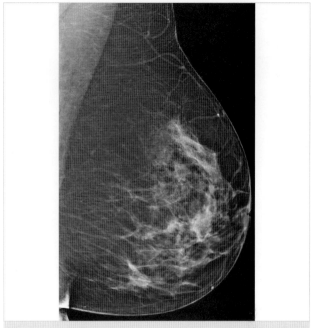

Fig. 62.2 Left mediolateral oblique (LMLO) mammogram.

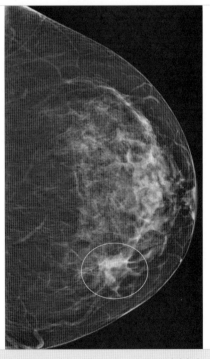

Fig. 62.3 Left craniocaudal (LCC) mammogram with label.

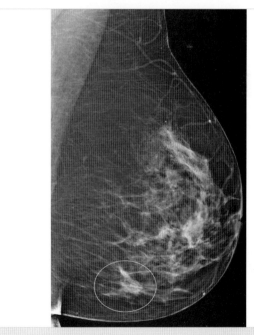

Fig. 62.4 Left mediolateral oblique (LMLO) mammogram with label.

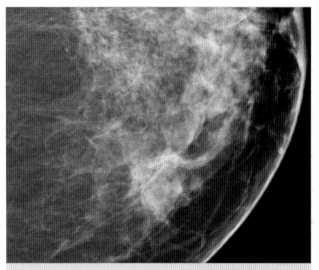

Fig. 62.5 Left craniocaudal (LCC) spot-compression mammogram.

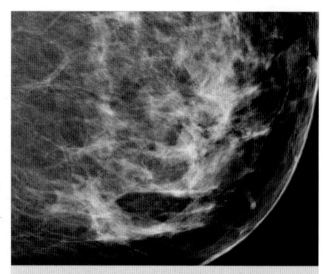

Fig. 62.6 Left mediolateral oblique (LMLO) spot-compression mammogram.

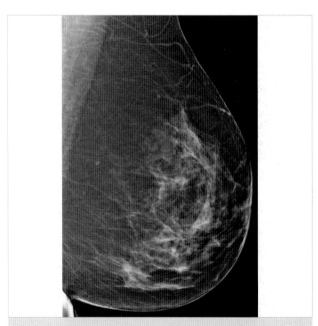

Fig. 62.7 Left mediolateral (LML) mammogram.

63 Architectural Distortion within Dense Breast Tissue

Tanya W. Moseley

63.1 Presentation and Presenting Images

(▶ Fig. 63.1, ▶ Fig. 63.2, ▶ Fig. 63.3, ▶ Fig. 63.4)

A 63-year-old female with a history of left breast cancer treated with segmentectomy and radiation therapy presents for routine screening mammography.

63.2 Key Images

(▶ Fig. 63.5, ▶ Fig. 63.6, ▶ Fig. 63.7, ▶ Fig. 63.8)

63.2.1 Breast Tissue Density

The breasts are heterogeneously dense, which may obscure small masses.

63.2.2 Imaging Findings

There is a possible 1-cm architectural distortion (*circle* in ▶ Fig. 63.5 and ▶ Fig. 63.7) in the posterior depth of the right breast's upper outer quadrant at the 11 o'clock location, 7 cm from the nipple. There is a postsurgical scar in the left breast denoted by a scar marker (*arrow* in ▶ Fig. 63.6 and ▶ Fig. 63.8). Clinical information regarding a prior procedure on the right breast would be helpful. The patient reports that she has not undergone any right breast procedures. Additional diagnostic mammography with possible ultrasound are recommended.

63.3 BI-RADS Classification and Action

Category 0: Mammography: Incomplete. Need additional imaging evaluation and/or prior mammograms for comparison.

63.4 Diagnostic Images

(▶ Fig. 63.9, ▶ Fig. 63.10, ▶ Fig. 63.11, ▶ Fig. 63.12, ▶ Fig. 63.13)

63.4.1 Imaging Findings

Slices from the digital breast tomosynthesis movies confirm architectural distortion (*circle* in ▶ Fig. 63.11 and ▶ Fig. 63.12) in the right breast at the 11 o'clock position in the posterior depth, 7 cm from the nipple.

Ultrasound shows a 1-cm hypoechoic area of architectural distortion that corresponds to the mammographic finding (▶ Fig. 63.13). This finding is suspicious and an ultrasound-guided biopsy was performed.

63.5 BI-RADS Classification and Action

Category 4B: Moderate suspicion for malignancy

63.6 Differential Diagnosis

1. *Focal fibrosis*: Focal fibrosis, also known as stromal fibrosis, has a variety of appearances.
2. *Radial scar*: Radial scars usually present as an area of architectural distortion.
3. *Postprocedure changes*: Postprocedure changes may present as areas of architectural distortion. The lack of prior procedures makes this an unlikely possibility.

63.7 Essential Facts

- Although its prevalence on mammography is small compared with masses or calcifications, architectural distortion may be more challenging to diagnose due to its subtle and variable appearance.
- Architectural distortion is a common finding in retrospective assessments of false-negative mammograms and may represent an early manifestation of breast cancer.
- Focal fibrosis is characterized by the proliferation of the stromal connective tissue with obliteration of the mammary ducts and lobules.
- Focal fibrosis has been called by many names, including stromal fibrosis, focal fibrous disease of the breast, fibrous mastopathy, fibrous tumor of the breast, and chronic indurative mastitis.
- On mammography and ultrasound, the appearance of focal fibrosis is variable from benign-appearing to suspicious-appearing.

63.8 Management and Digital Breast Tomosynthesis Principles

- Digital breast tomosynthesis (DBT) allows for improved visualization of architectural distortion over conventional mammography.
- In this case, the finding was seen well only on the craniocaudal (CC) view on conventional mammography but on both views with DBT.
- If the finding had been seen on only one view with DBT, its position in the orthogonal view could have been determined.
- Tomosynthesis-directed stereotactic biopsy could have been performed rather than ultrasound-guided biopsy. Ultrasound-guided biopsy is more convenient for many patients given that the biopsy can be performed without compression and with the patient in a recumbent position.

63.9 Further Reading

[1] Gaur S, Dialani V, Slanetz PJ, Eisenberg RL. Architectural distortion of the breast. AJR Am J Roentgenol. 2013; 201(5):W662-W670

[2] Rangayyan RM, Banik S, Desautels JEL. Computer-aided detection of architectural distortion in prior mammograms of interval cancer. J Digit Imaging. 2010; 23(5):611–631

[3] You JK, Kim E-K, Kwak JY, et al. Focal fibrosis of the breast diagnosed by a sonographically guided core biopsy of nonpalpable lesions: imaging findings and clinical relevance. J Ultrasound Med. 2005; 24(10):1377–1384

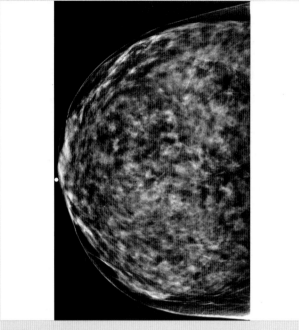

Fig. 63.1 Right craniocaudal (RCC) mammogram.

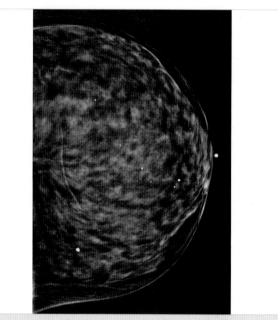

Fig. 63.2 Left craniocaudal (LCC) mammogram.

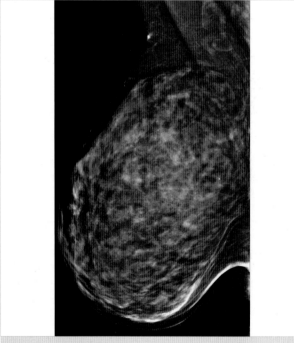

Fig. 63.3 Right mediolateral oblique (RMLO) mammogram.

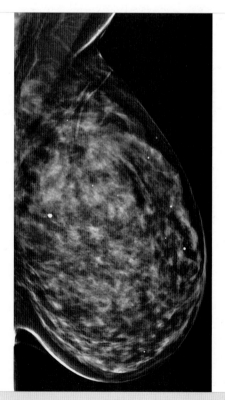

Fig. 63.4 Left mediolateral oblique (LMLO) mammogram.

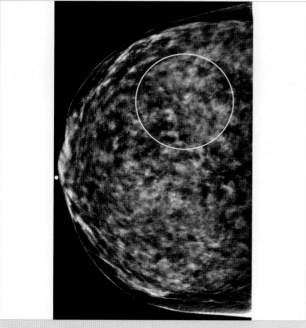

Fig. 63.5 Right craniocaudal (RCC) mammogram with label.

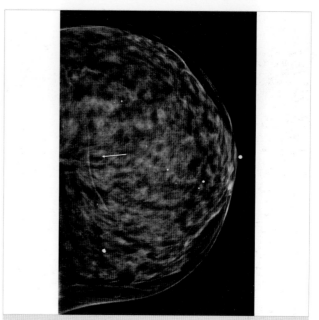

Fig. 63.6 Left craniocaudal (LCC) mammogram with label.

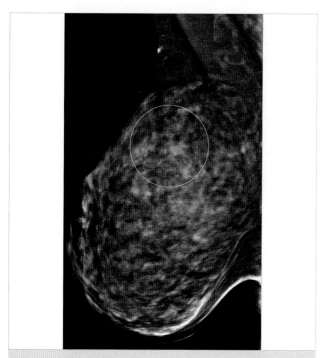

Fig. 63.7 Right mediolateral oblique (RMLO) mammogram with label.

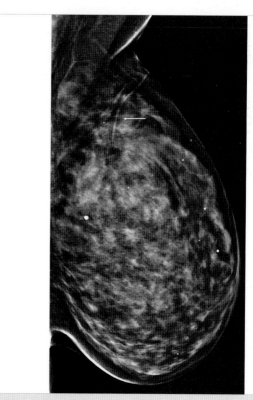

Fig. 63.8 Left mediolateral oblique (LMLO) mammogram with label.

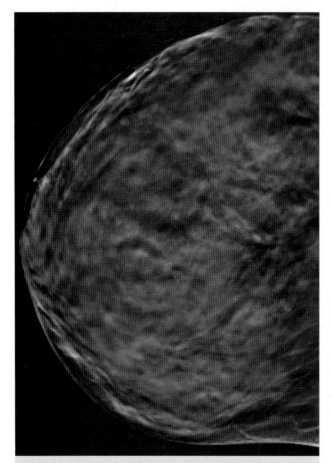

Fig. 63.9 Right craniocaudal digital breast tomosynthesis (RCC DBT), slice 22 of 68.

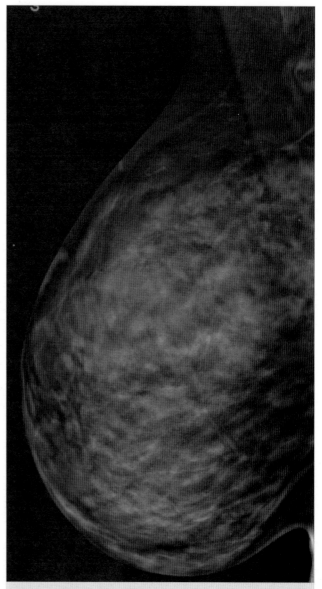

Fig. 63.10 Right lateromedial digital breast tomosynthesis (RLM DBT), slice 55 of 72.

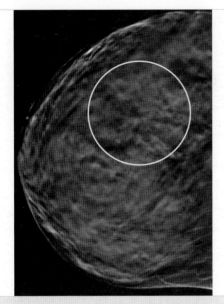

Fig. 63.11 Right craniocaudal digital breast tomosynthesis (RCC DBT), slice 22 of 68 with label.

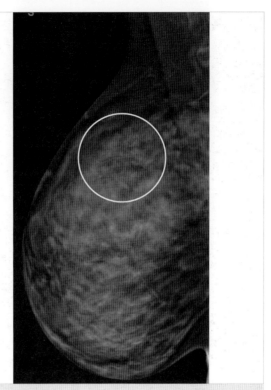

Fig. 63.12 Right lateromedial digital breast tomosynthesis (RLM DT), slice 55 of 72 with label.

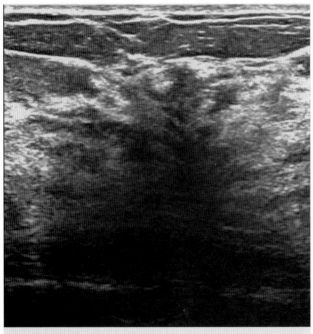

Fig. 63.13 Right breast ultrasound.

64 Architectural Distortion with Negative Ultrasound

Lonie R. Salkowski

64.1 Presentation and Presenting Images

(► Fig. 64.1, ► Fig. 64.2, ► Fig. 64.3)

A 40-year-old female presents for baseline screening mammography.

64.2 Key Images

(► Fig. 64.4, ► Fig. 64.5)

64.2.1 Breast Tissue Density

The breasts are heterogeneously dense, which may obscure small masses.

64.2.2 Imaging Findings

The patient had a conventional digital screening mammogram. There is a possible area of architectural distortion seen posteriorly and superiorly in the left breast around the 12 o'clock location (► Fig. 64.4 and ► Fig. 64.5).

64.3 BI-RADS Classification and Action

Category 0: Mammography: Incomplete. Need additional imaging evaluation and/or prior mammograms for comparison.

64.4 Diagnostic Images

(► Fig. 64.6, ► Fig. 64.7, ► Fig. 64.8, ► Fig. 64.9)

64.4.1 Imaging Findings

As part of the diagnostic imaging, the patient had digital breast tomosynthesis (DBT) of the left breast. Only the DBT images are shown here, and they demonstrate a focal area of architectural distortion (► Fig. 64.8 and ► Fig. 64.9). An ultrasound following the diagnostic imaging did not provide a sonographic correlate to the findings on DBT. The patient was biopsied with stereotactic guidance.

64.5 BI-RADS Classification and Action

Category 4B: Moderate suspicion for malignancy

64.6 Differential Diagnosis

1. **Radial scar**: Radial scars when seen mammographically most often present as architectural distortion. DBT is especially effective at identifying architectural distortion.
2. *Carcinoma*: Architectural distortion, although less common than other imaging findings, has a high probability of being carcinoma when identified mammographically. This would be considered a concordant diagnosis.
3. *Normal breast tissue*: Normal breast tissue does not typically appear as architectural distortion. Even on a baseline mammographic examination, architectural distortion should be completely evaluated and this may require a biopsy.

64.7 Essential Facts

- The estimated prevalence of architectural distortion on conventional screening digital mammography is 6%.
- *A CR BI-RADS Atlas, 5th edition*, defines architectural distortion as distortion of the parenchyma with no definite mass visible.
- Architectural distortion can be associated with an asymmetry or calcifications.
- Architectural distortion is often undetected on conventional digital mammography and is one of the main sources of false-negative mammograms.

64.8 Management and Digital Breast Tomosynthesis Principles

- Partyka and colleagues (2014) raised the possibility that areas of architectural distortion seen only on DBT and occult on conventional mammography and ultrasound are more likely to be a radial sclerosing lesion than carcinoma.
- DBT is expensive to add into a practice. The expense is not only in the mammography equipment, but also in the storage of large data files and the workstations that are needed to view the image sets.
- There is no uniform adoption of DBT into screening or diagnostic mammogram imaging protocols.

64.9 Further Reading

[1] Partyka L, Lourenco AP, Mainiero MB. Detection of mammographically occult architectural distortion on digital breast tomosynthesis screening: initial clinical experience. AJR Am J Roentgenol. 2014; 203(1):216–222

[2] Shaheen R, Schimmelpenninck CA, Stoddart L, Raymond H, Slanetz PJ. Spectrum of diseases presenting as architectural distortion on mammography: multimodality radiologic imaging with pathologic correlation. Semin Ultrasound CT MR. 2011; 32(4):351–362

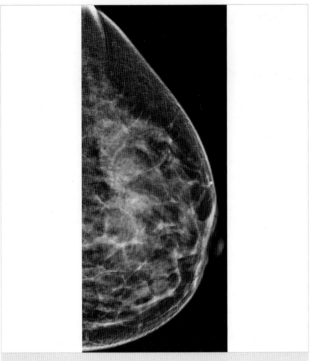

Fig. 64.1 Exaggerated left craniocaudal (XLCC) mammogram.

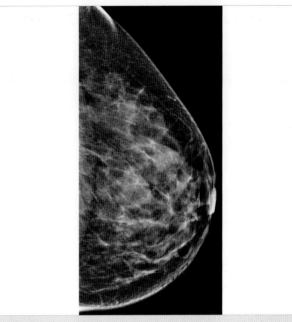

Fig. 64.2 Left craniocaudal (LCC) mammogram.

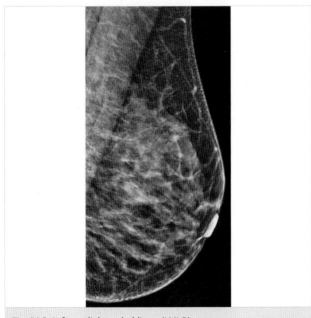

Fig. 64.3 Left mediolateral oblique (LMLO) mammogram.

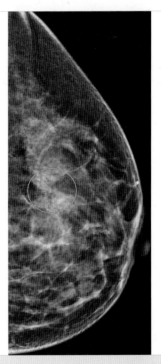

Fig. 64.4 Exaggerated left craniocaudal (XLCC) mammogram with label.

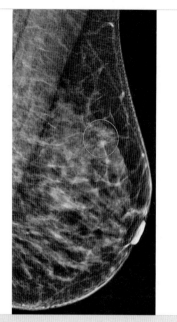

Fig. 64.5 Left mediolateral oblique (LMLO) mammogram with label.

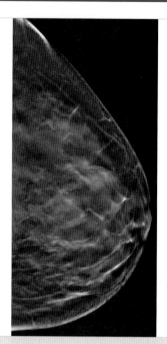

Fig. 64.6 Left craniocaudal digital breast tomosynthesis (LCC DBT), slice 31 of 58.

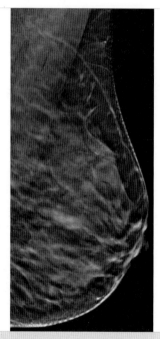

Fig. 64.7 Left mediolateral oblique digital breast tomosynthesis (LMLO DBT), slice 22 of 55.

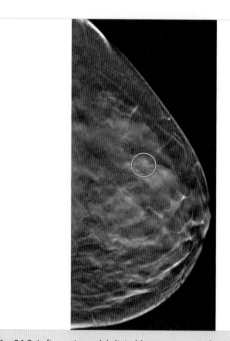

Fig. 64.8 Left craniocaudal digital breast tomosynthesis (LCC DBT), slice 31 of 58 with label.

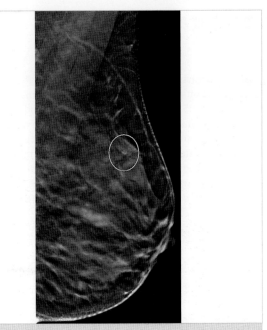

Fig. 64.9 Left mediolateral oblique digital breast tomosynthesis (LMLO DBT), slice 22 of 55 with label.

65 Focal Asymmetry with Architectural Distortion

Tanya W. Moseley

65.1 Presentation and Presenting Images

(▶ Fig. 65.1, ▶ Fig. 65.2)

A 69-year-old female presents for routine screening mammography.

65.2 Key Images

(▶ Fig. 65.3, ▶ Fig. 65.4)

65.2.1 Breast Tissue Density

The breasts are heterogeneously dense, which may obscure small masses.

65.2.2 Imaging Findings

The imaging of the right breast is normal (*not shown*). The left breast demonstrates a focal asymmetry at the 11 to 12 o'clock location in the middle depth, 6 cm from the nipple (*circle* in ▶ Fig. 65.3 and ▶ Fig. 65.4). There are coarse calcifications nearby but these calcifications have been stable for many years.

Because the screening mammogram was performed without digital breast tomosynthesis (DBT), DBT followed by ultrasound is the next step in the imaging evaluation. DBT can confirm a true mass lesion or determine if the screen-detected asymmetry is the result of parenchymal overlap. If the finding is a true lesion, sonography is recommended for further characterization and biopsy. If the mass is a true lesion and not identified by ultrasound, tomosynthesis-directed stereotactic-guided biopsy can be performed.

65.3 BI-RADS Classification and Action

Category 0: Mammography: Incomplete. Need additional imaging evaluation and/or prior mammograms for comparison.

65.4 Diagnostic Imaging

(▶ Fig. 65.5, ▶ Fig. 65.6, ▶ Fig. 65.7, ▶ Fig. 65.8, ▶ Fig. 65.9, ▶ Fig. 65.10, ▶ Fig. 65.11, ▶ Fig. 65.12, ▶ Fig. 65.13, ▶ Fig. 65.14, ▶ Fig. 65.15, ▶ Fig. 65.16)

65.4.1 Imaging Findings

Slices from the left DBT movies (▶ Fig. 65.5, ▶ Fig. 65.6, ▶ Fig. 65.7, ▶ Fig. 65.8, ▶ Fig. 65.9, ▶ Fig. 65.10, ▶ Fig. 65.11, and ▶ Fig. 65.12) demonstrate a focal asymmetry (*circle*) measuring 7 mm at the 12 o'clock location in the middle depth, 6 cm from the nipple. There is associated architectural distortion.

On left breast ultrasound, there is a subtle area of architectural distortion at the 11 to 12 o'clock location, 6 cm from the nipple (▶ Fig. 65.13 and ▶ Fig. 65.14), corresponding to the area of architectural distortion on the mammogram and DBT. Ultrasound-guided core needle biopsy is indicated and subsequently performed. Pathology was consistent with ductal carcinoma in situ (DCIS). A postbiopsy mammogram shows mammographic–sonographic correlation and adequate placement of the postbiopsy clip (*arrow* in ▶ Fig. 65.15 and ▶ Fig. 65.16).

65.5 BI-RADS Classification and Action

Category 5: Highly suggestive of malignancy

65.6 Differential Diagnosis

1. ***Breast cancer (ductal carcinoma in situ)***: D CIS most commonly presents as microcalcifications but may present as a mass, an architectural distortion, and as developing densities.
2. *Breast cancer (invasive carcinoma)*: Invasive ductal carcinoma is more likely than DCIS to present as a focal asymmetry. This would be a concordant diagnosis.
3. *Pseudomass*: DBT can confirm a true mass lesion or determine if the screen-detected asymmetry is the result of parenchymal overlap.

65.7 Essential Facts

- The incidence of DCIS rose from 1.87 per 100,000 in 1973 to 1975 to 32.5 in 2004. The increased use of mammography during this time period accounts for some but not all of the increase in incidence.
- DCIS typically presents as calcifications on mammography. The morphology of DCIS calcifications on mammography includes amorphous, coarse heterogeneous, fine pleomorphic, and fine-linear or fine-linear branching types.
- Not all cases of DCIS present as calcifications. Less common presentations include masses, asymmetries, architectural distortions, dilated retroareolar ducts, or developing asymmetries.
- Although unable to perform magnification views of calcifications suspicious for DCIS, DBT can detect, characterize, and localize the less common presentations of DCIS.

65.8 Management and Digital Breast Tomosynthesis Principles

- DBT has shown superior performance in the detection of masses and architectural distortions. In this case specifically, the architectural distortion associated with the focal asymmetry was undetected on the conventional two-dimensional

(2D) mammogram. DBT imaging can better characterize masses and architectural distortions due to the reduction in breast parenchymal overlap.

- Subtle lesions may only be identifiable on DBT and will require DBT-tomosynthesis-directed stereotactic-guided biopsy. Using the breast tomosynthesis unit, one DBT scan is performed, the lesion is targeted, and the x, y, z location of the lesion calculated directly from the three-dimensional (3D) image.

- Virnig and colleagues (2010) concluded that further investigation is needed to the determine which DCIS lesions are destined to become clinically problematic. DBT may be helpful in this investigation.

65.9 Further Reading

[1] Evans A, Pinder S, Wilson R, et al. Ductal carcinoma in situ of the breast: correlation between mammographic and pathologic findings. AJR Am J Roentgenol. 1994; 162(6):1307–1311

[2] Ikeda DM, Andersson I. Ductal carcinoma in situ: atypical mammographic appearances. Radiology. 1989; 172(3):661–666

[3] Mitnick JS, Roses DF, Harris MN, Feiner HD. Circumscribed intraductal carcinoma of the breast. Radiology. 1989; 170(2):423–425

[4] Virnig BA, Tuttle TM, Shamliyan T, Kane RL. Ductal carcinoma in situ of the breast: a systematic review of incidence, treatment, and outcomes. J Natl Cancer Inst. 2010; 102(3):170–178

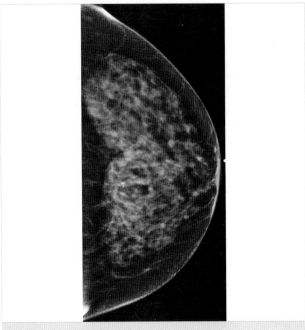

Fig. 65.1 Left craniocaudal (LCC) mammogram.

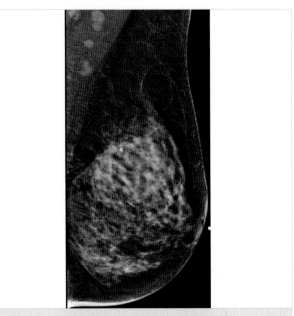

Fig. 65.2 Left mediolateral oblique (LMLO) mammogram.

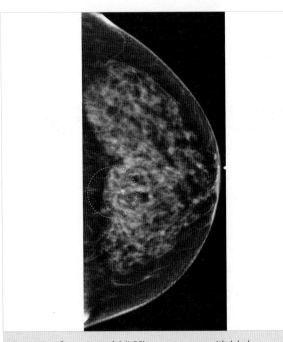

Fig. 65.3 Left craniocaudal (LCC) mammogram with label.

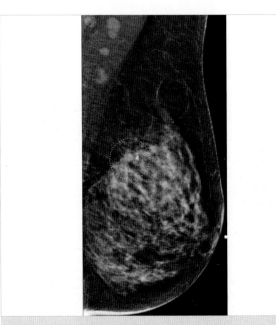

Fig. 65.4 Left mediolateral oblique (LMLO) mammogram with label.

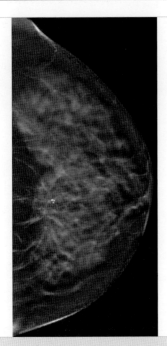

Fig. 65.5 Left craniocaudal digital breast tomosynthesis (LCC DBT), slice 40 of 66.

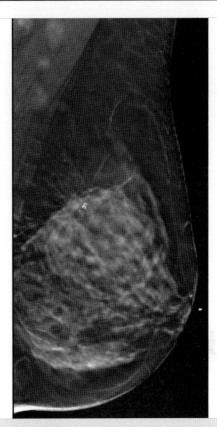

Fig. 65.6 Left mediolateral oblique digital breast tomosynthesis (LMLO DBT), slice 40 of 69.

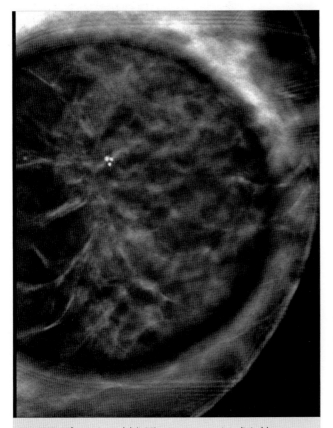

Fig. 65.7 Left craniocaudal (LCC) spot-compression digital breast tomosynthesis (DBT), slice 37 of 59.

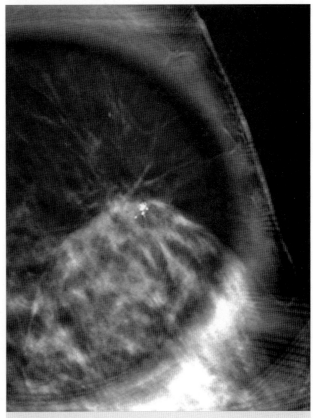

Fig. 65.8 Left lateromedial (LLM) spot-compression digital breast tomosynthesis (DBT), slice 24 of 58.

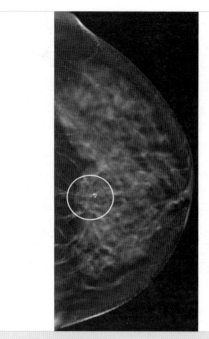

Fig. 65.9 Left craniocaudal digital breast tomosynthesis (LCC DBT), slice 40 of 66 with label.

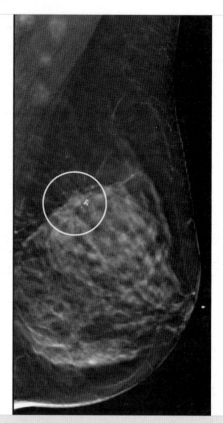

Fig. 65.10 Left mediolateral oblique digital breast tomosynthesis (LMLO DBT), slice 40 of 69 with label.

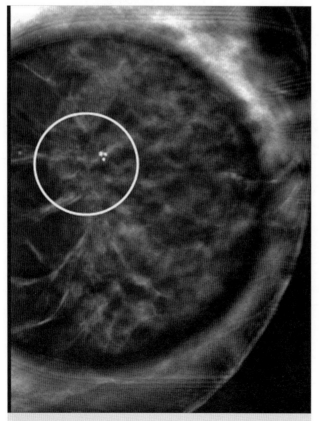

Fig. 65.11 Left craniocaudal (LCC) spot-compression digital breast tomosynthesis (DBT), slice 37 of 59 with label.

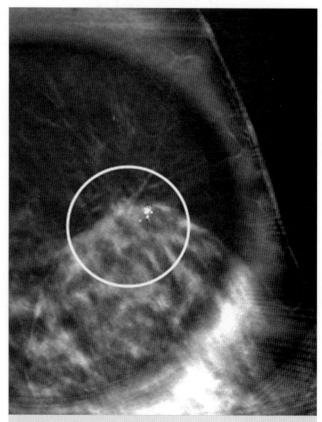

Fig. 65.12 Left lateromedial (LLM) spot-compression digital breast tomosynthesis (DBT), slice 24 of 58 with label.

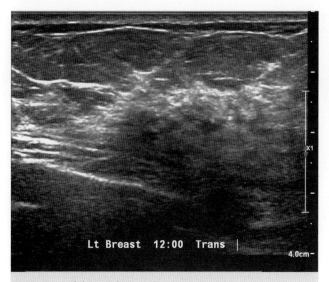

Fig. 65.13 Left breast ultrasound, transverse view.

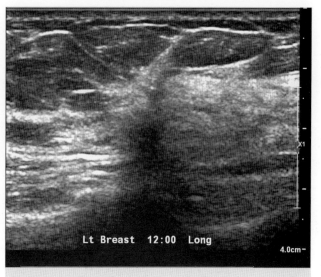

Fig. 65.14 Left breast ultrasound, longitudinal view.

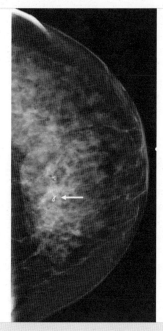

Fig. 65.15 Postbiopsy mammogram showing mammographic–sonographic correlation and adequate placement of the postbiopsy clip.

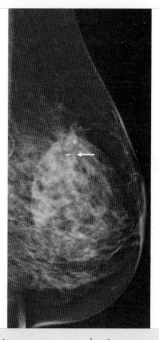

Fig. 65.16 Postbiopsy mammogram showing mammographic–sonographic correlation and adequate placement of the postbiopsy clip.

66 Focal Asymmetry—One or Two Lesions

Lonie R. Salkowski

66.1 Presentation and Presenting Images

(▶ Fig. 66.1, ▶ Fig. 66.2)

A 58-year-old female presents for asymptomatic screening mammography.

66.2 Key Images

(▶ Fig. 66.3, ▶ Fig. 66.4)

66.2.1 Breast Tissue Density

The breasts are heterogeneously dense, which may obscure small masses.

66.2.2 Imaging Findings

There is a 9-mm focal asymmetry in the left breast at the 11 o'clock location in the middle depth (▶ Fig. 66.3 and ▶ Fig. 66.4). It is best seen on the craniocaudal (CC) view (▶ Fig. 66.3). The mammogram of the right breast was normal (*not shown*).

66.3 BI-RADS Classification and Action

Category 0: Mammography: Incomplete. Need additional imaging evaluation and/or prior mammograms for comparison.

66.4 Diagnostic Images 1

(▶ Fig. 66.5, ▶ Fig. 66.6, ▶ Fig. 66.7, ▶ Fig. 66.8, ▶ Fig. 66.9, ▶ Fig. 66.10, ▶ Fig. 66.11)

66.4.1 Imaging Findings

The diagnostic imaging confirms a 10×4×9 mm round mass with spiculated margins at 11 o'clock in the anterior depth (▶ Fig. 66.5, ▶ Fig. 66.6, and ▶ Fig. 66.7). The targeted ultrasound demonstrates a 10×14×9 mm irregular mass located at 11 to 12 o'clock, 4 cm from the nipple (▶ Fig. 66.8 and ▶ Fig. 66.9). A biopsy was recommended. The ribbon clip placed at the time of biopsy is noted to be 10 mm lateral and 10 mm superior to the mammographic mass (▶ Fig. 66.10 and ▶ Fig. 66.11).

66.5 BI-RADS Classification and Action

Category 4C: High suspicion for malignancy

66.6 Diagnostic Images 2

(▶ Fig. 66.12, ▶ Fig. 66.13, ▶ Fig. 66.14, ▶ Fig. 66.15, ▶ Fig. 66.16, ▶ Fig. 66.17, ▶ Fig. 66.18, ▶ Fig. 66.19, ▶ Fig. 66.20)

66.6.1 Imaging Findings

The patient returned for additional evaluation. A craniocaudal (CC) and a mediolateral oblique (MLO) tomosynthesis combination examination was performed to localize both masses (▶ Fig. 66.12 and ▶ Fig. 66.13). The original mass seen on the screening mammogram is again identified (▶ Fig. 66.14 and ▶ Fig. 66.15) on the digital breast tomosynthesis (DBT) images. With the presence of the biopsy clip, the more superficial mass is also localized on the DBT images (▶ Fig. 66.16 and ▶ Fig. 66.17). A second ultrasound examination was performed and the smaller and deeper mass at the 11 o'clock location, 4 cm from the nipple, originally noted on the mammogram, is seen as a hypoechoic mass with indistinct margins (▶ Fig. 66.18). With further examination, the two masses can be seen in the same area on the ultrasound (the larger, more superficial mass has an echogenic clip present) (▶ Fig. 66.19). The patient underwent a magnetic resonance (MR) examination, which revealed the two masses seen on the mammogram and ultrasound imaging. Additional masses can be seen on the MR that were not appreciated on either examination (▶ Fig. 66.20).

66.7 Differential Diagnosis

1. ***Multifocal breast cancer***: Multifocal cancer is defined as multiple lesions within 4 to 5 cm of each other and often in the same quadrant. This case represents a multifocal cancer which at presentation was thought to be a single-focus cancer.
2. *Multicentric breast cancer*: Multicentric cancer involves lesions farther than 5 cm apart and in two distinct quadrants.
3. *Multiple fibroadenomas*: Although multiple fibroadenomas can exist, the imaging of these masses appears more suspicious. A biopsy yielding a fibroadenoma would be considered discordant.

66.8 Essential Facts

- This case demonstrates that care must be taken to correlate the location of lesions seen mammographically and sonographically. The initial mammographic lesion did not correlate with the sonographic lesion. The placement of the biopsy marker helped to detect that mismatch.
- A postprocedure mammogram is very helpful in demonstrating the presence of the biopsy marker clip and for future planning.
- The subsequent imaging confirmed the presence of at least two lesions, with the MRI confirming multiple additional foci.

- MRI identifies additional sites of cancer in the ipsilateral breast in 27% of patients with biopsy-proven breast cancer. Nearly three-quarters of these additional cancers are located in the same quadrant as the index (primary or presenting) cancer and about a quarter in another quadrant.
- Women with a family history of breast cancer are more likely to have multifocal or multicentric breast cancer compared to women without a family history of breast cancer.

66.9 Management and Digital Breast Tomosynthesis Principles

- DBT has the potential for assisting with the detection of multifocal and multicentric cancers.

- DBT's ability to reduce the anatomical noise of the breast tissue, and not be affected by the density of the breast tissue, affords it the ability to better perceive tumors. It may also help in recognizing complex tumor growth patterns including multiple tumors. Additional investigation is needed as use of DBT becomes more widespread.

66.10 Further Reading

[1] Förnvik D, Zackrisson S, Ljungberg O, et al. Breast tomosynthesis: Accuracy of tumor measurement compared with digital mammography and ultrasonography. Acta Radiol. 2010; 51(3):240–247

[2] Liberman L, Morris EA, Dershaw DD, Abramson AF, Tan LK. MR imaging of the ipsilateral breast in women with percutaneously proven breast cancer. AJR Am J Roentgenol. 2003; 180(4):901–910

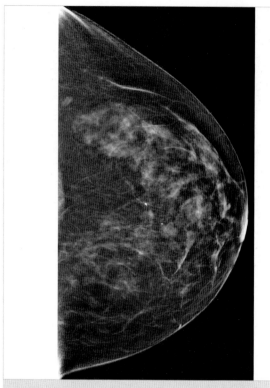

Fig. 66.1 Left craniocaudal (LCC) mammogram.

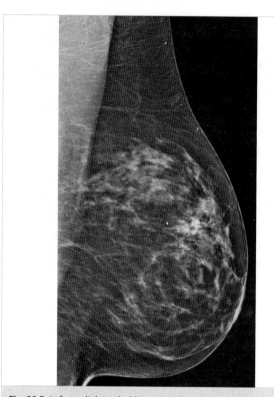

Fig. 66.2 Left mediolateral oblique (LMLO) mammogram.

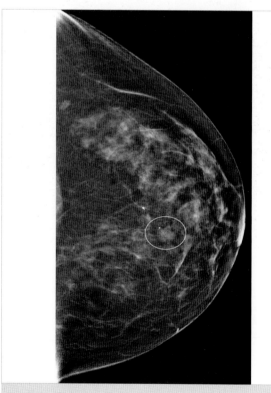

Fig. 66.3 Left craniocaudal (LCC) mammogram with label.

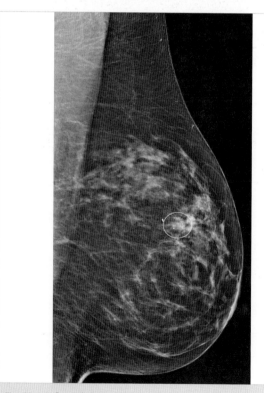

Fig. 66.4 Left mediolateral oblique (LMLO) mammogram with label.

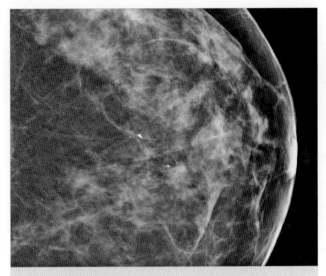

Fig. 66.5 Left craniocaudal (LCC) spot-compression mammogram.

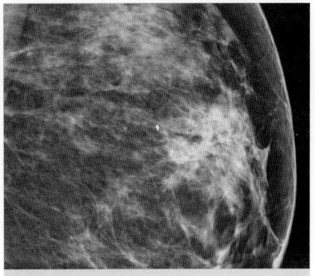

Fig. 66.6 Left mediolateral oblique (LMLO) spot-compression mammogram.

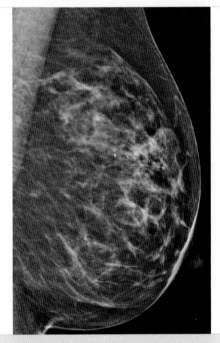

Fig. 66.7 Left mediolateral (LML) mammogram.

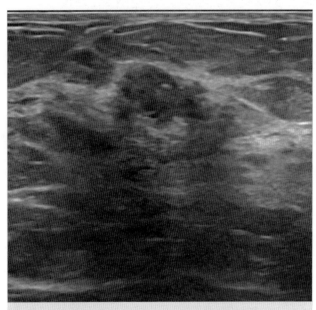

Fig. 66.8 Left breast ultrasound, transverse view.

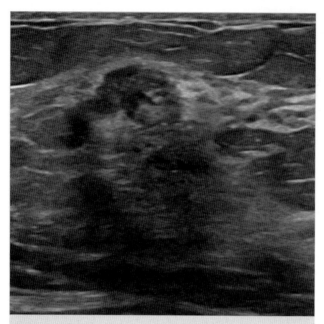

Fig. 66.9 Left breast ultrasound, longitudinal view.

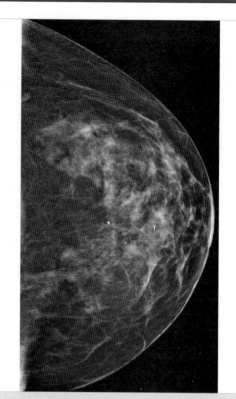

Fig. 66.10 Postbiopsy left craniocaudal (LCC) mammogram.

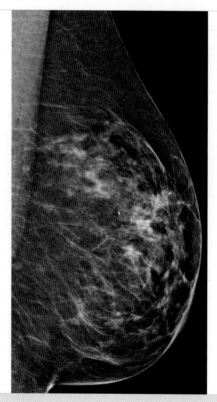

Fig. 66.11 Postbiopsy left mediolateral (LML) mammogram.

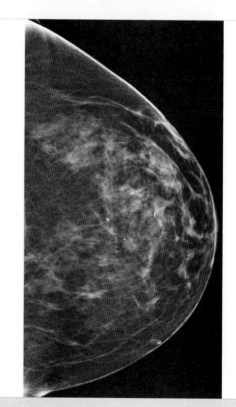

Fig. 66.12 Left craniocaudal (LCC) FFDM from combination digital breast tomosynthesis (DBT).

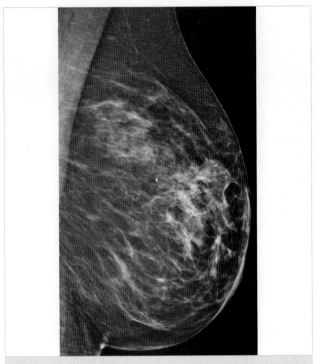

Fig. 66.13 Left mediolateral oblique (LMLO) FFDM from combination digital breast tomosynthesis (DBT).

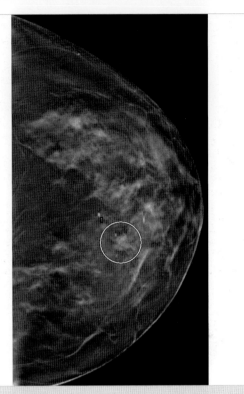

Fig. 66.14 Left craniocaudal digital breast tomosynthesis (LCC DBT), slice 47 of 81, with label.

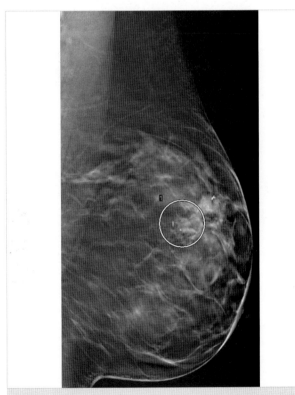

Fig. 66.15 Left mediolateral oblique digital breast tomosynthesis (LMLO DBT), slice 52 of 83, with label.

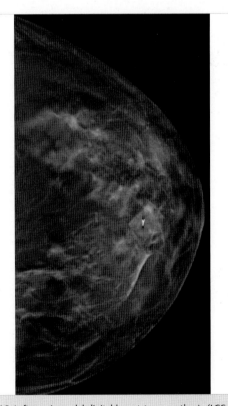

Fig. 66.16 Left craniocaudal digital breast tomosynthesis (LCC DBT), slice 57 of 81.

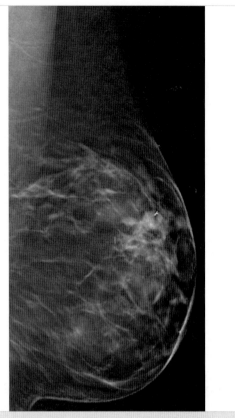

Fig. 66.17 Left mediolateral oblique digital breast tomosynthesis (LMLO DBT), slice 57 of 83.

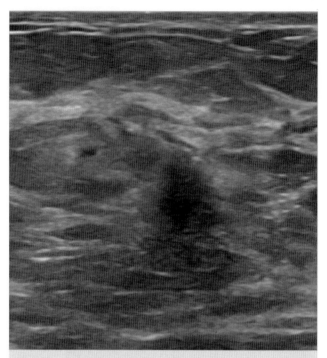

Fig. 66.18 Left breast ultrasound of smaller masses 4 cm from nipple.

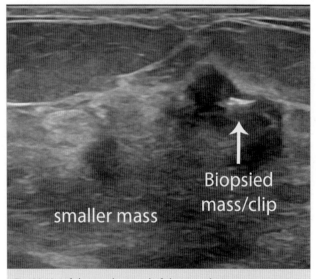

smaller mass

Biopsied mass/clip

Fig. 66.19 Left breast ultrasound of the two adjacent masses 4 cm from nipple.

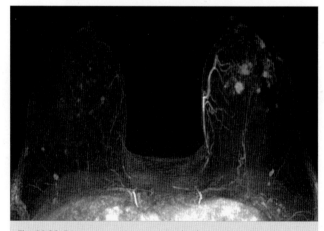

Fig. 66.20 Breast magnetic resonance (MR) maximum-intensity projection (MIP) image.

67 Asymmetry on the Craniocaudal View

Tanya W. Moseley

67.1 Presentation and Presenting Images

(▶ Fig. 67.1, ▶ Fig. 67.2, ▶ Fig. 67.3, ▶ Fig. 67.4, ▶ Fig. 67.5, ▶ Fig. 67.6)

A 65-year-old female with a history of a right mastectomy for intraductal and invasive ductal carcinoma presents for routine screening mammography.

67.2 Key Images

(▶ Fig. 67.7)

67.2.1 Breast Tissue Density

The breasts are heterogeneously dense, which may obscure small masses.

67.2.2 Imaging Findings

The patient had a right mastectomy. The left breast demonstrates a 1-cm asymmetry (*circle* in ▶ Fig. 67.7) seen only on the craniocaudal (CC) view. It is located in the posterior depth, 8.5 cm from the nipple. This represents a new finding since the prior mammogram. The two stereotactic clips (T-shaped and rod-shaped) denote the sites of prior benign biopsies.

67.3 BI-RADS Classification and Action

Category 0: Mammography: Incomplete. Need additional imaging evaluation and/or prior mammograms for comparison.

67.4 Diagnostic Images

(▶ Fig. 67.8, ▶ Fig. 67.9)

67.4.1 Imaging Findings

The finding is much less conspicuous with spot compression and has an appearance most consistent with undercompressed breast tissue (▶ Fig. 67.9). The spot-compression view and tomosynthesis confirm that the finding is secondary to overlapping breast tissue.

67.5 BI-RADS Classification and Action

Category 2: Benign

67.6 Differential Diagnosis

1. ***Overlapping breast tissue***: Undercompression can cause summation artifacts and pseudomasses.
2. *Fat necrosis*: This finding is in the immediate vicinity of one of the two stereotactic clips making fat necrosis a reasonable diagnostic consideration. This is unlikely because the finding is more conspicuous than noted on the prior study. Although fat necrosis can have a variety of appearances, it would be expected to become more lucent over time.
3. *Breast cancer*: Patients with a prior history of breast cancer are at an increased risk of developing another breast cancer. Cancers, specifically invasive lobular carcinomas, may present as a one-view finding.

67.7 Essential Facts

- Although the spot-compression view cleared the finding, the digital breast tomosynthesis (DBT) movie provided additional confirmation that the finding was the result of undercompression and overlapping breast tissue.
- Overlapping breast tissue is a common consequence of positioning and of compressing the breast to obtain a two-dimensional mammogram.
- Variability in positioning can have a greater effect on mammography than on other imaging modalities and produce summation artifacts seen on only one view.
- The most common cause of a one-view finding at screening mammography is overlapping breast tissue.
- Breast cancers may present as a subtle one-view finding or may go undetected on the second view.

67.8 Management and Digital Breast Tomosynthesis Principles

- Misinterpretation of one-view findings may lead to a missed or delayed cancer diagnosis.
- DBT reduces or eliminates the effect of overlapping breast tissue.
- DBT reduces the recall rate; however, the interpretation time for tomosynthesis is greater than the interpretation time for conventional mammography. This is the case with any new modality. In time, with use, the interpretation time should decrease.
- On the DBT movie, the area of the density was localized to the upper inner quadrant at the 10 to 11 o'clock location. Although it was not done in this case, a mediolateral (ML) tomosynthesis movie with attention to the superior breast could have been performed and would have provided additional evidence regarding the benignity of this finding.

67.9 Further Reading

[1] Giess CS, Frost EP, Birdwell RL. Interpreting one-view mammographic findings: minimizing callbacks while maximizing cancer detection. Radiographics. 2014; 34(4):928–940

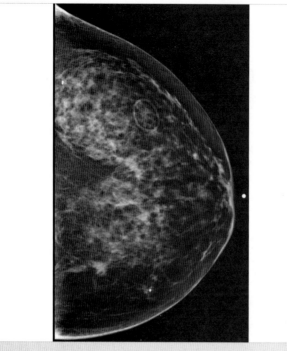

Fig. 67.1 Left craniocaudal (LCC) mammogram.

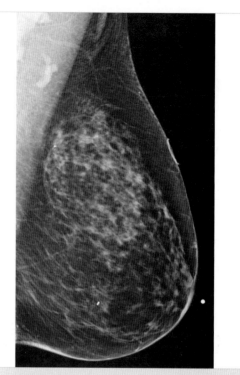

Fig. 67.2 Left mediolateral oblique (LMLO) mammogram.

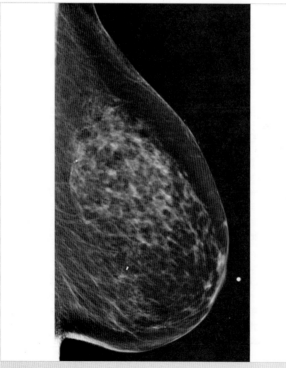

Fig. 67.3 Left lateromedial (LLM) mammogram.

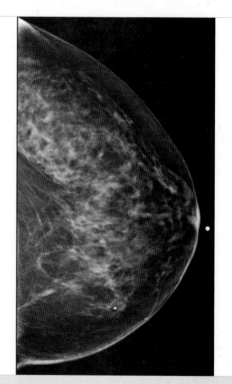

Fig. 67.4 Left craniocaudal (LCC) mammogram comparison.

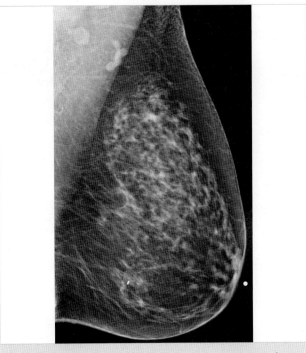

Fig. 67.5 Left mediolateral oblique LMLO mammogram comparison.

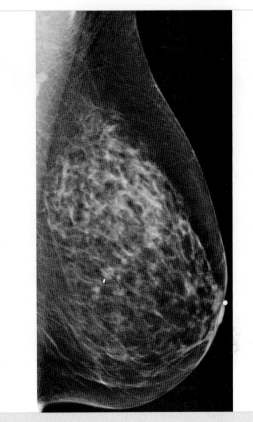

Fig. 67.6 Left lateromedial (LLM) mammogram comparison.

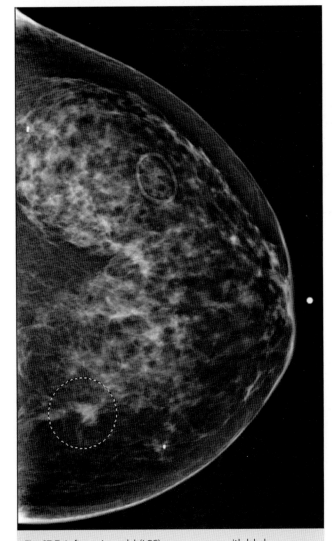

Fig. 67.7 Left craniocaudal (LCC) mammogram with label.

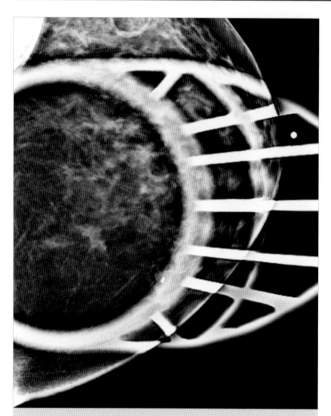

Fig. 67.8 Left craniocaudal (LCC) spot-compression mammogram.

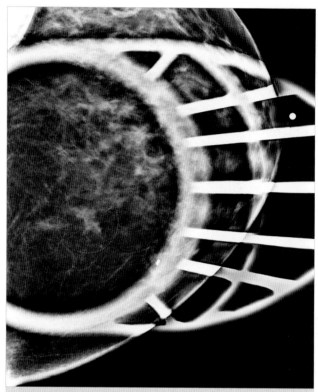

Fig. 67.9 Left craniocaudal (LCC) spot-compression mammogram with label.

68 Asymmetry on the Craniocaudal View

Lonie R. Salkowski

68.1 Presentation and Presenting Images

(▶ Fig. 68.1, ▶ Fig. 68.2)

A 64-year-old female presents for asymptomatic screening mammography.

68.2 Key Images

(▶ Fig. 68.3)

68.2.1 Breast Tissue Density

There are scattered areas of fibroglandular density.

68.2.2 Imaging Findings

The patient had a conventional digital screening mammogram. There is an asymmetry located just medial to the nipple in the middle depth on the craniocaudal (CC) view of the right breast (▶ Fig. 68.3). The left breast mammogram was normal. (*not shown*).

68.3 BI-RADS Classification and Action

Category 0: Mammography: Incomplete. Need additional imaging evaluation and/or prior mammograms for comparison.

68.4 Diagnostic Images 1

(▶ Fig. 68.4, ▶ Fig. 68.5, ▶ Fig. 68.6, ▶ Fig. 68.7, ▶ Fig. 68.8)

68.4.1 Imaging Findings

The main goal is to determine if this asymmetry is real and if it is, to localize it on the mediolateral oblique/ mediolateral (MLO/ML) projection. The rolled view confirms that the asymmetry is real (▶ Fig. 68.4 and ▶ Fig. 68.5). The repeat MLO and ML view (▶ Fig. 68.6 and ▶ Fig. 68.7) still does not define this asymmetry. The CC digital breast tomosynthesis (DBT) was performed to determine, by slice location, if it can be localized for further evaluation. The asymmetry is best seen on slice 36 of 57 (▶ Fig. 68.8), suggesting that it is near the middle but slightly superior to the middle.

68.5 Diagnostic Images 2

(▶ Fig. 68.9; ▶ Fig. 68.10; ▶ Fig. 68.11; ▶ Fig. 68.12; ▶ Fig. 68.13; ▶ Fig. 68.14)

68.5.1 Imaging Findings

The additional imaging does not define a clear lesion on the spot-compression MLO or ML views (▶ Fig. 68.10 and ▶ Fig. 68.11). Mammographically this mass is oval with indistinct and obscured margins and measures 9 mm in greatest dimension. The DBT images have determined that the mass is near the middle of the superior to inferior extent of the breast. This helps to localize the ultrasound search so that the reader can be confident that the area investigated on the ultrasound correlates to that of the finding on the mammogram. The ultrasound reveals a 9-mm oval hypoechoic mass with circumscribed and microlobulated margins located at the 3 o'clock location, 3 cm from the nipple (▶ Fig. 68.12). There is mild posterior enhancement on the right side of the mass. Although this mass may have several features that suggest it is benign, this mass was new on mammography, and so was biopsied by ultrasound. A ribbon clip was placed and a postbiopsy mammogram obtained (▶ Fig. 68.13 and ▶ Fig. 68.14).

(▶ Fig. 68.15)

68.6 BI-RADS Classification and Action

Category 4B: Moderate suspicion for malignancy

68.7 Differential Diagnosis

1. ***Invasive cancer (grade 3 invasive ductal carcinoma [IDC] with medullary features):*** Medullary carcinomas have a tendency to have benign imaging features. Historically these masses have been assessed as being benign by imaging, only to demonstrate an increase in size at follow-up.
2. *Fibroadenoma*: This mass had several benign attributes; however, this mass was new and warranted a biopsy. A biopsy result of fibroadenoma would not have been concordant.
3. *Complicated cyst*: Sonographically this mass could be mistaken for a cyst. However, the indistinct margins that were seen on the full-field digital mammography (FFDM) and digital breast tomosynthesis (DBT) images suggested that this mass should be biopsied.

68.8 Essential Facts

- Medullary carcinoma constitutes about 5% of breast cancers.
- Medullary carcinoma typically presents as a partially or well-circumscribed mass and, compared to other breast cancers, has benign features. It is often termed the circumscribed carcinoma.
- Mammographically, medullary carcinoma lesions appear as round or oval non-calcified masses.

- Sonographically, medullary carcinoma lesions are hypoechoic with mostly circumscribed margins and occasionally microlobulated margins. Often they have posterior acoustic enhancement, thus displaying a pseudocystic appearance.
- In medullary carcinoma, central necrosis is common in large tumors.
- Medullary carcinoma's benign imaging features can also be confused for lymphoma.
- Axillary adenopathy is common at presentation for medullary carcinoma. These appear to be reactive and not metastatic.

68.9 Management and Digital Breast Tomosynthesis Principles

- Step obliques and rolled views are diagnostic methods used to localize lesions that are often only seen on one view.
- DBT has the ability to localize a lesion from one view to its orthogonal location.
- The slider tool (► Fig. 68.15) that is present in some form on the imaging workstation allows the user to localize a mass by identifying the slice number of the one view in the stack, and by the orientation of the slider, can determine the head/foot or medial/lateral location of that view within the stack.
- As a result of localizing a one-view finding at a certain location within an image stack, the slider tool provides the reader the ability to triangulate the location in the other imaging plane. If the lesion is a mass, this localization can help focus a targeted ultrasound and improve correlation of the mammographic and sonographic findings.

68.10 Further Reading

[1] Cohen Y. Tomosynthesis assisting in localization of breast lesions for ultrasound targeting seen on one mammographic view only. AJR Am J Roentgenol. 2014; 203(5):W555–W555

[2] Meyer JE, Amin E, Lindfors KK, Lipman JC, Stomper PC, Genest D. Medullary carcinoma of the breast: mammographic and US appearance. Radiology. 1989; 170 1 Pt 1:79–82

[3] Yilmaz E, Lebe B, Balci P, Sal S, Canda T. Comparison of mammographic and sonographic findings in typical and atypical medullary carcinomas of the breast. Clin Radiol. 2002; 57(7):640–645

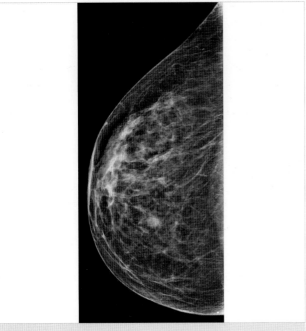

Fig. 68.1 Right craniocaudal (RCC) mammogram.

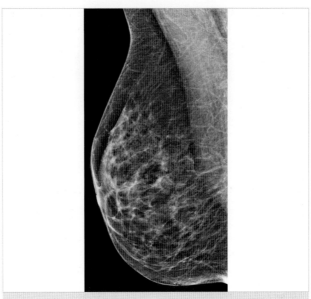

Fig. 68.2 Right mediolateral oblique (RMLO) mammogram.

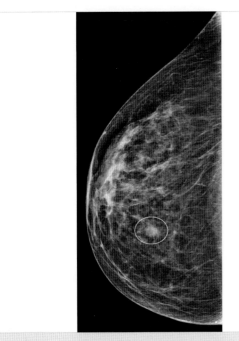

Fig. 68.3 Right craniocaudal (RCC) mammogram with label.

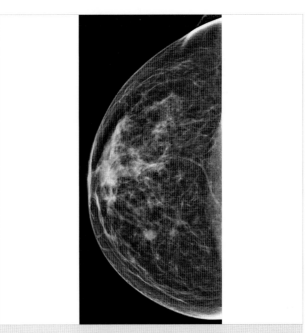

Fig. 68.4 Right craniocaudal (RCC) rolled medial mammogram.

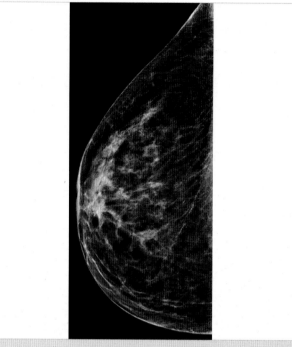

Fig. 68.5 Right craniocaudal RCC rolled lateral mammogram.

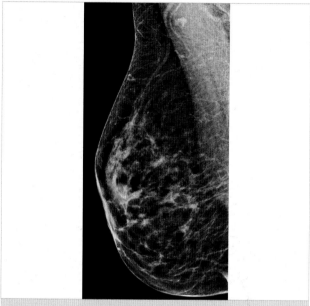

Fig. 68.6 Repeat right mediolateral oblique (RMLO) mammogram.

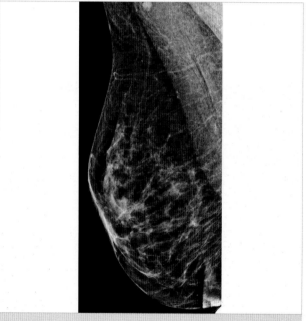

Fig. 68.7 Right mediolateral (RML) mammogram.

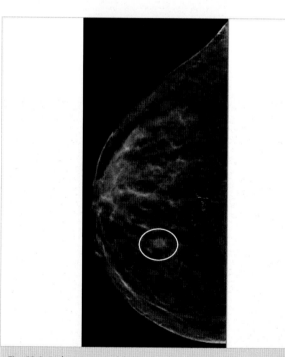

Fig. 68.8 Right craniocaudal digital breast tomosynthesis (RCC DBT), slice 36 of 57 with label.

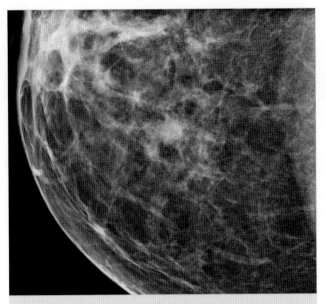

Fig. 68.9 Right craniocaudal (RCC) spot-compression mammogram.

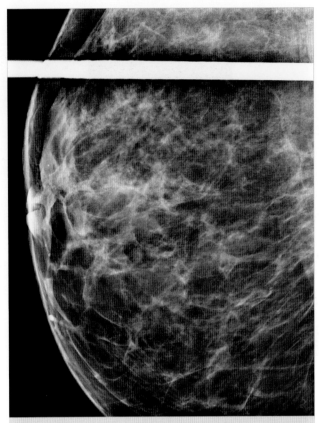

Fig. 68.10 Right mediolateral oblique (RMLO) spot-compression mammogram.

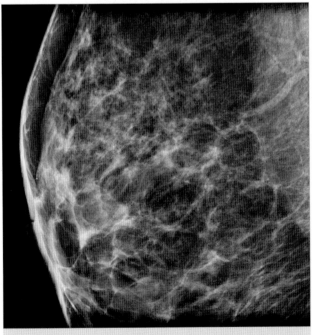

Fig. 68.11 Right mediolateral (RML) spot-compression mammogram.

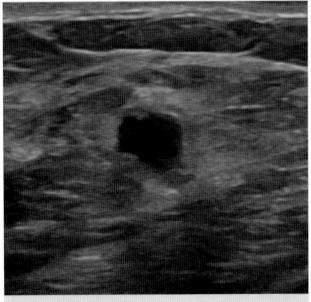

Fig. 68.12 Right breast ultrasound.

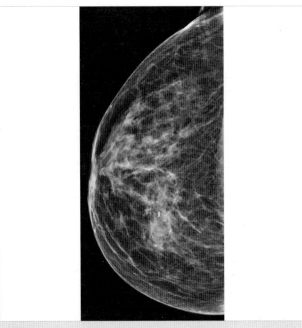

Fig. 68.13 Postbiopsy right craniocaudal (RCC) mammogram.

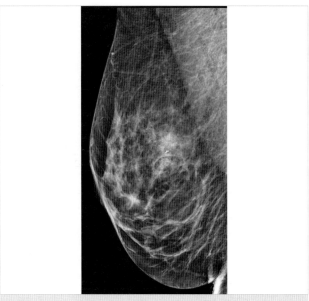

Fig. 68.14 Postbiopsy right mediolateral (RML) mammogram.

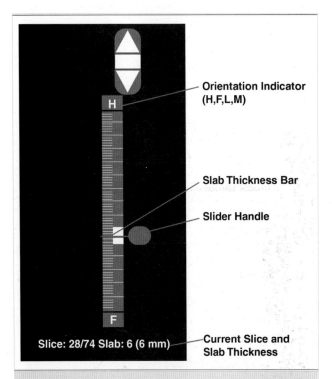

Fig. 68.15 Slider tool on DBT workstation for viewing digital breast tomosynthesis (DBT) images (slices). (Reproduced with permission from Cohen Y. Tomosynthesis assisting in localization of breast lesions for ultrasound targeting seen on one mammographic view only. AJR Am J Roentgenol 2014;203(5): W555–W555.)

69 Small Adjacent Masses

Tanya W. Moseley

69.1 Presentation and Presenting Images

(▶ Fig. 69.1, ▶ Fig. 69.2)

A 57-year-old female with a family history of breast cancer (paternal aunt diagnosed at age 39). Her Gail model risk assessment estimates a 5-year risk for breast cancer of 1.3% with a lifetime risk of 9.3%. She presents for routine screening mammography.

69.2 Key Images

(▶ Fig. 69.3, ▶ Fig. 69.4)

69.2.1 Breast Tissue Density

There are scattered areas of fibroglandular density.

69.2.2 Imaging Findings

There are two adjacent oval masses in the posterior upper outer region of the left breast (▶ Fig. 69.3 and ▶ Fig. 69.4). Both masses are in the posterior depth at the 3 to 4 o'clock location. One mass (*broken arrow*) is 10 cm from the nipple and the other mass (*solid arrow*) is 12 cm from the nipple.

69.3 BI-RADS Classification and Action

Category 0: Mammography: Incomplete. Need additional imaging evaluation and/or prior mammograms for comparison.

69.4 Diagnostic Images 1

(▶ Fig. 69.5, ▶ Fig. 69.6, ▶ Fig. 69.7, ▶ Fig. 69.8, ▶ Fig. 69.9, ▶ Fig. 69.10)

69.4.1 Imaging Findings

Digital breast tomosynthesis (DBT) shows the masses to be well circumscribed and low density (▶ Fig. 69.8, ▶ Fig. 69.9, and ▶ Fig. 69.10). A fatty cleft suggestive of a fatty hilum is not seen within either mass. Sonography is necessary to further characterize the masses.

69.5 Diagnostic Images 2

(▶ Fig. 69.11, ▶ Fig. 69.12, ▶ Fig. 69.13)

69.5.1 Imaging Findings

Ultrasound imaging demonstrates mammographic-sonographic correlation and characterizes both as fibrocystic changes.

69.6 BI-RADS Classification and Action

(▶ Fig. 69.11, ▶ Fig. 69.12, ▶ Fig. 69.13)

Category 2: Benign

69.7 Differential Diagnosis

1. *Fibrocystic changes*: On mammography, solid and cystic masses may have a similar appearance. Sonography demonstrates features consistent with fibrocystic changes.
2. *Lymph nodes*: This is an excellent location for lymph nodes; however, sonography does not support this diagnosis. A fatty hilum is absent from both masses.
3. *Breast cancer*: This would be an example of a multifocal malignancy; however, sonography does not support this diagnosis. The sonographic features are benign.

69.8 Essential Facts

- DBT shows the masses to be well circumscribed and low density. A fatty cleft suggestive of a fatty hilum is not seen within either mass on conventional mammography or on DBT imaging. Sonography is necessary to further characterize the masses.
- Cysts result from distension of the terminal duct lobular units (TDLU) due to progressive filling with fluid.
- Breast clustered microcysts are relatively common, seen in about 6% of breast sonograms. Clustered microcysts may be followed with annual surveillance (BI-RADS Category 2), or, if the diagnosis is uncertain, short-interval follow-up (BI-RADS Category 3) may be performed. At our institution we consider them a BI-RADS Category 2 finding.

69.9 Management and Digital Breast Tomosynthesis Principles

- DBT is considerably more dose-efficient than tomography, due to the fact that a complete three-dimensional (3D) image can be reconstructed from a single scan.

- On two-dimensional (2D) mammograms, findings may be difficult to see because of the anatomical noise from objects above and below. This is because the signal detected at a location on the film cassette or digital detector is dependent upon the total attenuation of all the tissues above the location.
- DBT technology compiles 3D images of the breast and can therefore detect masses masked by overlapping tissue.

69.10 Further Reading

[1] Berg WA. Sonographically depicted breast clustered microcysts: is follow-up appropriate? AJR Am J Roentgenol. 2005;185(4):952–959

[2] Berg WA, Sechtin AG, Marques H, Zhang Z. Cystic breast masses and the ACRIN 6666 experience. Radiol Clin North Am. 2010; 48(5):931–987

[3] Souchay H, Carton A-K, Iordache R. Boosting dose efficiency with digital breast tomosynthesis. GE white paper. Accessed 12/25/2015. Available at: https://www.google.co.in/url?sa=t&rct=j&q=&esrc=s&source=web&cd=1&-cad=rja&uact=8&ved=0ahUKEwiA587BpuPMAhXLgI8KHe9HC3IQFggc-MAA&url=http%3A%2F%2Fwww3.gehealthcare.com.br%2F~%2Fmedia%2Fdownloads%2Fbr%2Fsenoclaire_dose_white_paper_-_doc1403841.pdf%3FParent%3D%257B10196544-07D9-4A31-95BB-DD2D94F05C16%257D&usg=AFQjCNEZqb51t7uNyS1TGyT2S_kzhrHkJA&bvm=bv.122129774,d.c2I

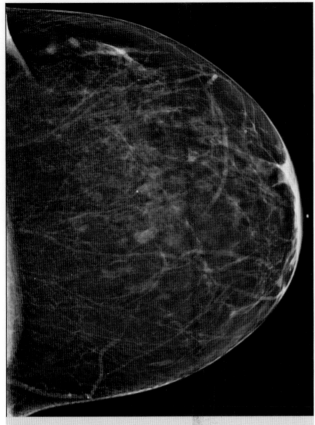

Fig. 69.1 Left craniocaudal (LCC) mammogram.

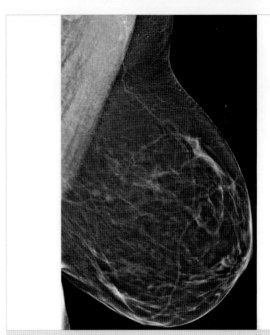

Fig. 69.2 Left mediolateral oblique (LMLO) mammogram.

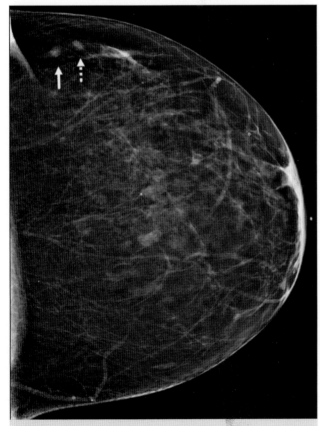

Fig. 69.3 Left craniocaudal (LCC) mammogram with label.

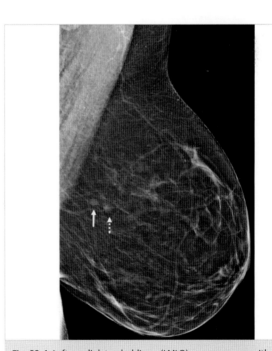

Fig. 69.4 Left mediolateral oblique (LMLO) mammogram with label.

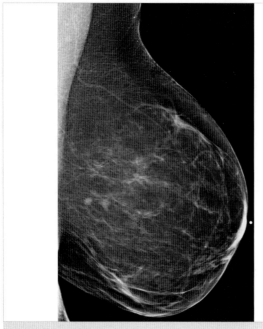

Fig. 69.5 Left lateromedial (LLM) mammogram.

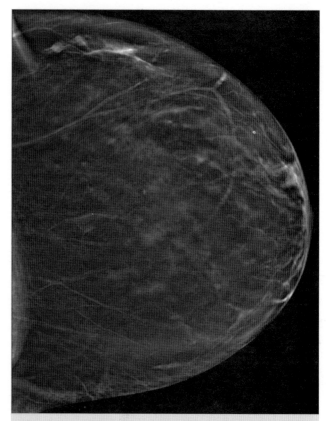

Fig. 69.6 Left craniocaudal digital breast tomosynthesis (LCC DBT), slice 16 of 64.

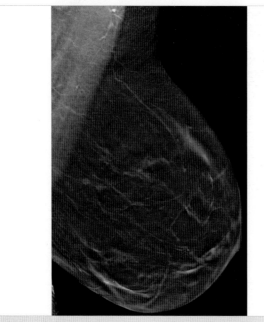

Fig. 69.7 Left lateromedial digital breast tomosynthesis (LLM LLM DBT), slice 9 of 72.

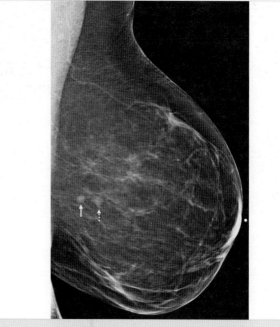

Fig. 69.8 Left lateromedial (LLM) mammogram with label.

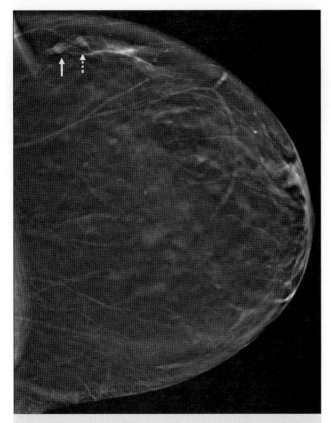

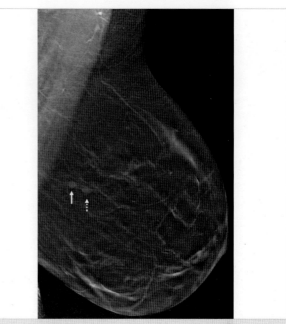

Fig. 69.10 Left lateromedial digital breast tomosynthesis (RLM DBT), slice 9 of 72 with label.

Fig. 69.9 Left craniocaudal (LCC DBT), slice 16 of 64 with label.

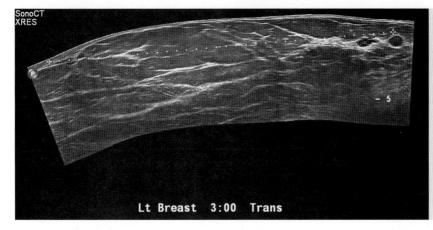

Fig. 69.11 Left breast ultrasound.

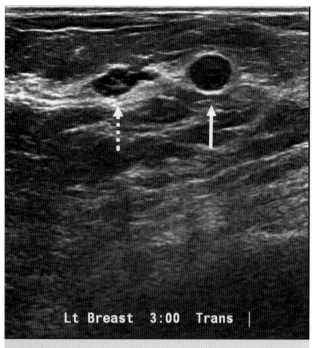

Fig. 69.12 left breast ultrasound with Label.

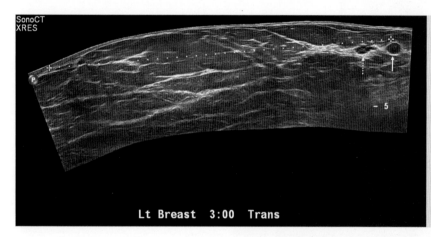

Fig. 69.13 Left breast ultrasound with label.

70 Oval Mass at 6 O'Clock

Tanya W. Moseley

70.1 Presentation and Presenting Images

(▸ Fig. 70.1, ▸ Fig. 70.2, ▸ Fig. 70.3, ▸ Fig. 70.4, ▸ Fig. 70.5, ▸ Fig. 70.6, ▸ Fig. 70.7)

A 38-year-old female with an abnormal baseline mammogram at an outside institution presents for diagnostic mammography.

70.2 Key Images

(▸ Fig. 70.8, ▸ Fig. 70.9, ▸ Fig. 70.10, ▸ Fig. 70.11, ▸ Fig. 70.12, ▸ Fig. 70.13, ▸ Fig. 70.14)

70.2.1 Breast Tissue Density

There are scattered areas of fibroglandular density.

70.2.2 Imaging Findings

The imaging of the right breast is normal (*not shown*). The left breast demonstrates a 1-cm isodense oval mass in the posterior depth of the left breast at the 6 to 7 o'clock location, 10 cm from the nipple (▸ Fig. 70.8, ▸ Fig. 70.9, ▸ Fig. 70.10). A fatty hilum is suggested on the lateromedial (LM) spot-compression digital breast tomosynthesis (DBT) slice 37 of 41 (▸ Fig. 70.12 and ▸ Fig. 70.14) and the craniocaudal (CC) spot-compression DBT slice 19 of 69 (▸ Fig. 70.11 and ▸ Fig. 70.13). A skin marker (*arrow*) denotes an unrelated skin lesion.

70.3 BI-RADS Classification and Action

Category 2: Benign; resume routine mammography

70.4 Differential Diagnosis

1. ***Intramammary lymph node***: Although this is an uncommon location for an intramammary lymph node, the fatty hilum helps to make the diagnosis.
2. *Cyst*: Cysts are often multiple, usually bilateral, and may be painful and fluctuate in size. They are most common in 30- to 50-year-old patients. The fatty hilum makes a cyst an unlikely possibility.
3. *Fibroadenoma*: Fibroadenomas are the most common benign masses in young women. They are multiple in 10 to 15% of patients. The fatty hilum makes a fibroadenoma an unlikely possibility.

70.5 Essential Facts

- A normal intramammary lymph node is a well-circumscribed, slightly lobulated mass which is most instances contains a radiolucent cleft, which represents fat in the hilum of the node.
- A fatty hilum is suggested with the mass in this case; however, this mass is not in the typical location for an intramammary lymph node—the upper outer quadrant. Meyer et al (1993) suggests that no further work-up is necessary for a typical-appearing lymph node in an abnormal location.
- DBT evaluation demonstrating the fatty hilum helps to make this diagnosis.

70.6 Management and Digital Breast Tomosynthesis Principles

- DBT of the entire breast or spot compression (as in this example) may be performed. All views performed with conventional two-dimensional (2D) mammography may be performed with DBT except spot-magnification views.
- Distant metastases are the major cause of mortality and morbidity in breast cancer patients. Axillary node metastases have proven to be the most important prognostic indicator, and are significantly associated with decreased disease-free survival and overall survival time after diagnosis. Intramammary nodes are seen on all breast imaging modalities, but the clinical significance of a metastatic intramammary node is not well established.
- The preoperative detection and accurate characterization of intramammary lymph nodes is vital to stage and plan treatment for these patients, particularly for patients with axillary-lymph-node–negative disease. A metastatic intramammary lymph node upgrades the disease and warrants further axillary dissection at the time of surgery and these patients may be candidates for neoadjuvant systemic therapy.

70.7 Further Reading

[1] Hogan BV, Peter MB, Shenoy H, Horgan K, Shaaban A. Intramammary lymph node metastasis predicts poorer survival in breast cancer patients. Surg Oncol. 2010;19(1):11–16

[2] Mahajan A, Udare A, Shet T, Juvekar S, Thakur M. Diagnosis of a malignant intramammary node retrospectively aided by mastectomy specimen MRI-Is the search worth it? A case report and review of current literature. Korean J Radiol. 2013; 14(4):576–580

[3] Meyer JE, Ferraro FA, Frenna TH, DiPiro PJ, Denison CM. Mammographic appearance of normal intramammary lymph nodes in an atypical location. AJR Am J Roentgenol. 1993; 161(4):779–780

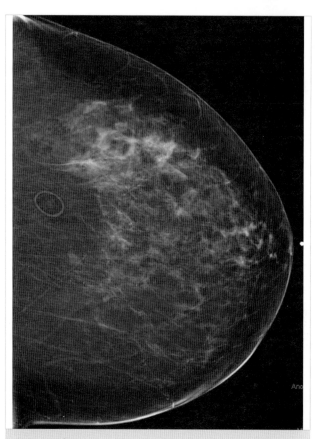

Fig. 70.1 Left craniocaudal (LCC) mammogram.

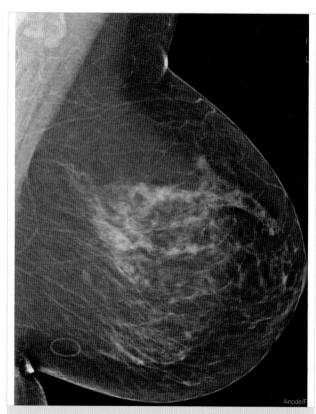

Fig. 70.2 Left mediolateral oblique (LMLO) mammogram.

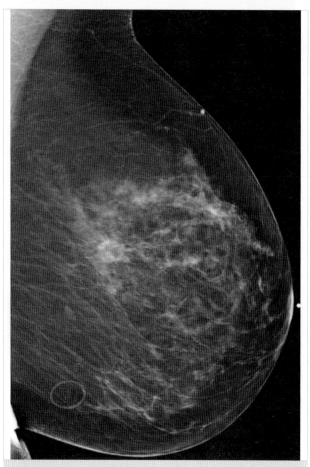

Fig. 70.3 Left lateromedial (LLM) mammogram.

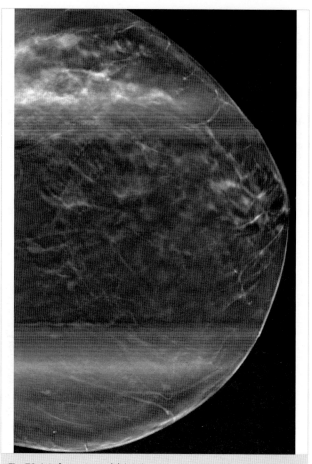

Fig. 70.4 Left craniocaudal (LCC) spot-compression digital breast tomosynthesis (DBT) slice 19 of 69.

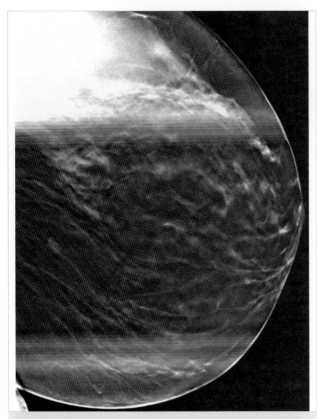

Fig. 70.5 Left lateromedial (LLM) spot-compression digital breast tomosynthesis (DBT), slice 37 of 41.

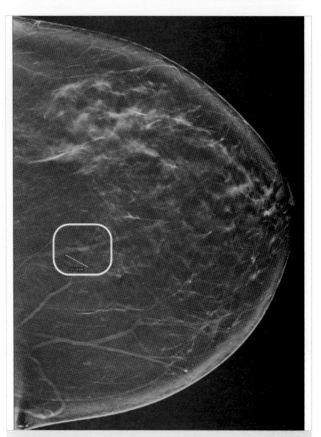

Fig. 70.6 Left craniocaudal (LCC) synthetic mammogram comparison, with label.

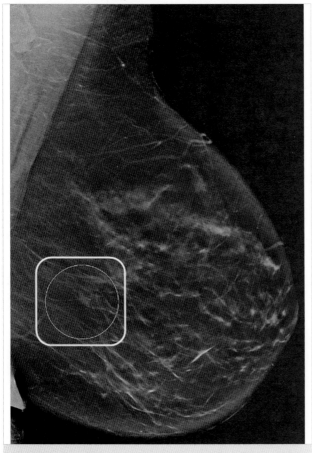

Fig. 70.7 Left mediolateral oblique (LMLO) synthetic mammogram comparison, with label.

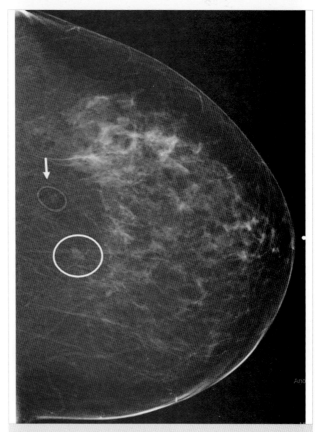

Fig. 70.8 Left craniocaudal (LCC) mammogram with label.

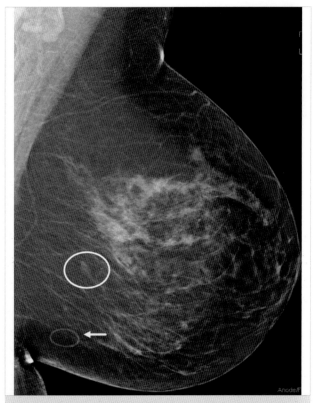

Fig. 70.9 Left mediolateral oblique (LMLO) mammogram with label.

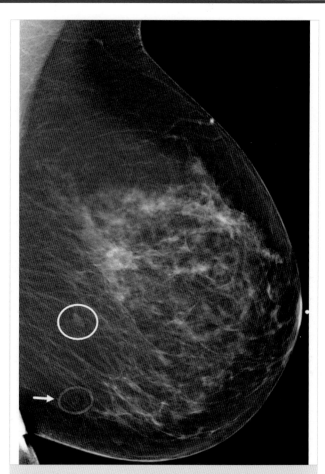

Fig. 70.10 Left lateromedial (LLM) mammogram with label.

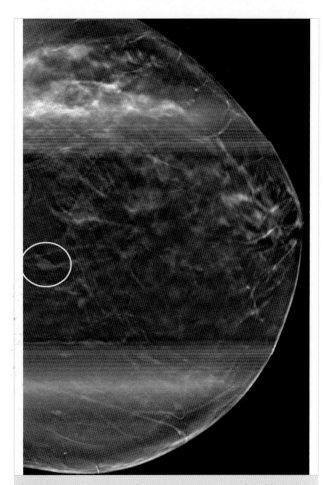

Fig. 70.11 Left craniocaudal (LCC) spot-compression digital breast tomosynthesis (DBT), slice 19 of 69 with label.

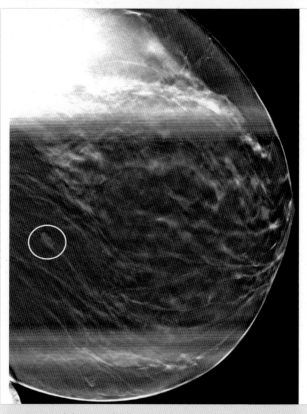

Fig. 70.12 Left lateromedial (LLM) spot-compression digital breast tomosynthesis (DBT), slice 37 of 41 with label.

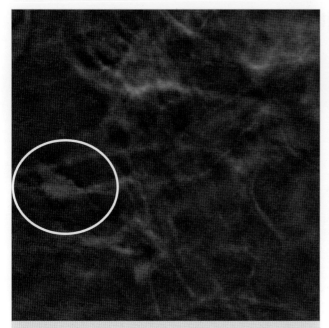

Fig. 70.13 Close-up of left craniocaudal (LCC) spot-compression digital breast tomosynthesis (DBT), slice 19 of 69 with label.

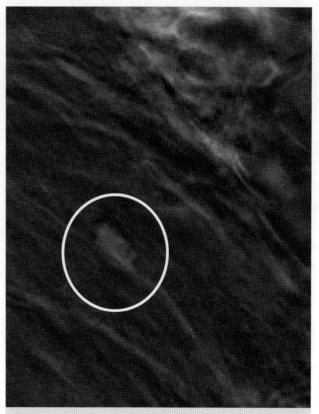

Fig. 70.14 Close-up of left lateromedial (LLM) spot-compression digital breast tomosynthesis (DBT), slice 37 of 41 with label.

71 Architectural Distortion with Calcifications

Lonie R. Salkowski

71.1 Presentation and Presenting Images

(▶ Fig. 71.1, ▶ Fig. 71.2)

A 75-year-old female presents for asymptomatic screening mammography.

71.2 Key Image

(▶ Fig. 71.3)

71.2.1 Breast Tissue Density

There are scattered areas of fibroglandular density.

71.2.2 Imaging Findings

The patient had a conventional digital screening mammogram. There is architectural distortion possibly associated with calcifications in the lateral aspect in the middle depth on the craniocaudal (CC) view of the right breast (▶ Fig. 71.3). The mammogram of the left breast was normal (*not shown*).

71.3 BI-RADS Classification and Action

Category 0: Mammography: Incomplete. Need additional imaging evaluation and/or prior mammograms for comparison.

71.4 Diagnostic Images

(▶ Fig. 71.4, ▶ Fig. 71.5, ▶ Fig. 71.6, ▶ Fig. 71.7, ▶ Fig. 71.8, ▶ Fig. 71.9, ▶ Fig. 71.10, ▶ Fig. 71.11, ▶ Fig. 71.12, ▶ Fig. 71.13, ▶ Fig. 71.14)

71.4.1 Imaging Findings

The architectural distortion could be reproduced on the CC spot-compression image (▶ Fig. 71.4 and ▶ Fig. 71.5). However, there was still confusion about the location in the lateral view. Thus, combination CC and mediolateral (ML) full-field digital mammogram (FFDM) with digital breast tomosynthesis (DBT) imaging was obtained (▶ Fig. 71.6, ▶ Fig. 71.7, ▶ Fig. 71.8, and ▶ Fig. 71.9). These images support an architectural distortion correlate in the lateral projection. There are scattered calcifications in the breast; however, there is a group of coarse heterogeneous calcifications that appear to follow the architectural distortion (▶ Fig. 71.10 and ▶ Fig. 71.11). This area was localized to the upper outer quadrant around the 10 o'clock location. An ultrasound was then performed.

The targeted ultrasound revealed a very subtle irregular hypoechoic mass with indistinct margins located at the 10 o'clock location, 9 cm from the nipple (▶ Fig. 71.12). This lesion was biopsied with ultrasound guidance. The clip on the post-procedure mammogram appears to be located at the sight of the architectural distortion (▶ Fig. 71.13 and ▶ Fig. 71.14). If the clip was not located at this site, it would be reasonable to biopsy this finding with stereotactic technique and use the calcifications as the target.

71.5 BI-RADS Classification and Action

Category 4B: Moderate suspicion for malignancy

71.6 Differential Diagnosis

1. ***Invasive ductal carcinoma (IDC)***: IDC can present as an architectural distortion with or without associated calcifications. Architectural distortion is not very common, but when present has a high predictive value for carcinoma. Biopsy of this lesion was grade 1 IDC with DCIS.
2. *Ductal carcinoma in situ (DCIS)* : The calcifications could be associated with DCIS. Invasive cancer is more likely to be associated with architectural distortion than DCIS. If DCIS is identified on image-guided biopsy, it is possible that an upgrade to invasive cancer could be found at surgical excision.
3. *Sclerosing adenosis*: Sclerosing adenosis is a great mimicker of carcinoma. If the lesion seen on imaging is comparable to the size of the lesion seen at pathology, it could be considered concordant.

71.7 Essential Facts

- Mammographic features alone cannot be used to differentiate benign from malignant causes of architectural distortion.
- The positive predictive value (PPV) of architectural distortion for cancer is 74.5%.
- Architectural distortion with calcifications and without calcifications do not have significant differences in their rates of malignancy.
- If the architectural distortion seen mammographically or on digital breast tomosynthesis (DBT) does not appear to have a sonographic correlate, the presence of calcifications can aid in targeting the biopsy with traditional stereotactic techniques.
- Architectural distortion also can be biopsied with the new DBT-guided stereotactic biopsy.
- Due to its high PPV for cancer, architectural distortion does not fit the criteria for observation.

71.8 Management and Digital Breast Tomosynthesis Principles

- Architectural distortion and asymmetries seen on conventional mammography are often proven to be overlapping tissue on DBT.
- Architectural distortion is less likely to be a malignancy if detected on screening mammography, and more likely if seen on diagnostic mammography.
- Early studies suggest that architectural distortion seen on DBT without a sonographic correlate is more likely to be a radial scar than a malignancy. Further studies are needed to determine if architectural distortion seen only on DBT without an ultrasound correlate can be followed or requires biopsy.
- The cancer detection rate for architectural distortion seen on DBT that is mammographically occult has been reported to be 21.1% and 47.2%.

71.9 Further Reading

[1] Bahl M, Baker JA, Kinsey EN, Ghate SV. Architectural Distortion on Mammography: Correlation With Pathologic Outcomes and Predictors of Malignancy. AJR Am J Roentgenol. 2015; 205(6):1339–1345

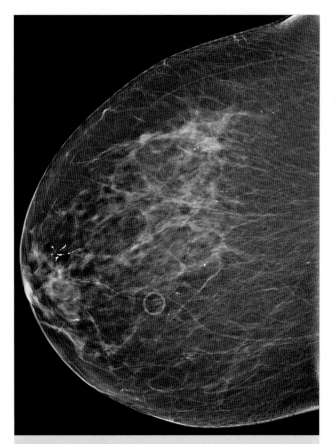

Fig. 71.1 Right craniocaudal (RCC) mammogram.

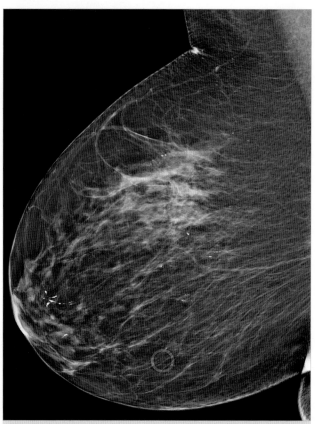

Fig. 71.2 Right mediolateral oblique (RMLO) mammogram.

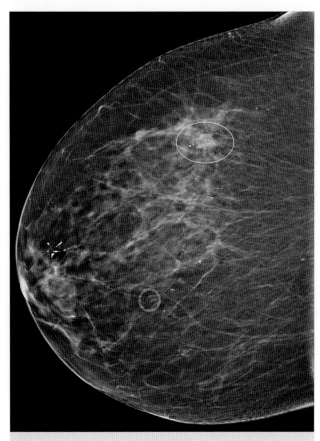

Fig. 71.3 Right craniocaudal (RCC) mammogram with label.

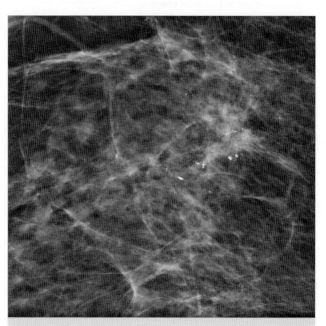

Fig. 71.4 Right craniocaudal (RCC) spot-compression. mammogram

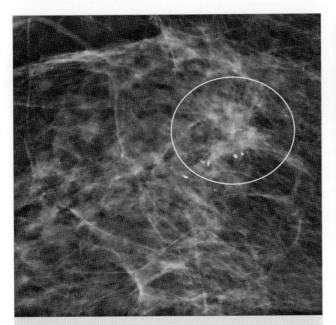

Fig. 71.5 Right craniocaudal (RCC) spot-compression mammogram with label.

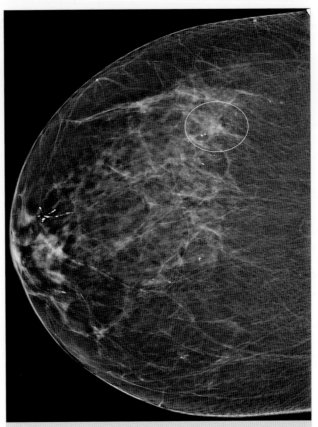

Fig. 71.6 Right craniocaudal (RCC) mammogram, with label.

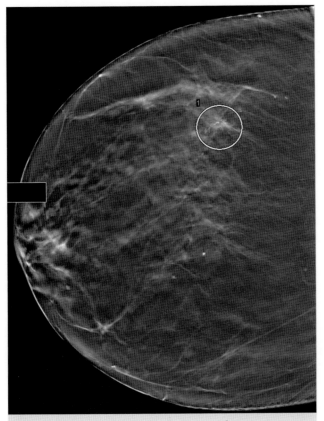

Fig. 71.7 Right craniocaudal digital breast tomosynthesis (RCC DBT), slice 29 of 69, with label.

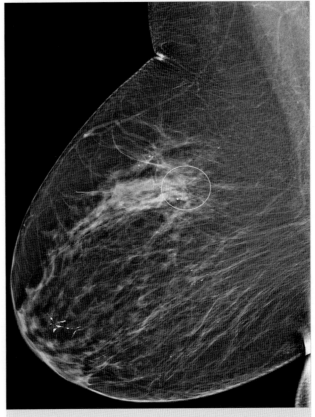

Fig. 71.8 Right mediolateral (RML) mammogram, with label.

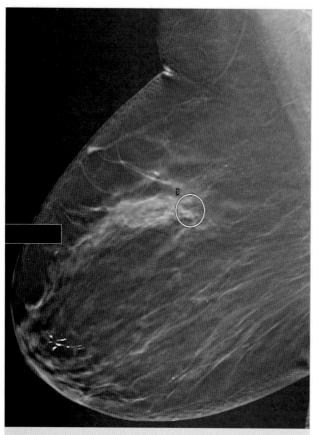

Fig. 71.9 Right mediolateral digital breast tomosynthesis (RML DBT), slice 27 of 81, with label.

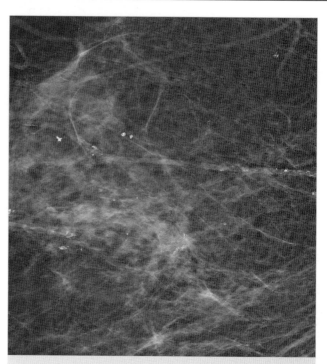

Fig. 71.10 Right mediolateral (RML) spot-compression mammogram.

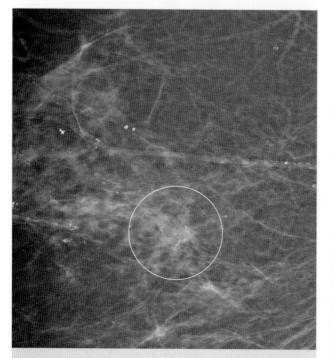

Fig. 71.11 Right mediolateral (RML) spot-compression mammogram with label.

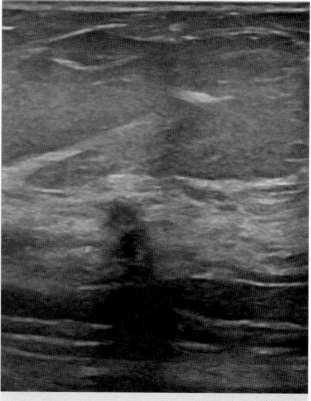

Fig. 71.12 Right breast ultrasound, transverse view.

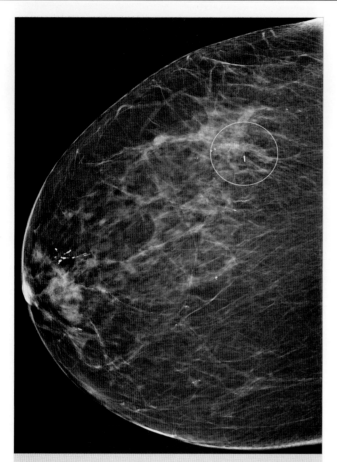

Fig. 71.13 Postbiopsy right craniocaudal (RCC) mammogram, with label.

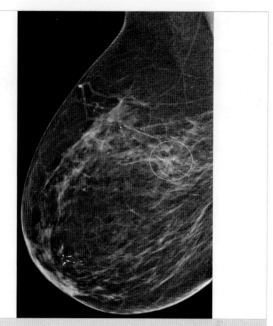

Fig. 71.14 Postbiopsy right mediolateral (RML) mammogram, with label.

72 Focal Asymmetry

Tanya W. Moseley

72.1 Presentation and Presenting Images

(▶ Fig. 72.1, ▶ Fig. 72.2, ▶ Fig. 72.3, ▶ Fig. 72.4)

A 45-year-old female presents for routine screening mammography.

72.2 Key Images

(▶ Fig. 72.5, ▶ Fig. 72.6)

72.2.1 Breast Tissue Density

There are scattered areas of fibroglandular density.

72.2.2 Imaging Findings

The imaging of the right breast is normal (*not shown*). The left breast demonstrates a focal asymmetry (*circle* in ▶ Fig. 72.5 and ▶ Fig. 72.6) measuring 2 cm located at 12 o'clock, 9 cm from the nipple.

72.3 BI-RADS Classification and Action

Category 0: Incomplete. Need additional imaging evaluation and/or prior mammograms for comparison.

72.4 Diagnostic Images

(▶ Fig. 72.7, ▶ Fig. 72.8)

72.4.1 Imaging Findings

Additional clinical information revealed that the patient has lost 150 pounds. Additional evaluation was performed for the focal asymmetry in the left breast at the 12 o'clock position. This finding is less prominent (▶ Fig. 72.7 and ▶ Fig. 72.8) than on the screening mammogram. In light of the patient's weight loss since the comparison mammogram, this finding is most consistent with an island of breast parenchyma. Sonography is recommended to confirm benignity. Normal breast parenchyma is seen on ultrasound (*not shown*). The triangular marker on the left diagnostic images denotes a palpable asymmetry felt by the patient (▶ Fig. 72.7 and ▶ Fig. 72.8). No abnormality is seen on the digital breast tomosynthesis (DBT) images. Normal breast parenchyma is seen on ultrasound (*not shown*).

72.5 BI-RADS Classification and Action

Category 3: Probably benign

72.6 Differential Diagnosis

1. ***Normal breast tissue***: Additional imaging showed the finding to be less conspicuous than on the screening mammogram.
2. *Breast cancer*: This asymmetry has a small likelihood of malignancy and is not likely breast cancer.
3. *Fibrocystic changes*: Fibrocystic changes may present as a focal asymmetry; however, the fact that there is no sonographic correlate makes this an unlikely possibility.

72.7 Essential Facts

- In this case there were no additional findings at diagnostic mammography and no sonographic correlate so the likelihood of malignancy for this focal asymmetry is greater than 0% and less than 2%.
- There are four types of asymmetries described in *ACR BI-RADS Atlas, 5th edition* : asymmetry, focal asymmetry, developing asymmetry, and global asymmetry.
  - An asymmetry is a finding seen on only one mammographic view.
  - A focal asymmetry is a nonmass lesion visible on at least two mammographic views that occupies less than a quadrant.
  - A developing asymmetry is a focal asymmetry that is new, larger, or more conspicuous than noted previously. The risk of malignancy is 15% at screening mammography and 25% at diagnostic mammography, making this a suspicious finding.
  - A global asymmetry is a nonmass lesion visible on at least two mammographic views and occupies at least a quadrant.

72.8 Management and Digital Breast Tomosynthesis Principles

- The ability of DBT to eliminate the obscuration of overlapping breast tissue demonstrates no associated suspicious findings, further supporting the benignity of the this finding.
- If DBT had identified associated or adjacent suspicious findings and these findings were not visible sonographically, biopsy could be performed using tomosynthesis-directed stereotactic biopsy.

72.9 Further Reading

[1] Leung JWT, Sickles EA. Developing asymmetry identified on mammography: correlation with imaging outcome and pathologic findings. AJR Am J Roentgenol. 2007; 188(3):667–675

[2] Sickles EA, D'Orsi CJ, Bassett LW, et al. ACR BI-RADS Mammography. In: ACR BI-RADS Atlas, 5th edition. Reston, VA: American College of Radiology; 2013.

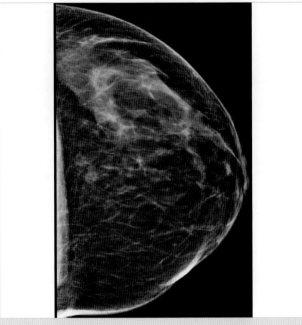

Fig. 72.1 Left craniocaudal (LCC) mammogram.

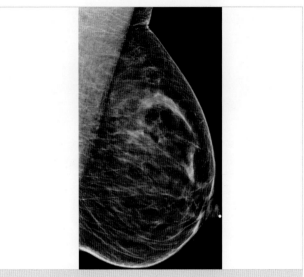

Fig. 72.2 Left mediolateral oblique (LMLO) mammogram.

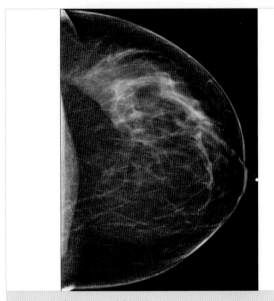

Fig. 72.3 Left craniocaudal (LCC) mammogram comparison.

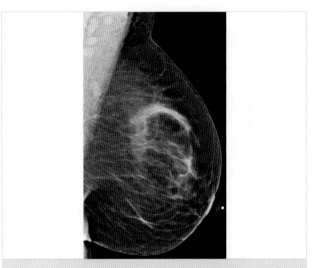

Fig. 72.4 Left mediolateral oblique (LMLO) mammogram comparison.

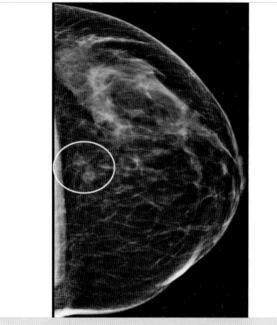

Fig. 72.5 Left craniocaudal (LCC) mammogram with label.

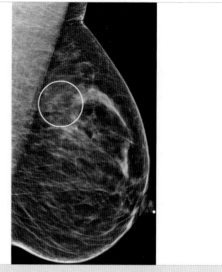

Fig. 72.6 Left mediolateral oblique (LMLO) mammogram with label.

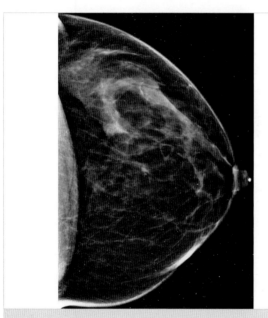

Fig. 72.7 Left craniocaudal (LCC) mammogram.

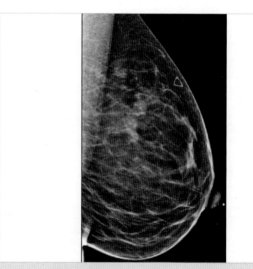

Fig. 72.8 Left lateromedial (LLM) mammogram.

73 Architectural Distortion

Tanya W. Moseley

73.1 Presentation and Presenting Images

(▶ Fig. 73.1, ▶ Fig. 73.2, ▶ Fig. 73.3, ▶ Fig. 73.4)

A 50-year-old female presents for routine screening mammography.

73.2 Key Images

(▶ Fig. 73.5, ▶ Fig. 73.6)

73.2.1 Breast Tissue Density

The breasts are heterogeneously dense, which may obscure small masses.

73.2.2 Imaging Findings

The imaging of the right breast is normal (*not shown*). The left breast demonstrates possible architectural distortion (*circle* in ▶ Fig. 73.5 and ▶ Fig. 73.6), which may have been present on earlier based on comparison studies (▶ Fig. 73.3 and ▶ Fig. 73.4). and may not have appreciably changed. The possible 1.5-cm architectural distortion is in the upper inner quadrant at the 10 o'clock location, 8 cm from the nipple. The *asterisks* on the prior study (▶ Fig. 73.4) are computer-aided detection (CAD) marks unrelated to the possible architectural distortion. The circle marker (*arrow*) on the current study marks a skin mole.

73.3 BI-RADS Classification and Action

Category 0: Mammography: Incomplete. Need additional imaging evaluation and/or prior mammograms for comparison.

73.4 Diagnostic Images

(▶ Fig. 73.7, ▶ Fig. 73.8, ▶ Fig. 73.9, ▶ Fig. 73.10, ▶ Fig. 73.11, ▶ Fig. 73.12, ▶ Fig. 73.13)

73.4.1 Imaging Findings

Digital breast tomosynthesis confirms the architectural distortion on slice 52 of 104 (▶ Fig. 73.7) on the left craniocaudal (CC) DBT movie and slice 26 of 98 (▶ Fig. 73.8) on the left lateromedial (LM) DBT movie. Retrospectively, after DBT, the finding can be seen on the left lateromedial mammogram (▶ Fig. 73.9). Ultrasound was performed and showed a corresponding area of architectural distortion (*circle* in ▶ Fig. 73.10 and ▶ Fig. 73.11). The lesion on ultrasound is hypoechoic with indistinct margins. A core needle biopsy was performed and postbiopsy mammograms showed adequate placement of the postbiopsy clip (*box* in ▶ Fig. 73.12 and ▶ Fig. 73.13).

73.5 BI-RADS Classification and Action

Category 4B: Moderate suspicion for malignancy

73.6 Differential Diagnosis

1. ***Ductal carcinoma in situ (DCIS) involving a radial scar***: Architectural distortion is an uncommon presentation for DCIS. DCIS most commonly presents as microcalcifications. DCIS may be associated with radial scars, either involving the radial scar in this case or adjacent to a radial scar.
2. *Radial scar*: This finding was believed to have been present on the comparison mammogram and not appreciably changed, which makes a radial scar a reasonable possibility.
3. *Summation artifact*: The imaging finding persists on the DBT images and thus the imaging finding should not be dismissed.

73.7 Essential Facts

- Mammography gives radiologists the opportunity to detect noninvasive breast cancer.
- Ductal carcinoma in situ (DCIS) is noninvasive breast cancer: it is the proliferation of neoplastic cells of ducts of the breast without invasion of the parenchyma. The survival rate is almost 100% 10 years after diagnosis.
- DCIS typically presents as calcifications. Sometimes mammography can "predict" the histology of DCIS. Linearly distributed calcifications are usually consistent with poorly differentiated DCIS; whereas calcifications with amorphous morphology are usually consistent with well-differentiated DCIS.
- Radial scars have been shown to have a variable appearance on conventional mammography, presumably due to their planar configuration. The ability of DBT to improve lesion conspicuity reduces the effects of the planar configuration and allows detection of the radial scars.
- Many radial scars will be visible on sonography and, when visible, may be indistinguishable from breast cancer. Radial scars are often more conspicuous on sonography than on mammography. When radial scars are visible on only one mammographic view and cannot be localized with certainty, sonography can be helpful to further evaluate these lesions. Now, that DBT can accurately localize one-view findings, it can better guide targeted ultrasound examinations.
- The management and treatment of radial scars is controversial and varies from institution to institution.

73.8 Management and Digital Breast Tomosynthesis Principles

- DBT acquires multiple images of the breast at multiple angles. The individual images are reconstructed into a series of thin slices typically 1 mm thick, which can be viewed in the same manner as computed tomography (CT) or magnetic resonance (MR) images, as single slices or as a dynamic cine on the workstation.
- The ability to view images as a single slice or in dynamic mode eliminates the effects of overlapping breast tissue, which allows for better visualization and characterization of masses and architectural distortions.
- The three-dimensional (3D) images of DBT eliminate the overlapping breast tissue, making lesions more conspicuous.

In this case, the architectural distortion suspected on conventional mammographic imaging was confirmed on DBT.

- Although it was not done in this case, DBT postbiopsy imaging could have been performed to further confirm that the architectural distortion was biopsied. Surgical excision was performed and no DCIS was identified in the surgical specimens.

73.9 Further Reading

[1] Cohen MA, Sferlazza SJ. Role of sonography in evaluation of radial scars of the breast. AJR Am J Roentgenol. 2000; 174(4):1075–1078

[2] Ikeda DM, Andersson I. Ductal carcinoma in situ: atypical mammographic appearances. Radiology. 1989; 172(3):661–666

[3] Leonard GD, Swain SM. Ductal carcinoma in situ, complexities and challenges. J Natl Cancer Inst. 2004; 96(12):906–920

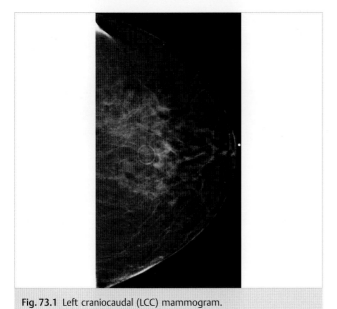

Fig. 73.1 Left craniocaudal (LCC) mammogram.

Fig. 73.2 Left mediolateral oblique (LMLO) mammogram.

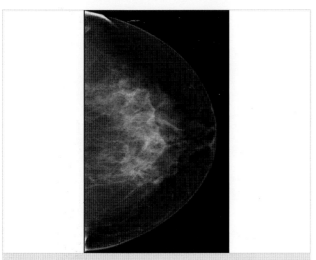

Fig. 73.3 Left craniocaudal (LCC) mammogram comparison.

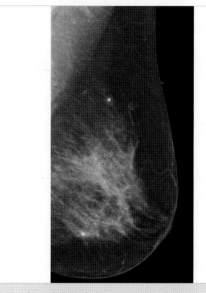

Fig. 73.4 Left mediolateral oblique (LMLO) mammogram comparison.

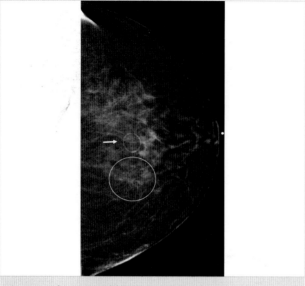

Fig. 73.5 Left craniocaudal (LCC) mammogram with label.

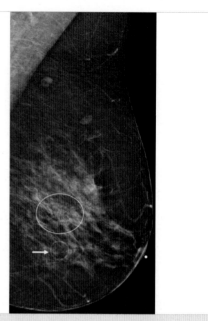

Fig. 73.6 Left mediolateral oblique (LMLO) mammogram with label.

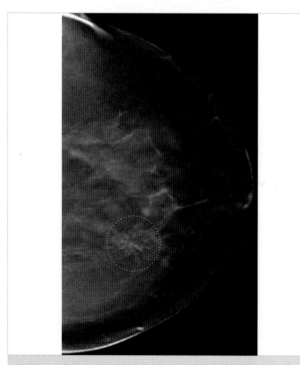

Fig. 73.7 Left craniocaudal digital breast tomosynthesis (LCC DBT), slice 52 of 104 with label.

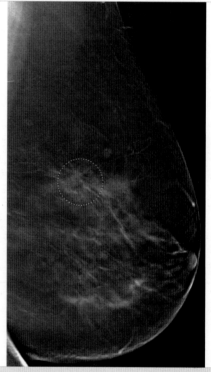

Fig. 73.8 Left lateromedial digital breast tomosynthesis (LLM DBT), slice 26 of 98 with label.

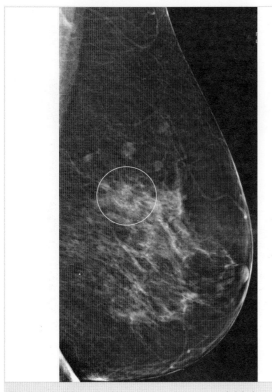

Fig. 73.9 Left lateromedial (LLM) mammogram with label.

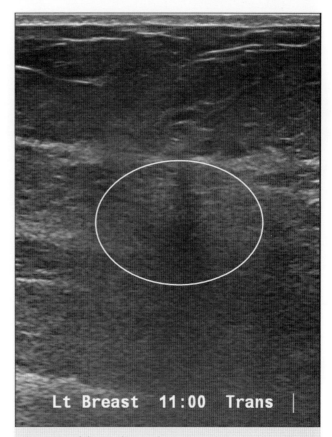

Fig. 73.10 Left breast ultrasound, transverse view.

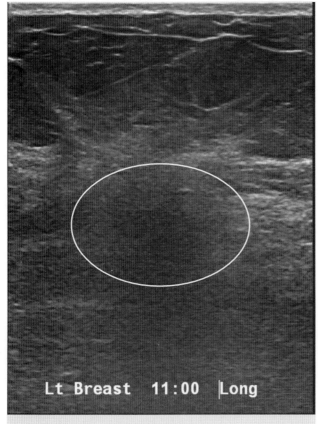

Fig. 73.11 Left breast ultrasound, longitudinal view.

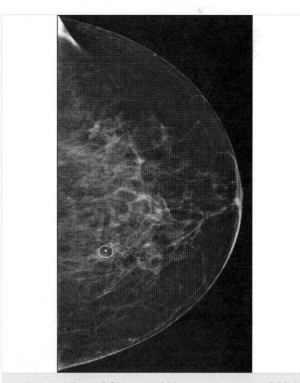

Fig. 73.12 Postbiopsy left craniocaudal (LCC) mammogram with label.

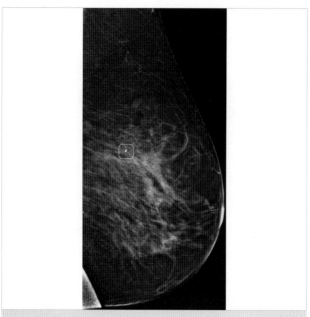

Fig. 73.13 Postbiopsy left lateromedial (LLM) mammogram with label.

74 Calcifications with Architectural Distortion

Tanya W. Moseley

74.1 Presentation and Presenting Images

(▶ Fig. 74.1, ▶ Fig. 74.2, ▶ Fig. 74.3, ▶ Fig. 74.4, ▶ Fig. 74.5, ▶ Fig. 74.6)

A 43-year-old female with a history of an abnormal mammogram performed at an outside institution presents for diagnostic mammographic evaluation.

74.2 Key Images

(▶ Fig. 74.7, ▶ Fig. 74.8, ▶ Fig. 74.9, ▶ Fig. 74.10, ▶ Fig. 74.11, ▶ Fig. 74.12)

74.2.1 Breast Tissue Density

The breasts are heterogeneously dense, which may obscure small masses.

74.2.2 Imaging Findings

The imaging of the right breast is normal (*not shown*). The prior study performed at the outside institution is unavailable (*not shown*). The left breast demonstrates a 1.5-cm group of pleomorphic calcifications with a linear distribution at the 2 to 3 o'clock location in middle depth, 5 cm from the nipple (▶ Fig. 74.7, ▶ Fig. 74.8, ▶ Fig. 74.9, ▶ Fig. 74.11, and ▶ Fig. 74.12). Due to patient anxiety, only lateromedial (LM) digital breast tomosynthesis (DBT) was then performed and it demonstrated possible architectural distortion associated with the pleomorphic calcifications (▶ Fig. 74.10). Lymph nodes (*arrow*) are incompletely visualized on the mediolateral oblique (MLO) view (▶ Fig. 74.8).

74.3 BI-RADS Classification and Action

Category 5: Highly suggestive of malignancy

74.4 Differential Diagnosis

1. ***In situ and invasive ductal carcinoma***: The combination of calcifications and architectural distortion is concerning for in situ and invasive ductal carcinoma. The incompletely visualized lymph nodes raise concern for invasive disease.

2. *In situ carcinoma (DCIS)*: Although most commonly presenting as calcifications, DCIS may present as a mass with calcifications.

3. *Fat necrosis:* Fat necrosis has many appearances that overlap with the appearance of malignancy.

74.5 Essential Facts

- *ACR BI-RADS* (Breast Imaging Reporting and Data System) *Atlas, 5th edition*, describes architectural distortion as distortion of the normal architecture of the breast with no discernible mass.
- The differential diagnosis of architectural distortion includes both benign and malignant entities. The differential diagnosis of architectural distortion with associated calcifications also includes both benign and malignant entities.
- In this case the suspicious calcifications, but not the architectural distortion, were identified on the conventional mammogram. The architectural distortion was unmasked at the time of DBT imaging. Identifying the architectural distortion increases the diagnostic suspicion for invasive malignancy in this case and leads to an upgrade of the BIRADS classification.

74.6 Management and Digital Breast Tomosynthesis Principles

- DBT is excellent for identifying and characterizing findings other than calcifications. It is less effective than conventional mammography for identifying and characterizing calcifications.
- Magnification views are vital to completely assess the morphology of calcifications. DBT cannot perform magnification views. The tomosynthesis system must support both mammographic imaging and tomosynthesis imaging.
- With early tomosynthesis systems, large calcifications could cause considerable artifacts. Newer systems have software that reduce artifacts. These calcifications are very small and would not cause a significant artifact.

74.7 Further Reading

[1] Gaur S, Dialani V, Slanetz PJ, Eisenberg RL. Architectural distortion of the breast. AJR Am J Roentgenol. 2013;201(5):W662-W670

[2] Sickles EA, D'Orsi CJ, Bassett LW, et al. ACR BI-RADS Mammography. In: ACR BI-RADS® Atlas, 5th edition. Reston, VA: American College of Radiology; 2013.

[3] Spangler ML, Zuley ML, Sumkin JH, et al. Detection and classification of calcifications on digital breast tomosynthesis and 2D digital mammography: a comparison. AJR Am J Roentgenol. 2011; 196(2):320–324

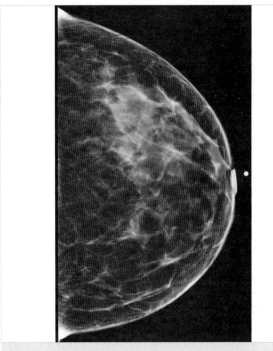

Fig. 74.1 Left craniocaudal (LLC) mammogram.

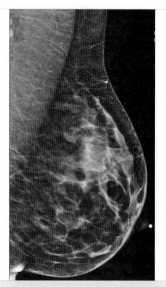

Fig. 74.2 Left mediolateral oblique (LMLO) mammogram.

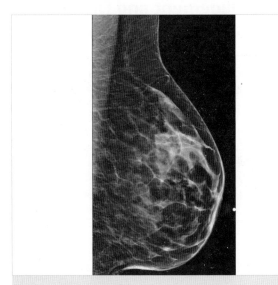

Fig. 74.3 Left lateromedial (LLM) mammogram.

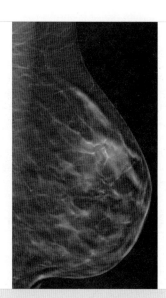

Fig. 74.4 Left lateromedial digital breast tomosynthesis (LLM DBT), slice 37 of 54.

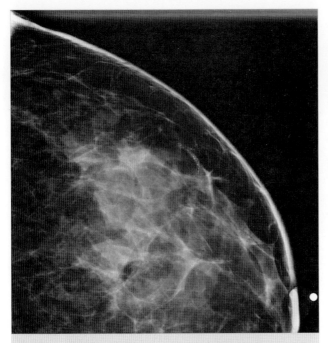

Fig. 74.5 Left craniocaudal (LCC) spot-magnification mammogram.

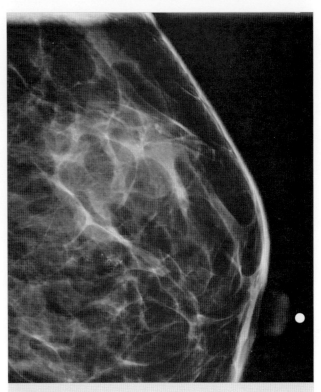

Fig. 74.6 Left lateromedial (LLM) spot-magnification mammogram.

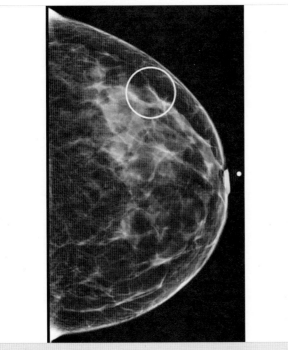

Fig. 74.7 Left craniocaudal (LCC) mammogram with label.

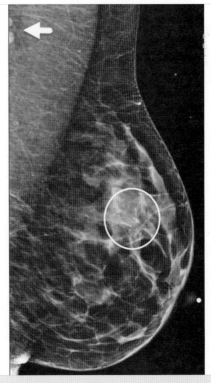

Fig. 74.8 Left mediolateral oblique (LMLO) mammogram with label.

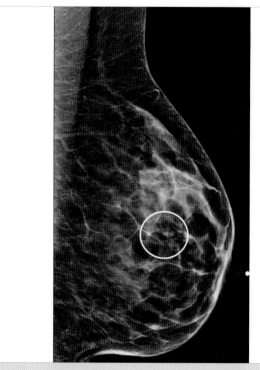

Fig. 74.9 Left lateromedial (LLM) mammogram with label.

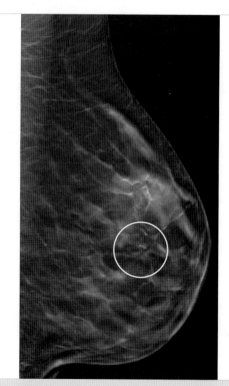

Fig. 74.10 Left lateromedial digital breast tomosynthesis (LLM DBT) slice 37 of 54 with label.

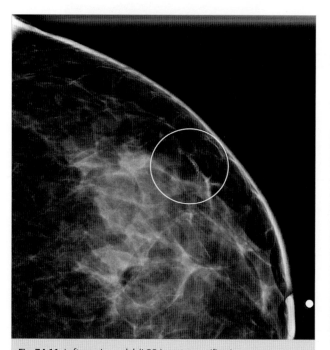

Fig. 74.11 Left craniocaudal (LCC) spot-magnification mammogram with label.

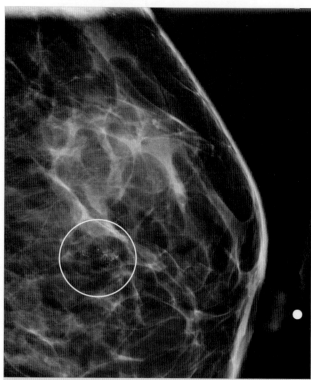

Fig. 74.12 Left lateromedial (LLM) spot-magnification mammogram with label.

75 Asymmetry on the Craniocaudal View

Tanya W. Moseley

75.1 Presentation and Presenting Images

(► Fig. 75.1, ► Fig. 75.2)

A 47-year-old female whose Gail model risk assessment estimates her 5-year risk for breast cancer is 1.7% and her lifetime risk is 16.7%. presents for routine screening mammography.

75.2 Key Images

(► Fig. 75.3)

75.2.1 Breast Tissue Density

There are scattered areas of fibroglandular density.

75.2.2 Imaging Findings

The imaging of the right breast is normal (*not shown*). There is an asymmetry (*circle*) seen in the craniocaudal (CC) view only in the lateral aspect of the left breast (► Fig. 75.3). There is no comparison imaging.

75.3 BI-RADS Classification and Action

Category 0: Mammography: Incomplete. Need additional imaging evaluation and/or prior mammograms for comparison.

75.4 Diagnostic Images

(► Fig. 75.4, ► Fig. 75.5)

75.4.1 Imaging Findings

A repeat left CC view with adequate compression and a left CC digital breast tomosynthesis (DBT) image demonstrate normal breast tissue without an associated mass lesion (► Fig. 75.4 and ► Fig. 75.5). Ultrasound was performed (*not shown*) and demonstrated normal fibroglandular tissue, confirming benignity.

75.5 BI-RADS Classification and Action

Category 2: Benign

75.6 Differential Diagnosis

1. ***Overlapping parenchyma or summation artifact***: DBT obtained at the diagnostic evaluation demonstrated that this asymmetry is created by overlapping tissue.
2. *Breast cancer*: Breast cancer may present as asymmetry; however, this finding did not persist on tomosynthesis imaging. Suspicious findings would be confirmed on sonography.
3. *Fibrocystic changes*: Fibrocystic changes may present as an asymmetry on mammography. The ultrasound was negative and did not reveal any cysts or changes of fibrocystic disease.

75.7 Essential Facts

- This finding was the result of a summation artifact secondary to a lack of compression. Attention to proper technique with adequate compression can avoid recalls for pseudolesions.
- A pseudolesion may be misinterpreted as a true lesion and lead to a biopsy.
- The combination of conventional mammography and DBT improves the diagnostic performance, reduces recall rates, and increases cancer detection.
- The Gail model estimates the risk of developing breast cancer over the next 5 years and over a lifetime. A 5-year risk of 1.7% or higher means there is an increased risk of developing breast cancer.
- This patient is at increased risk of developing breast cancer in the next 5 years and has a lifetime risk of 16.7%.

75.8 Management and Digital Breast Tomosynthesis Principles

- Rather than depending on the high likelihood that a one-view finding is a false-positive, radiologists should determine which asymmetries may have clinical significance.
- Asymmetries associated with clinical findings, architectural distortion, or calcifications are of likely clinical significance and warrant further imaging evaluation and/or biopsy.
- Asymmetries seen with DBT may be biopsied using tomosynthesis-directed stereotactic-guided biopsy.
- Since early-stage breast cancer can have a subtle presentation, radiologists must consistently and carefully scrutinize mammograms to detect early breast cancer.

75.9 Further Reading

[1] Brenner RJ. Asymmetric densities of the breast: strategies for imaging evaluation. Semin Roentgenol. 2001; 36(3):201–216
[2] Giess CS, Frost EP, Birdwell RL. Interpreting one-view mammographic findings: minimizing callbacks while maximizing cancer detection. Radiographics. 2014; 34(4):928–940

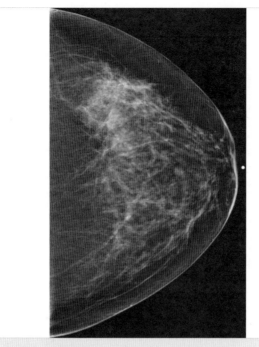

Fig. 75.1 Left craniocaudal (LLC) mammogram.

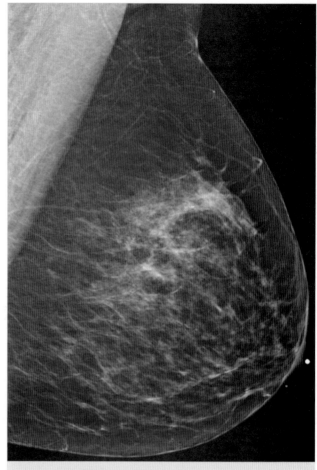

Fig. 75.2 Left mediolateral oblique (LMLO) mammogram.

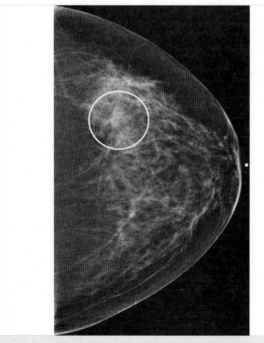

Fig. 75.3 Left craniocaudal (LCC) mammogram with label.

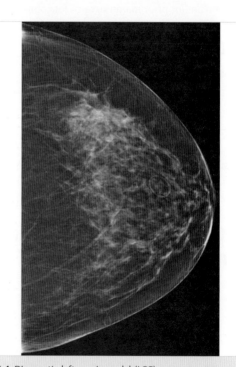

Fig. 75.4 Diagnostic left craniocaudal (LCC) mammogram.

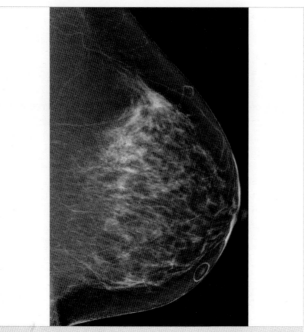

Fig. 75.5 Diagnostic left lateromedial (LLM) mammogram.

76 Linear Asymmetry

Tanya W. Moseley

76.1 Presentation and Presenting Images

(▶ Fig. 76.1, ▶ Fig. 76.2, ▶ Fig. 76.3)

A 70-year-old female with a history of left mastectomy for papillary carcinoma 4 years ago, presents for routine screening mammography of her right breast.

76.2 Key Images

(▶ Fig. 76.4, ▶ Fig. 76.5)

76.2.1 Breast Tissue Density

There are scattered areas of fibroglandular density

76.2.2 Imaging Findings

A linear density (*oval*) is seen on the mediolateral (MLO) view (▶ Fig. 76.4) and the lateromedial (LM) view (▶ Fig. 76.5), but not on the craniocaudal (CC) view. The CC view is normal. This density was not seen on prior mammograms (*not shown*).

76.3 BI-RADS Classification and Action

Category 0: Mammography: Incomplete. Need additional imaging evaluation and/or prior mammograms for comparison.

76.4 Diagnostic Images

(▶ Fig. 76.6, ▶ Fig. 76.7, ▶ Fig. 76.8)

76.4.1 Imaging Findings

A linear density (*oval*) is seen on the MLO spot-compression view (▶ Fig. 76.7). The patient had a repeat MLO view (▶ Fig. 76.8) and an LM digital breast tomosynthesis (DBT) view. The additional imaging showed no suspicious findings. The patient may return to annual mammography. The appropriate management would have been to repeat the MLO view rather than performing a MLO spot-compression view.

76.5 BI-RADS Classification and Action

Category 1: Negative

76.6 Differential Diagnosis

1. ***Pseudolesion, or summation artifact, due to undercompression***: In this case, the finding is noted in the MLO and LM views but not in the CC view. The length of the finding is less on the LM view than the MLO view, consistent with a pseudolesion due to undercompression. The finding is not reproduced on the DBT movie.
2. *Postreduction scar*: The finding is linear; however, the location is too high for a postreduction scar. The finding is not reproduced on the DBT movie.
3. *Foreign body*: The finding is not well seen on all views and is not reproduced on the tomosynthesis movie.

76.7 Essential Facts

- Although, breast cancer may present as a one-view mammographic finding, frequently one-view findings are due to overlapping breast tissue secondary to poor positioning and undercompression.
- One-view findings are commonly a summation artifact.
- With compression of the three-dimensional (3D) breast on a two-dimensional (2D) view, overlap is inevitable. Overlap occurs in breasts of all densities but is more common in dense breasts.
- Sometimes when the standard two mammographic breast views are compared, the radiologists can ascertain that the asymmetry spreads out in the other view in what Brenner has termed the "schmear" sign.

76.8 Management and Digital Breast Tomosynthesis Principles

- With DBT, the image data set is less vulnerable to summation artifacts than conventional mammography.
- The use of both conventional mammography and DBT has been shown to reduce recall rates for women without breast cancer. DBT would have prevented additional imaging in this case.
- DBT has been shown to be less likely than conventional mammography to require recall for asymmetries, focal asymmetries, and architectural distortions. This is due to DBT's ability to eliminate overlap.

76.9 Further Reading

[1] Brenner RJ. Asymmetric densities of the breast: strategies for imaging evaluation. Semin Roentgenol. 2001; 36(3):201–216
[2] Ciatto S, Houssami N, Bernardi D, et al. Integration of 3D digital mammography with tomosynthesis for population breast-cancer screening (STORM): a prospective comparison study. Lancet Oncol. 2013; 14(7):583–589
[3] Giess CS, Frost EP, Birdwell RL. Interpreting one-view mammographic findings: minimizing callbacks while maximizing cancer detection. Radiographics. 2014; 34(4):928–940

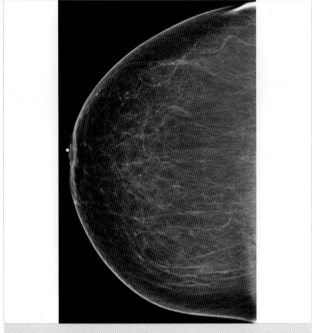

Fig. 76.1 Right craniocaudal (RCC) mammogram.

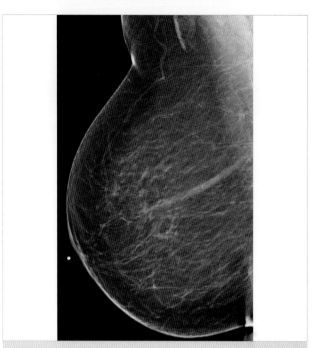

Fig. 76.2 Right mediolateral oblique (RMLO) mammogram.

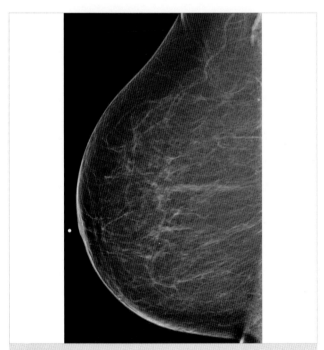

Fig. 76.3 Right lateromedial (RLM) mammogram.

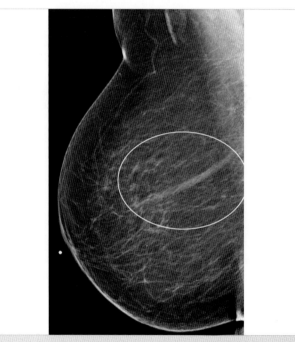

Fig. 76.4 Right mediolateral oblique (RMLO) mammogram with label.

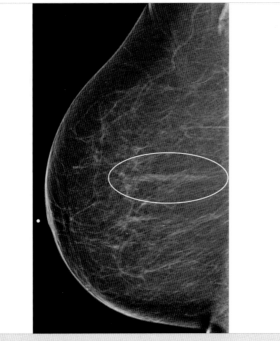

Fig. 76.5 Right lateromedial (RLM) mammogram with label.

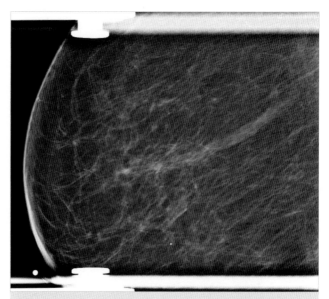

Fig. 76.6 Right mediolateral oblique (RMLO) spot-compression mammogram.

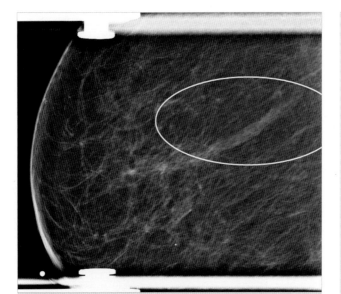

Fig. 76.7 Right mediolateral oblique (RMLO) spot-compression mammogram with label.

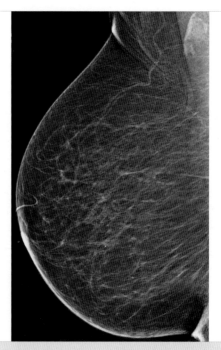

Fig. 76.8 Repeat right mediolateral oblique (RMLO) mammogram.

77 Architectural Distortion

Lonie R. Salkowski

77.1 Presentation and Presenting Images

(▶ Fig. 77.1, ▶ Fig. 77.2)

A 74-year-old female presents for screening mammography.

77.2 Key Images

(▶ Fig. 77.3, ▶ Fig. 77.4)

77.2.1 Breast Tissue Density

The breasts are almost entirely fatty.

77.2.2 Imaging Findings

The patient had conventional digital screening mammography. In the lower inner quadrant of the right breast at the 5 o'clock location, there is an area of architectural distortion (*circle* in ▶ Fig. 77.3 and ▶ Fig. 77.4). The mammogram of the left breast is normal (*not shown*).

77.3 BI-RADS Classification and Action

Category 0: Mammography: Incomplete. Need additional imaging evaluation and/or prior mammograms for comparison.

77.4 Diagnostic Images

(▶ Fig. 77.5, ▶ Fig. 77.6, ▶ Fig. 77.7, ▶ Fig. 77.8, ▶ Fig. 77.9, ▶ Fig. 77.10, ▶ Fig. 77.11, ▶ Fig. 77.12, ▶ Fig. 77.13)

77.4.1 Imaging Findings

The diagnostic imaging (▶ Fig. 77.5, ▶ Fig. 77.6, ▶ Fig. 77.8, ▶ Fig. 77.9, and ▶ Fig. 77.11) demonstrates a persistent 1.5-cm area of architectural distortion located at the 5 o'clock location, which is also seen on the corresponding spot-compression digital breast tomosynthesis (DBT) images (▶ Fig. 77.7 and ▶ Fig. 77.10). An ultrasound was performed and no correlating abnormality was identified. The patient underwent stereotactic biopsy. The postbiopsy images demonstrate the biopsy clip at the location of the architectural distortion (▶ Fig. 77.12 and ▶ Fig. 77.13).

77.5 BI-RADS Classification and Action

Category 4B: Moderate suspicion for malignancy

77.6 Differential Diagnosis

1. **Sclerosing adenosis**: Sclerosing adenosis is the great mimicker of carcinoma. It can present as calcifications, a mass, and architectural distortion.

2. *Carcinoma*: Architectural distortion has a high positive predictive value (PPV) for carcinoma. This would be considered a concordant diagnosis for this lesion.
3. *Radial scar*: Radial scars typically present as an architectural distortion. This would be considered a concordant diagnosis for an image-guided biopsy provided that the histopathology expected for a radial scar is the dominant feature of the biopsy and not a small incidental finding.

77.7 Essential Facts

- Sclerosing adenosis (SA) is a proliferation of the epithelium and myoepithelium that originates in the glandular lobules and is accompanied by desmoplasia.
- SA can be associated with benign breast disorders, atypical lobular hyperplasia, and lobular carcinoma in situ.
- SA can mimic carcinoma grossly and microscopically, and also on sonographic and mammographic imaging.
- SA has variable appearances on imaging: calcifications, a mass, and architectural distortion. It is most commonly seen as calcifications. This case demonstrates a case of SA as architectural distortion.

77.8 Management and Digital Breast Tomosynthesis Principles

- Architectural distortion seen on mammography has a high positive predictive value (PPV) for carcinoma (74.5%). Thus, it is important to sample the tissue. If the lesion is not seen on ultrasound (as in this case), then stereotactic biopsy or needle localization and excision should be performed to ensure that the lesion is not carcinoma.
- DBT improves visualization of architectural distortion that is seen on conventional mammography, and in addition, identifies architectural distortion that is occult on conventional mammography.
- The identification of occult architectural distortion by DBT accounts for the 12 to 45% of missed breast cancers.
- DBT can improve the detection of architectural distortion; however, it cannot determine if the architectural distortion is of benign or malignant origin. A biopsy is required to make that determination.

77.9 Further Reading

[1] Bahl M, Baker JA, Kinsey EN, Ghate SV. Architectural Distortion on Mammography: Correlation With Pathologic Outcomes and Predictors of Malignancy. AJR Am J Roentgenol. 2015; 205(6):1339–1345

[2] Günhan-Bilgen I, Memiş A, Ustün EE, Ozdemir N, Erhan Y. Sclerosing adenosis: mammographic and ultrasonographic findings with clinical and histopathological correlation. Eur J Radiol. 2002; 44(3):232–238

[3] Partyka L, Lourenco AP, Mainiero MB. Detection of mammographically occult architectural distortion on digital breast tomosynthesis screening: initial clinical experience. AJR Am J Roentgenol. 2014; 203(1):216–222

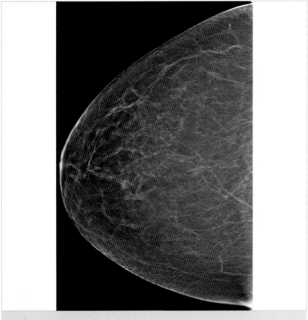

Fig. 77.1 Right craniocaudal (RCC) mammogram.

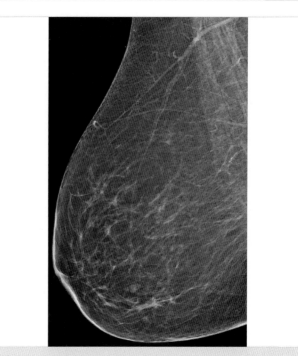

Fig. 77.2 Right mediolateral oblique (RMLO) mammogram.

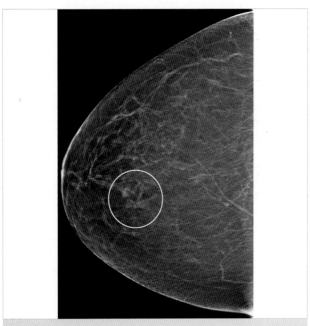

Fig. 77.3 Right craniocaudal (RCC) mammogram with label.

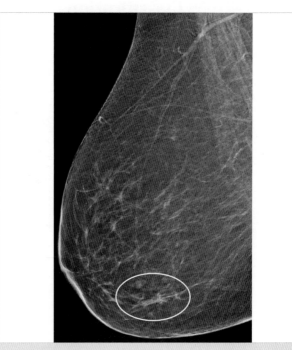

Fig. 77.4 Right mediolateral oblique (RMLO) mammogram with label.

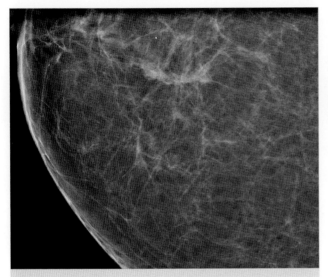

Fig. 77.5 Right craniocaudal (RCC) spot-compression mammogram.

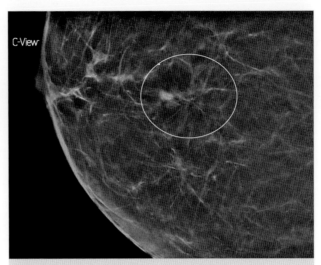

Fig. 77.6 Right craniocaudal (RCC) synthetic spot-compression mammogram, with label.

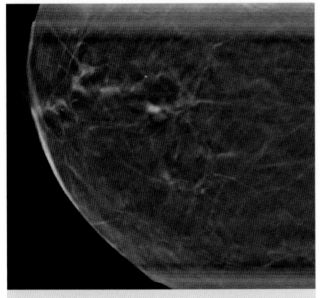

Fig. 77.7 Right craniocaudal (RCC) spot-compression digital breast tomosynthesis (DBT), slice 9 of 47.

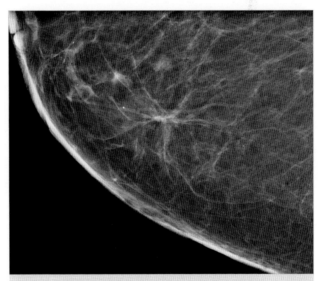

Fig. 77.8 Right mediolateral oblique (RMLO) spot-compression mammogram.

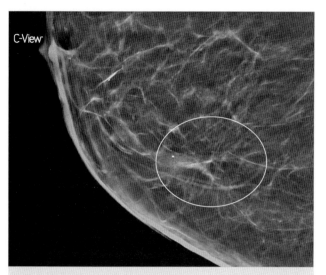

Fig. 77.9 Right mediolateral oblique (RMLO) synthetic spot-compression mammogram, with label.

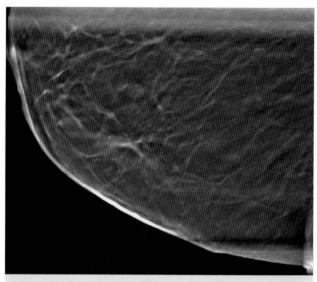

Fig. 77.10 Right mediolateral oblique (RMLO) spot-compression digital breast tomosynthesis (DBT), slice 22 of 53.

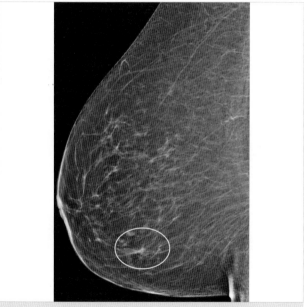

Fig. 77.11 Right craniocaudal (RCC) spot-compression mammogram, with label.

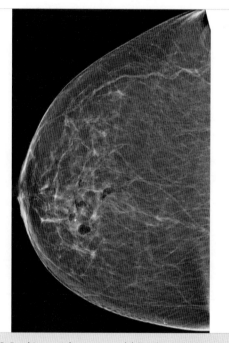

Fig. 77.12 Postbiopsy right craniocaudal (RCC) mammogram.

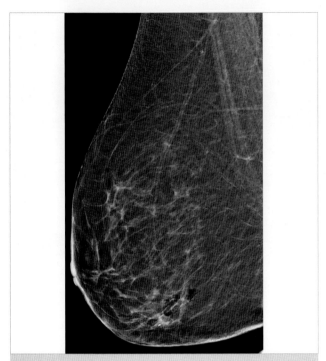

Fig. 77.13 Postbiopsy right mediolateral (RML) mammogram.

Part VI

Cases with Diagnostic Tomosynthesis Evaluation Presenting with Clinical Indication

VI

78 Right Axillary Palpable Finding and Left Breast Pain

Tanya W. Moseley

78.1 Presentation and Presenting Images

(▶ Fig. 78.1, ▶ Fig. 78.2, ▶ Fig. 78.3, ▶ Fig. 78.4, ▶ Fig. 78.5)

A 35-year-old female with a palpable finding in the axillary tail of the right breast and left breast pain presents for diagnostic mammography.

78.2 Key Images

(▶ Fig. 78.6, ▶ Fig. 78.7, ▶ Fig. 78.8, ▶ Fig. 78.9, ▶ Fig. 78.10)

78.2.1 Breast Tissue Density

The breasts are heterogeneously dense, which may obscure small masses.

78.2.2 Imaging Findings

There was no mammographic finding corresponding to the palpable finding reported in the right axillary tail that is noted by the triangular skin marker (*arrow* in ▶ Fig. 78.6 and ▶ Fig. 78.8). The left breast demonstrates a 5-cm well-circumscribed, fat-containing mass central in the breast and located 3 cm from the nipple (▶ Fig. 78.7 and ▶ Fig. 78.9). Only the craniocaudal (CC) digital breast tomosynthesis (DBT) movie was done and demonstrates the finding it best on slice 26 of 83 (▶ Fig. 78.10).

78.3 BI-RADS Classification and Action

Category 0: Mammography: Incomplete. Need additional imaging evaluation and/or prior mammograms for comparison.

78.4 Diagnostic Images

(▶ Fig. 78.11, ▶ Fig. 78.12, ▶ Fig. 78.13, ▶ Fig. 78.14)

78.4.1 Imaging Findings

Ultrasound showed a mixed echoic encapsulated mass corresponding to the left breast mammographic finding (▶ Fig. 78.11 and ▶ Fig. 78.12). There was no sonographic correlate for the right axillary tail palpable finding (*not shown*).

The palpable finding was of great clinical concern so magnetic resource imaging (MRI) was also performed. The MRI showed no correlate for the right axillary tail palpable finding (*not shown*). Normal tissue was seen and clinical correlation was recommended. The mammographic and sonographic mass seen centrally in the left breast corresponds to an encapsulated mass containing both fat and breast tissue on MR (▶ Fig. 78.13 and ▶ Fig. 78.14). It has the classic appearance of a "breast within a breast."

78.5 BI-RADS Classification and Action

Category 2: Benign

78.6 Differential Diagnosis

1. ***Hamartoma***: The appearance of hamartomas depends on the fat to parenchyma ratio. Lesions with a greater amount of fat can mimic lipomas, those with a greater amount of parenchyma can mimic fibroadenomas.
2. *Galactocele*: The appearance depends upon the amount of fat and proteinaceous material and the viscosity of the fluid. Galactoceles are most commonly seen after the cessation of breast-feeding.
3. *Lipoma*: A lipoma usually presents on mammography as a well-circumscribed uniformly radiolucent mass.

78.7 Essential Facts

- Hamartomas were first described as lipofibroadenomas, fibroadenolipomas or adenolipomas, based on the predominant component of the mass.
- Hamartomas of the breast are uncommon masses with a reported incidence of 0.7% of all benign breast masses in females.
- On physical examination, hamartomas may be occult or may present as mobile, soft-to-firm palpable masses.
- Although not microscopically encapsulated, hamartomas have the appearance of a capsule or pseudocapsule on mammography and DBT.
- Hamartomas have been described as a "breast within a breast" because mammographically they are commonly seen as a well-circumscribed round to oval mass surrounded by a thin capsule and composed of fat and breast tissue.

78.8 Management and Digital Breast Tomosynthesis Principles

- DBT greatly reduces the effect of overlapping breast tissue, which results in the better visualization of mass margins than on conventional mammography.
- Fat, even when not appreciated on conventional mammography, is seen in benign and malignant masses with DBT.
- The greater detail seen with DBT imaging allows for definitive classification of encapsulated fat-containing masses.
- The majority of encapsulated fat-containing masses found on mammography and DBT are benign.

78.9 Further Reading

[1] Arrigoni MG, Dockerty MB, Judd ES. The identification and treatment of mammary hamartoma. Surg Gynecol Obstet. 1971; 133(4):577–582

[2] Freer PE, Wang JL, Rafferty EA. Digital breast tomosynthesis in the analysis of fat-containing lesions. Radiographics. 2014; 34(2):343–358

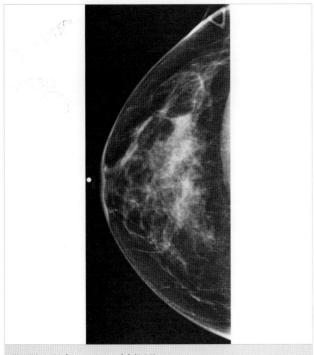

Fig. 78.1 Right craniocaudal (RCC) mammogram.

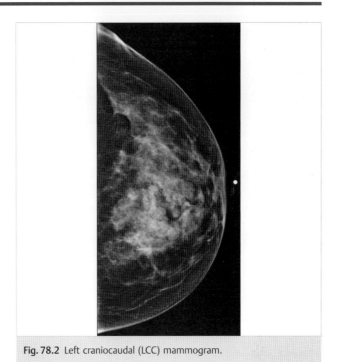

Fig. 78.2 Left craniocaudal (LCC) mammogram.

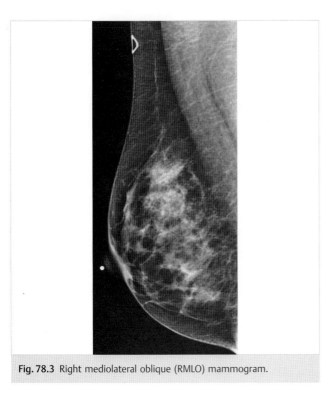

Fig. 78.3 Right mediolateral oblique (RMLO) mammogram.

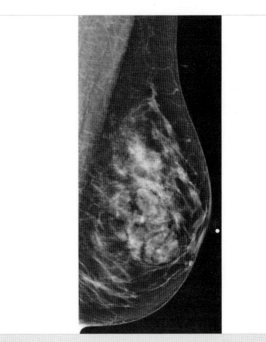

Fig. 78.4 Left mediolateral oblique (LMLO) mammogram.

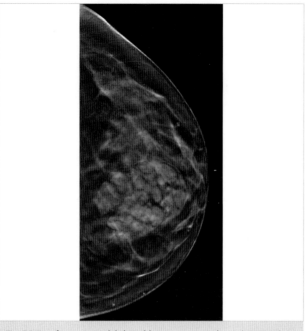

Fig. 78.5 Left craniocaudal digital breast tomosynthesis (LCC DBT), slice 26 of 63.

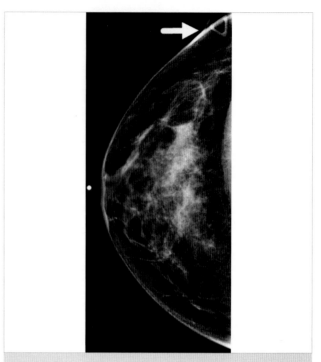

Fig. 78.6 Right craniocaudal (RCC) mammogram with label.

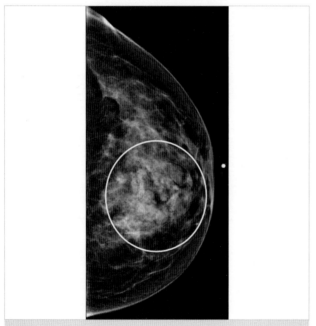

Fig. 78.7 Left craniocaudal (LCC) mammogram with label.

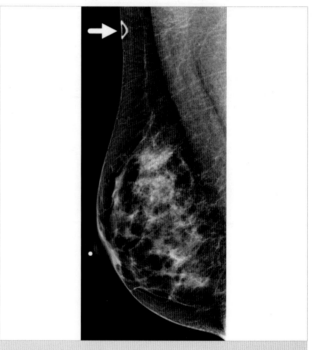

Fig. 78.8 Right mediolateral oblique (RMLO) mammogram with label.

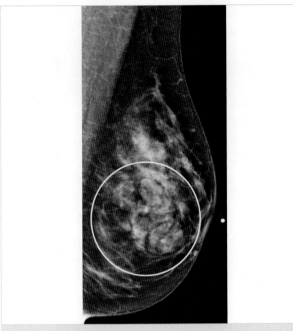

Fig. 78.9 Left mediolateral oblique (LMLO) mammogram with label.

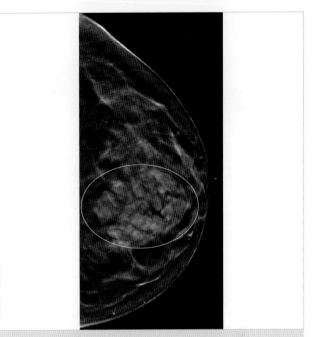

Fig. 78.10 Left craniocaudal digital breast tomosynthesis (LCC DBT), slice 26 of 63 with label.

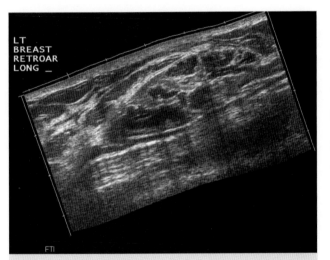

Fig. 78.11 Left breast ultrasound.

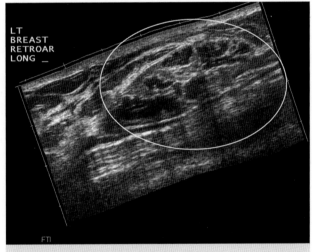

Fig. 78.12 Left breast ultrasound with label.

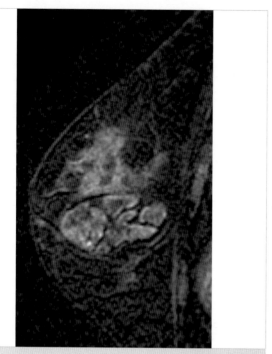

Fig. 78.13 Sagittal subtraction dynamic contrast-enhanced magnetic resonance image (CE MR).

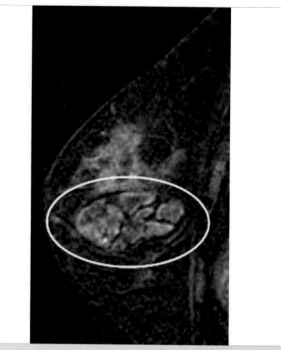

Fig. 78.14 Sagittal subtraction dynamic contrast-enhanced magnetic resonance image (CE MR) with label.

79 Palpable Masses with No Mammographic Correlate

Lonie R. Salkowski

79.1 Presentation and Presenting Images

(▶ Fig. 79.1, ▶ Fig. 79.2, ▶ Fig. 79.3, ▶ Fig. 79.4, ▶ Fig. 79.5, ▶ Fig. 79.6, ▶ Fig. 79.7, ▶ Fig. 79.8, ▶ Fig. 79.9)

A 47-year-old female with two palpable abnormalities marked with BBs presents for mammographic evaluation. She has a history of a benign left breast duct excision.

79.1.1 Breast Tissue Density

There are scattered areas of fibroglandular density.

79.1.2 Imaging Findings

The conventional digital mammograms and digital breast tomosynthesis (DBT) images did not reveal any findings to correspond to the two palpable findings marked with BBs at the 12 o'clock and 5 o'clock locations on the left breast (▶ Fig. 79.1, ▶ Fig. 79.2, ▶ Fig. 79.3, ▶ Fig. 79.4, ▶ Fig. 79.5, ▶ Fig. 79.6, ▶ Fig. 79.7, ▶ Fig. 79.8, and ▶ Fig. 79.9). The DBT images demonstrate an area of architectural distortion at the 10 o'clock location (▶ Fig. 79.5 and ▶ Fig. 79.6). An ultrasound was recommended to further evaluate the palpable findings and the area of architectural distortion at the 10 o'clock location.

79.2 Diagnostic Images

(▶ Fig. 79.10; ▶ Fig. 79.11; ▶ Fig. 79.12; ▶ Fig. 79.13; ▶ Fig. 79.14; ▶ Fig. 79.15; ▶ Fig. 79.16)

79.2.1 Imaging Findings

The ultrasound of the palpable findings at the 12 o'clock and 5 o'clock locations revealed normal breast tissue (*not shown*). Corresponding to the area of architectural distortion noted at the 10 o'clock location on the DBT images, there is 8 mm × 8 mm × 7 mm irregular mass with angular margins and posterior shadowing, 5 cm from the nipple (▶ Fig. 79.10 and ▶ Fig. 79.11). Due to the complexity of the imaging findings, the clinical history of a prior surgical excision, and the palpable findings, a BB marker was placed on the skin overlying the area of ultrasound abnormality. A repeat CC image was taken with the nipple in profile. The BB marker appears to correlate to the area of architectural distortion on the DBT (▶ Fig. 79.12). The lesion was biopsied with ultrasound guidance. The ribbon biopsy marker clip is located in the area of architectural distortion best seen on DBT (▶ Fig. 79.13 and ▶ Fig. 79.14). Enlarging the area of concern on the initial DBT images suggests that the architectural distortion is fatty, or radiolucent, in the center (▶ Fig. 79.15 and ▶ Fig. 79.16).

79.3 BI-RADS Classification and Action

Category 4C: High suspicion for malignancy

79.4 Differential Diagnosis

1. ***Invasive ductal carcinoma(IDC)***: The architectural distortion and irregular mass with indistinct margins are worrisome for an invasive carcinoma. The biopsy yielded grade 2 IDC with lobular features.
2. *Radial scar/radial sclerosing lesion*: The central area of the architectural distortion is more radiolucent, which has been reported as a sign in radial sclerosing lesions. This finding is not unique to radial scars. A biopsy is warranted.
3. *Postoperative scar*: The patient has had a prior duct excision. The skin marker denotes the surgical scar. This scar is in the inferior region of the breast and the area of concern is located in the upper inner quadrant; thus, the surgical scar is a much less likely cause of the finding. It is important to correlate skin incision scars and surgical reports to the imaging findings.

79.5 Essential Facts

- Positioning remains important even for DBT. The initial craniocaudal (CC) view with the nipple not in profile obscures the visualization of this lesion (▶ Fig. 79.1). The repeat CC view without DBT demonstrates the lesion better (▶ Fig. 79.12). This lesion may have been better seen on a repeat CC DBT.
- When a patient presents with a palpable finding or other clinical concern, it is important to evaluate that concern completely. However, it is just as important to evaluate the rest of the mammographic imaging and not become distracted by the area of clinical concern. This includes both breasts if both were imaged.
- The presence or absence of fat within a lesion on DBT is not predictive of benignity or malignancy.
- Cancers, due to their much faster growth rates compared to other tissue, may engulf fat as they grow and thus contain fat. This is in contrast to fat-containing benign masses, which are composed of fat and are surrounded by a thin capsule or pseudocapsule.
- It is important to evaluate the margins of a mass on DBT.

79.6 Management and Digital Breast Tomosynthesis Principles

- DBT's ability to reconstruct the breast tissue into slices provides a look inside of masses.
- DBT may reveal the presence of fat within a lesion that is not detected on conventional mammography.
- Both benign and malignant masses may contain fat. With DBT, it may be possible to make a clearer distinction and thus avoid unnecessary biopsies, only biopsying those lesions that warrant it.

- All spiculated fat-containing masses detected on DBT should be evaluated. The range of diagnosis for this finding is carcinoma, surgical scars, and fat necrosis. Historical information from the patient will be helpful in narrowing the diagnosis.

79.7 Further Reading

[1] Freer PE, Wang JL, Rafferty EA. Digital breast tomosynthesis in the analysis of fat-containing lesions. Radiographics. 2014; 34(2):343–358

[2] Noroozian M, Hadjiiski L, Rahnama-Moghadam S, et al. Digital breast tomosynthesis is comparable to mammographic spot views for mass characterization. Radiology. 2012; 262(1):61–68

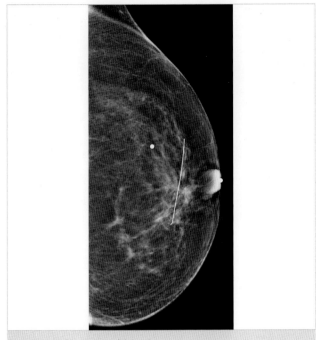

Fig. 79.1 Left craniocaudal (LCC) mammogram.

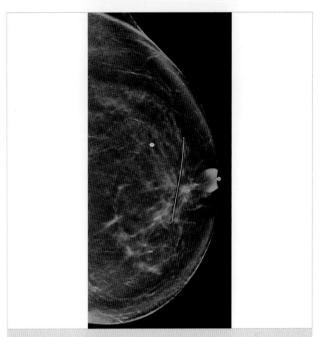

Fig. 79.2 Left craniocaudal (LCC) synthetic mammogram.

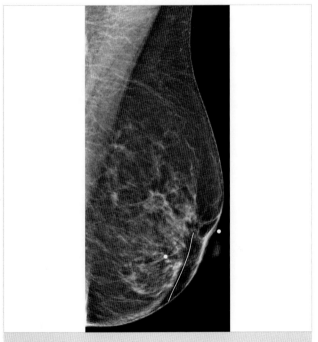

Fig. 79.3 Left mediolateral oblique (LMLO) mammogram.

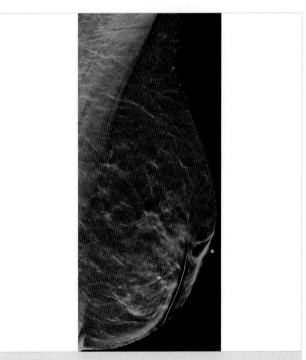

Fig. 79.4 Left mediolateral oblique (LMLO) synthetic mammogram.

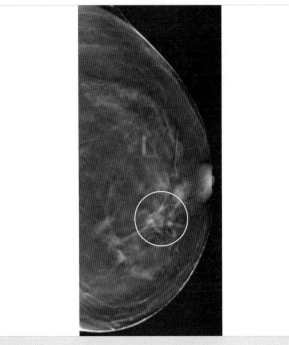

Fig. 79.5 Left craniocaudal digital breast tomosynthesis (LCC DBT), slice 34 of 77, with label.

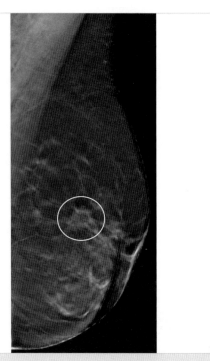

Fig. 79.6 Left mediolateral oblique digital breast tomosynthesis (LMLO DBT), slice 40 of 72.

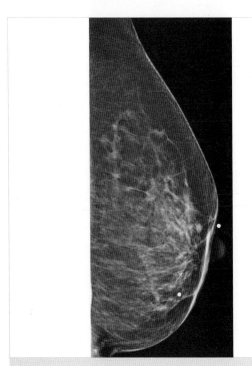

Fig. 79.7 Left mediolateral (LML) mammogram.

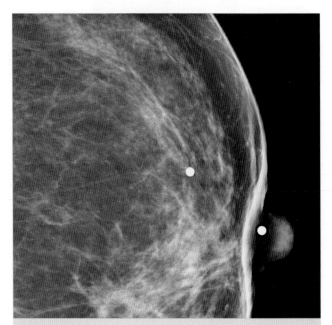

Fig. 79.8 Left craniocaudal (LCC) spot-compression mammogram.

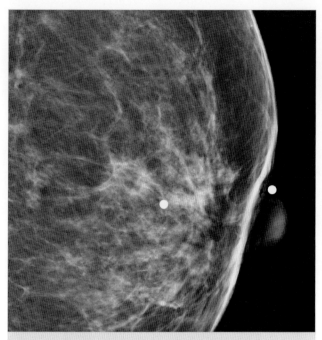

Fig. 79.9 Left mediolateral oblique (LMLO) spot-compression mammogram.

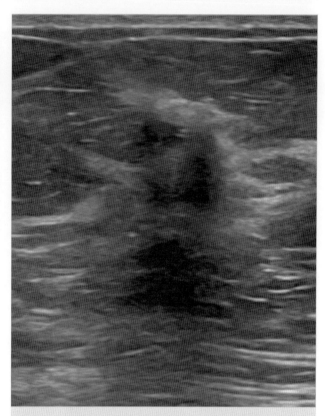

Fig. 79.10 Left breast ultrasound, transverse view of the 10 o'clock lesion.

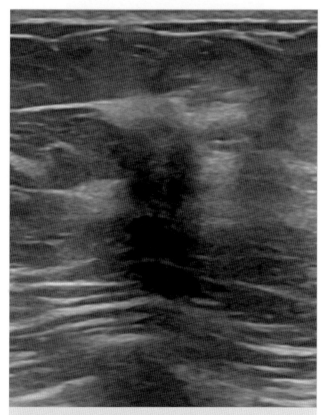

Fig. 79.11 Left breast ultrasound, longitudinal view of the 10 o'clock lesion.

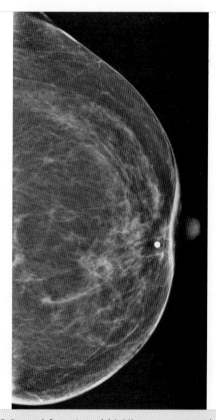

Fig. 79.12 Repeat left craniocaudal (LCC) mammogram with nipple in profile and BB marker on ultrasound finding.

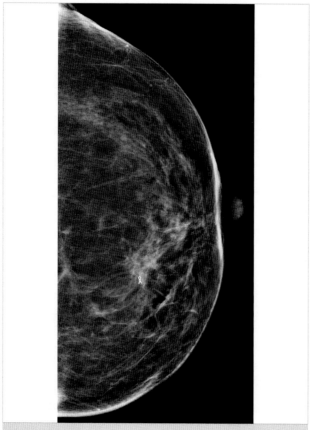

Fig. 79.13 Postbiopsy left craniocaudal (LCC) mammogram.

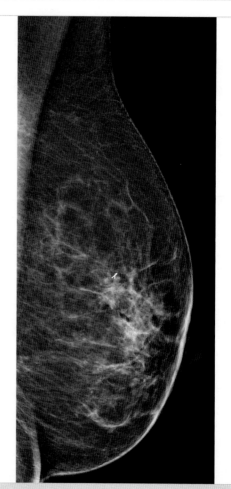

Fig. 79.14 Postbiopsy left mediolateral (LML) mammogram.

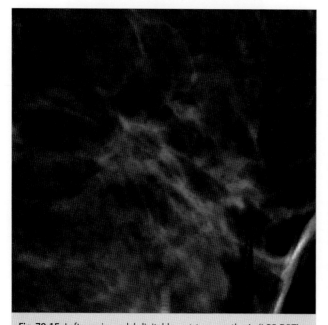

Fig. 79.15 Left craniocaudal digital breast tomosynthesis (LCC DBT), close-up slice 34 of 77.

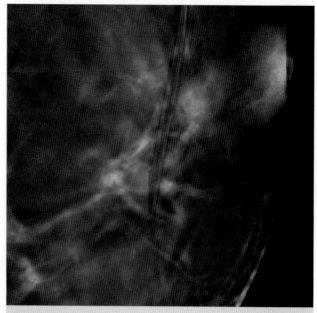

Fig. 79.16 Left mediolateral oblique digital breast tomosynthesis (LMLO DBT), close-up slice 40 of 72.

80 Palpable Breast Masses

Tanya W. Moseley

80.1 Presentation and Presenting Images

(▶ Fig. 80.1, ▶ Fig. 80.2, ▶ Fig. 80.3, ▶ Fig. 80.4, ▶ Fig. 80.5, ▶ Fig. 80.6)

A 31-year-old female with bilateral palpable breast masses presents for mammographic evaluation.

80.2 Key Images

(▶ Fig. 80.7, ▶ Fig. 80.8, ▶ Fig. 80.9, ▶ Fig. 80.10, ▶ Fig. 80.11, ▶ Fig. 80.12, ▶ Fig. 80.13, ▶ Fig. 80.14)

80.2.1 Breast Tissue Density

The breasts are heterogeneously dense, which may obscure small masses.

80.2.2 Imaging Findings

The patient has palpable abnormalities denoted by triangular markers (*arrows* in ▶ Fig. 80.7, ▶ Fig. 80.8, ▶ Fig. 80.9, and ▶ Fig. 80.10) in the upper outer quadrants of both breasts (1 o'clock location in left breast and 11 o'clock location in right breast). The triangular markers are not well seen on the right mediolateral oblique (MLO) and right lateromedial (LM) views (▶ Fig. 80.3 and ▶ Fig. 80.5). Historically the patient has solid masses in the right breast at the 3 o'clock location and the 10 o'clock location. These have been previously biopsied; however, biopsy clips were not placed at the time of the outside biopsies. The right 10 o'clock mass (*circle* in ▶ Fig. 80.13 and ▶ Fig. 80.14) is a oval hypoechoic mass, which is a fibroadenomatous change, and the right 3 o'clock mass (*circle* in ▶ Fig. 80.11 and ▶ Fig. 80.12) is an oval mixed echoic mass, which is a fibroadenoma. There are no correlates on conventional mammography or digital breast tomosynthesis for the current bilateral palpable abnormalities or the known right breast masses. The ultrasound of the current bilateral palpable areas (*triangle markers*) were consistent with benign breast parenchyma (*not shown*).

80.3 BI-RADS Classification and Action

Category 2: Benign

80.4 Differential Diagnosis

1. **Normal breast tissue**: Normal breast tissue is a common cause of palpable breast masses.
2. *Cysts*: Cysts are often multiple, usually bilateral, and may be palpable and/or painful and fluctuate in size. They are most common in 30- to 50-year-old patients.
3. *Fibroadenomas*: Fibroadenomas are the most common benign masses in young women. They are multiple in 10 to 15% of patients with them. Fibroadenomas may be palpable.

80.5 Essential Facts

- Palpable breast masses are common and usually benign, but accurate evaluation and prompt diagnosis are necessary to rule out malignancy.
- Additional supporting imaging or clinical information is helpful in diagnosis and management.
- In this case, there are no imaging correlates noted on conventional mammography or DBT for the bilateral palpable abnormalities or the known right breast masses.
- The biopsy-proven benign masses at the 3 o'clock and 10 o'clock positions of the right breast were unchanged in size by ultrasound.

80.6 Management and Digital Breast Tomosynthesis Principles

- There will be tomosynthesis-occult lesions. Further research is needed to determine which lesions are more likely to be tomosynthesis occult.
- There is a paucity of literature regarding lesions that are occult on tomosynthesis.
- Palpable findings without a mammographic or tomosynthesis correlate must be evaluated with ultrasound.
- The work-up of a palpable finding cannot stop with the absence of a mammographic or tomosynthesis finding. The palpable mass may be mammographically or tomosynthesis occult, as in this case. Palpable masses must be evaluated completely with ultrasound. If there is no ultrasound correlate, further work-up should be based upon the clinical suspicion.

80.7 Further Reading

[1] Klein S. Evaluation of palpable breast masses. Am Fam Physician. 2005; 71(9): 1731–1738
[2] Kopans DB. Digital breast tomosynthesis: a better mammogram. Radiology. 2013; 267(3):968–969

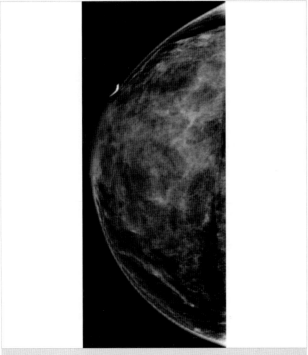

Fig. 80.1 Right craniocaudal (RCC) mammogram.

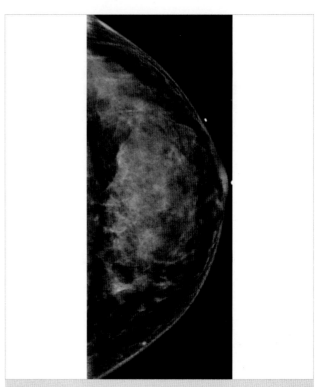

Fig. 80.2 Left craniocaudal (LCC) mammogram.

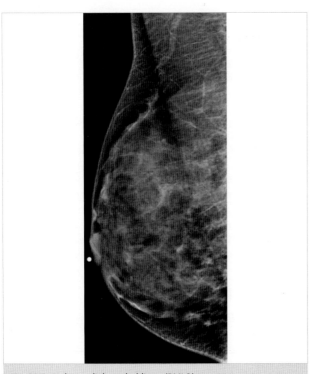

Fig. 80.3 Right mediolateral oblique (RMLO) mammogram.

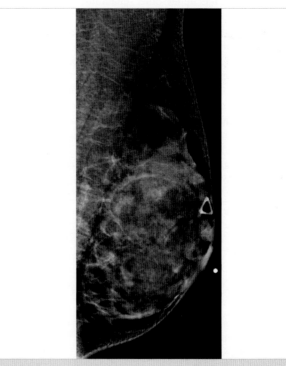

Fig. 80.4 Left mediolateral oblique (LMLO) mammogram.

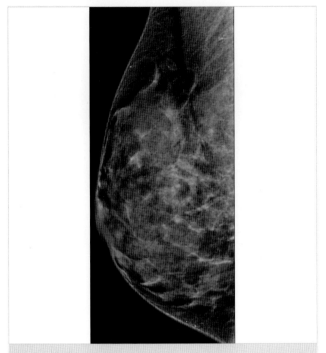

Fig. 80.5 Right lateromedial (RLM) mammogram.

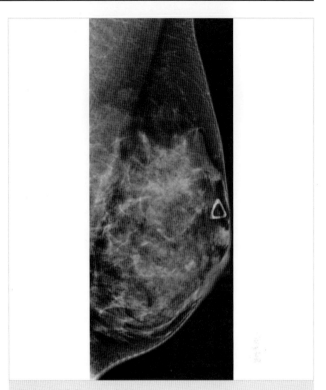

Fig. 80.6 Left lateromedial (LLM) mammogram.

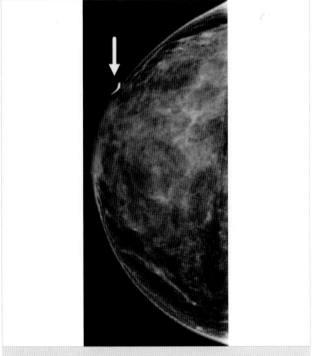

Fig. 80.7 Right craniocaudal (RCC) mammogram with label.

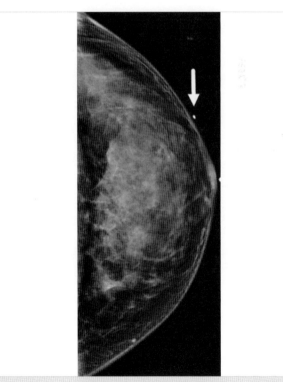

Fig. 80.8 Left craniocaudal (LCC) mammogram with label.

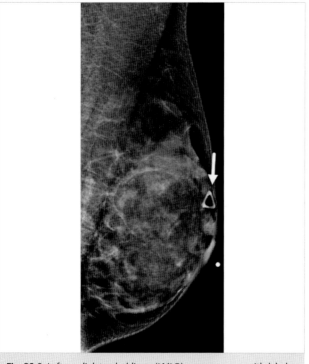

Fig. 80.9 Left mediolateral oblique (LMLO) mammogram with label.

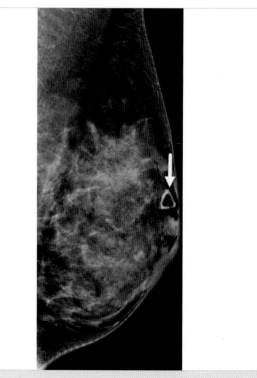

Fig. 80.10 Left lateromedial (LLM) mammogram with label.

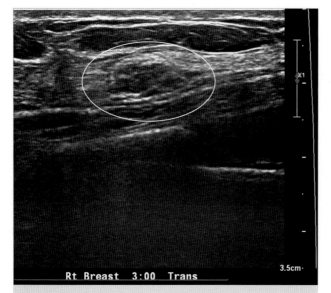

Fig. 80.11 Right breast ultrasound, transverse view of 3 o'clock mass.

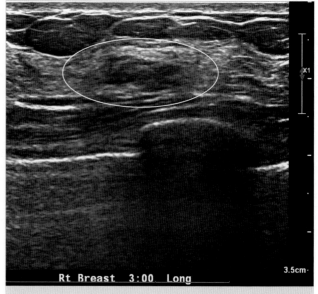

Fig. 80.12 Right breast ultrasound, longitudinal view of 3 o'clock mass.

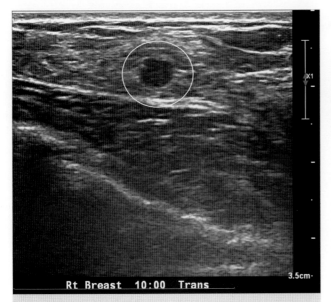

Fig. 80.13 Right breast ultrasound, transverse view of 10 o'clock mass.

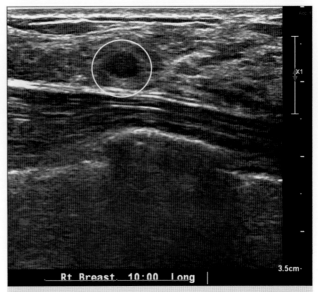

Fig. 80.14 Right breast ultrasound, longitudinal view of 10 o'clock mass.

81 Asymmetric Breast Tissue or Mass

Tanya W. Moseley

81.1 Presentation and Presenting Images

(▶ Fig. 81.1, ▶ Fig. 81.2, ▶ Fig. 81.3, ▶ Fig. 81.4, ▶ Fig. 81.5, ▶ Fig. 81.6, ▶ Fig. 81.7, ▶ Fig. 81.8, ▶ Fig. 81.9)

A 57-year-old male with a history of follicular lymphoma had a routine follow-up chest computed tomogram (CT), which revealed a mass in the retroareolar right breast. He presents for diagnostic mammographic evaluation.

81.2 Key Images

(▶ Fig. 81.10, ▶ Fig. 81.11, ▶ Fig. 81.12)

81.2.1 Breast Tissue Density

Breast tissue density is not typically evaluated in male patients.

81.2.2 Imaging Findings

The chest CT shows an asymmetrical soft tissue lesion in the right retroareolar region that is larger when compared to the prior CT (▶ Fig. 81.1, ▶ Fig. 81.2, ▶ Fig. 81.3). Conventional mammographic imaging of the right breast confirms the CT findings and demonstrates asymmetric breast tissue on the right breast compared to the left (▶ Fig. 81.10, ▶ Fig. 81.11, ▶ Fig. 81.12). Digital breast tomosynthesis (DBT) imaging reveals only breast tissue and no underlying mass lesions.

81.3 BI-RADS Classification and Action

Category 2: Benign

81.4 Differential Diagnosis

1. *Gynecomastia*: Gynecomastia, defined as benign proliferation of male breast glandular tissue, is usually caused by increased estrogen activity or decreased testosterone activity or is secondary to numerous medications.
2. *Breast cancer*: Breast cancer in men occurs approximately 100 times less than in women. The lifetime risk of having breast cancer is 1 in 1,000 for men.

3. *Lymphoma*: Primary lymphoma is less common than secondary lymphoma and is typically a B-cell type of non-Hodgkin's lymphoma (NHL). Primary non-Hodgkin's lymphoma of the breast represents only ~ 0.25% (range 0.12–0.53%) of all reported malignant breast tumors.

81.5 Essential Facts

- CT can identify incidental breast lesions when performed for cardiopulmonary evaluation. Indeterminate and suspicious CT-identified breast lesions should be further evaluated with mammography.
- This is a male patient and although breast cancer is rare in males, mammography should be performed to further evaluate CT-identified breast lesions in males.
- Gynecomastia is described as hyperplasia of the ductal and stromal elements of the male breast. It typically presents as a soft, mobile, painful mass.
- There is an association between gynecomastia, decreased testosterone, and increased estradiol. The increased estradiol–testosterone ratio may result from physiological changes at puberty and senescence or may be secondary to endocrine and hormonal disorders, neoplasms, and certain drugs and medications.

81.6 Management and Digital Breast Tomosynthesis Principles

- DBT may be safely performed on male patients.
- DBT's ability to remove overlapping tissue allows for evaluation of dense subareolar breast tissue.

81.7 Further Reading

[1] Appelbaum AH, Evans GFF, Levy KR, Amirkhan RH, Schumpert TD. Mammographic appearances of male breast disease. Radiographics. 1999; 19(3):559–568

[2] Braunstein GD. Clinical practice. Gynecomastia. N Engl J Med. 2007; 357(12): 1229–1237

[3] Moyle P, Sonoda L, Britton P, Sinnatamby R. Incidental breast lesions detected on CT: what is their significance? Br J Radiol. 2010; 83(987):233–240

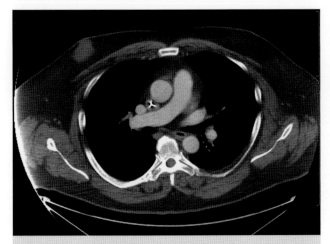

Fig. 81.1 Axial contrast-enhanced computed tomogram (CE-CT) of the chest on soft tissue window.

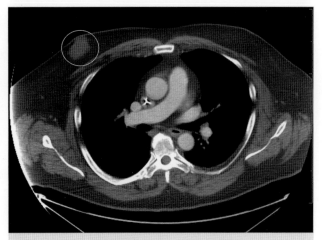

Fig. 81.2 Axial contrast-enhanced computed tomogram (CE-CT) of the chest on soft tissue window with label.

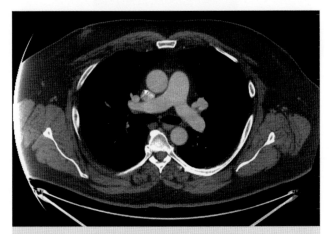

Fig. 81.3 Axial contrast-enhanced computed tomogram (CE-CT) of the chest on soft tissue window comparison.

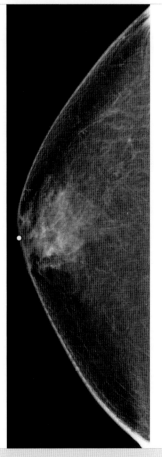

Fig. 81.4 Right craniocaudal (RCC) mammogram.

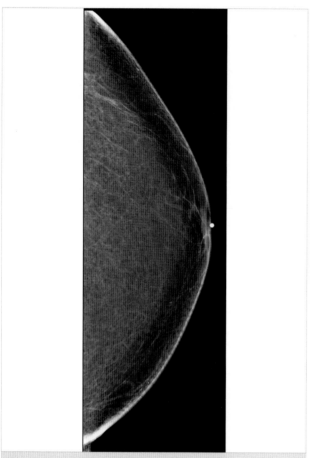

Fig. 81.5 Left craniocaudal (LCC) mammogram.

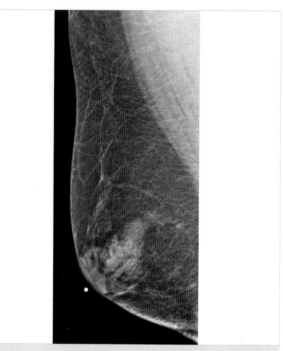

Fig. 81.6 Right mediolateral oblique (RMLO) mammogram.

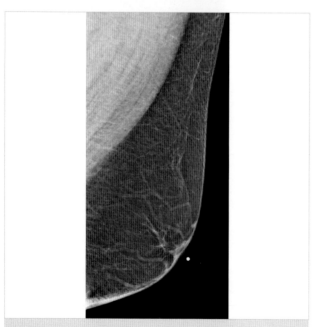

Fig. 81.7 Left mediolateral oblique (LMLO) mammogram.

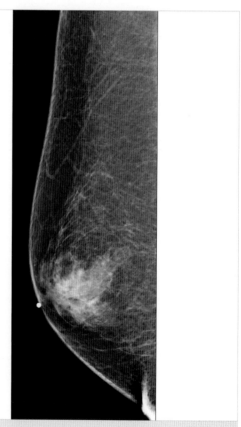

Fig. 81.8 Right lateromedial (RLM) mammogram.

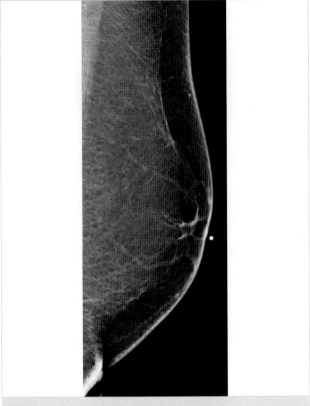

Fig. 81.9 Left lateromedial (LLM) mammogram.

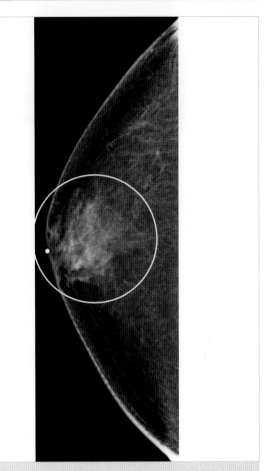

Fig. 81.10 Right craniocaudal (RCC) mammogram with label.

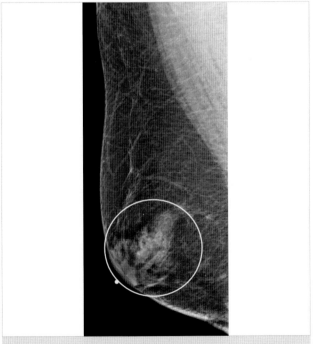

Fig. 81.11 Right mediolateral oblique (RMLO) mammogram with label.

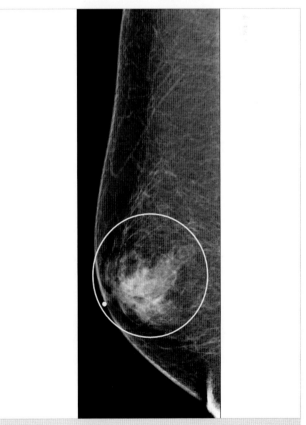

Fig. 81.12 Right lateromedial (RLM) mammogram with label.

82 New Palpable Finding at Site of a Remote Benign Image-Guided Biopsy

Lonie R. Salkowski

82.1 Presentation and Presenting Images

(▶ Fig. 82.1, ▶ Fig. 82.2, ▶ Fig. 82.3, ▶ Fig. 82.4, ▶ Fig. 82.5, ▶ Fig. 82.6, ▶ Fig. 82.7, ▶ Fig. 82.8, ▶ Fig. 82.9)

A 60-year-old female with a history of a benign stereotactic biopsy 15 years ago diagnosed as sclerosing adenosis, presents with a new palpable abnormality marked with a BB.

82.1.1 Breast Tissue Density

The breasts are heterogeneously dense, which may obscure small masses.

82.1.2 Imaging Findings

The two-view diagnostic conventional digital mammogram and the digital breast tomosynthesis (DBT) images (▶ Fig. 82.1, ▶ Fig. 82.2, ▶ Fig. 82.3 and ▶ Fig. 82.4) reveal that the palpable mass, marked with a BB, corresponds to an irregular high-density mass with spiculated margins at the 11 o'clock location, 2 cm from the nipple (▶ Fig. 82.5 and ▶ Fig. 82.6). This mass measures 3.3 × 1.3 × 1.7 cm, and there is associated nipple retraction (▶ Fig. 82.5 and ▶ Fig. 82.7). A clip is present from a prior stereotactic biopsy. The calcifications (▶ Fig. 82.7 and ▶ Fig. 82.8) have remained stable for the last 8 years (*not shown*). An ultrasound was recommended for further evaluation.

82.2 Diagnostic Images

(▶ Fig. 82.10, ▶ Fig. 82.11, ▶ Fig. 82.12, ▶ Fig. 82.13, ▶ Fig. 82.14, ▶ Fig. 82.15, ▶ Fig. 82.16)

82.2.1 Imaging Findings

The targeted ultrasound of the palpable mammographic finding reveals a 1.9 × 2.1 × 0.8 cm hypoechoic irregular mass with spiculated and angulated margins (▶ Fig. 82.10 and ▶ Fig. 82.11). This mass was biopsied with ultrasound guidance along with a suspicious axillary lymph node (*not shown*). The postprocedure mammogram (▶ Fig. 82.12 and ▶ Fig. 82.13) demonstrates the coil biopsy marker very close to the prior biopsy marker. To evaluate the extent of disease, magnetic resonance imaging (MRI) was performed that revealed a larger mass than noted on DBT or ultrasound, measuring 3.8 × 2.5 × 3.3 cm (▶ Fig. 82.14). Note that the signal void from the biopsy clip is in the center of the mass (▶ Fig. 82.15 and ▶ Fig. 82.16).

82.3 BI-RADS Classification and Action

Category 5: Highly suggestive of malignancy

82.4 Differential Diagnosis

1. ***Invasive lobular carcinoma (ILC)***: This mass appeared to incorporate itself into the breast tissue present. At the time of diagnosis, when it became symptomatic, it was quite large. These characteristics are compatible with an invasive lobular carcinoma. Pathology revealed a grade 2 invasive lobular carcinoma that was 3.5 cm.
2. *Invasive ductal carcinoma (IDC)*: Due to the overlap in imaging features, invasive ductal carcinoma would be a concordant diagnosis.
3. *Sclerosing adenosis*: Sclerosing adenosis can present as a mass, an architectural distortion, or calcifications. A biopsy result for this lesion revealing sclerosing adenosis would be considered discordant despite the prior biopsy of sclerosing adenosis. The imaging features suggest a much more aggressive process.

82.5 Essential Facts

- The mammogram demonstrated increased density within the dense breast tissue in the area of clinical concern. The DBT better revealed the mass located within this dense breast tissue. An ultrasound would have been done due to the palpable nature of the mass; however, the DBT was able to evaluate the size and margins of the lesion.
- ILC accounts for 10 to 15% of breast cancers.
- Similar to IDC, the most prognostic factor for ILC is lymph node status. This patient did have axillary metastases.
- ILC has a high tendency of positive margins at surgical excision; thus, MRI is often helpful to assess the extent of disease to optimize surgical resection.
- Compared to IDC, ILC has a higher tendency to be multifocal, multicentric, or bilateral.
- Stage for stage, ILC and IDC have similar prognoses.

82.6 Management and Digital Breast Tomosynthesis Principles

- DBT in diagnostic mammography provides an opportunity to evaluate all of the breast tissue for related pathology. The spot-compression mammographic views are helpful to assess a focal issue; however, DBT may provide a better overview of the clinical process.
- DBT may allow for better assessment of lesion size compared to FFDM (especially when the lesion is located in dense tissue) and provide a better estimate of pathologic size. This may afford more accurate preoperative tumor staging.
- The lesion size in this case was very similar on DBT (maximum 3.3 cm) and MRI (maximum 3.8 cm) compared to the final pathology size of 3.5 cm. Ultrasound underestimated the tumor size (maximum 2.1 cm).

- DBT can significantly reduce the anatomical noise that obscures small lesions. But DBT offers only marginal improvement in visualizing problematic growth patterns of large tumors including multifocality, diffuse infiltration, architectural distortion without evident tumor mass, and grade 3 tumors with nonspecific features that make them difficult to differentiate from normal breast tissue.

82.7 Further Reading

[1] Förnvik D, Zackrisson S, Ljungberg O, et al. Breast tomosynthesis: Accuracy of tumor measurement compared with digital mammography and ultrasonography. Acta Radiol. 2010; 51(3):240–247

[2] Lopez JK, Bassett LW. Invasive lobular carcinoma of the breast: spectrum of mammographic, US, and MR imaging findings. Radiographics. 2009; 29(1): 165–176

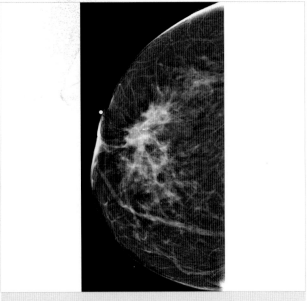

Fig. 82.1 Right craniocaudal (RCC) mammogram.

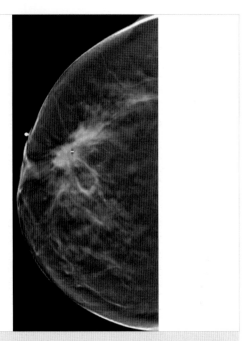

Fig. 82.2 Right craniocaudal digital breast tomosynthesis (RCC DBT), slice 33 of 76.

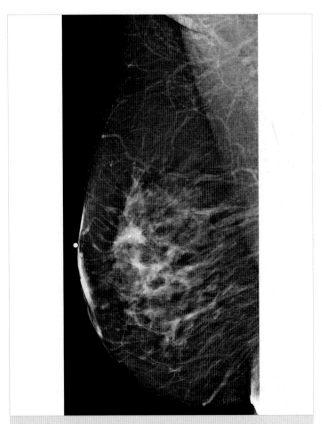

Fig. 82.3 Right mediolateral oblique (RMLO) mammogram.

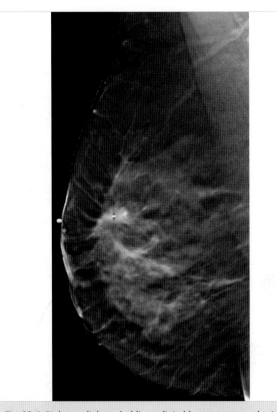

Fig. 82.4 Right mediolateral oblique digital breast tomosynthesis (RMLO DBT), slice 34 of 76.

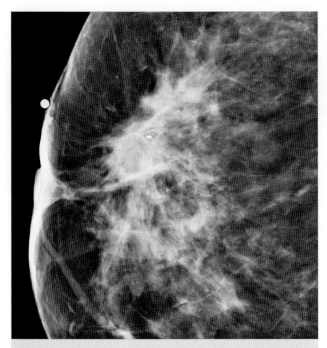

Fig. 82.5 Right craniocaudal (RCC) spot-compression mammogram.

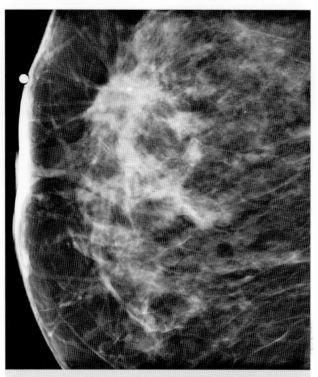

Fig. 82.6 Right mediolateral oblique (RLMO) spot-compression mammogram.

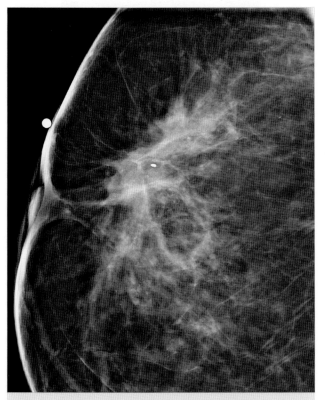

Fig. 82.7 Right craniocaudal (RCC) spot-magnification mammogram.

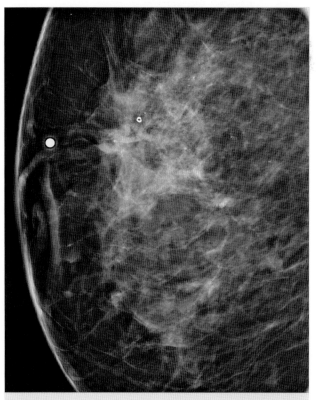

Fig. 82.8 Right mediolateral (RML) spot-magnification mammogram.

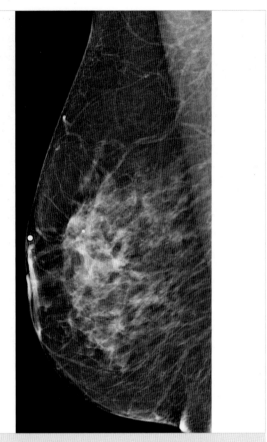

Fig. 82.9 Right mediolateral (RML) mammogram.

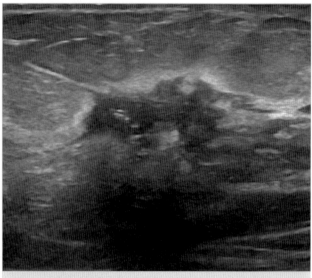

Fig. 82.10 Right breast ultrasound, radial view.

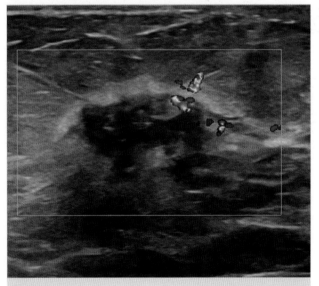

Fig. 82.11 Right breast Doppler ultrasound, radial view.

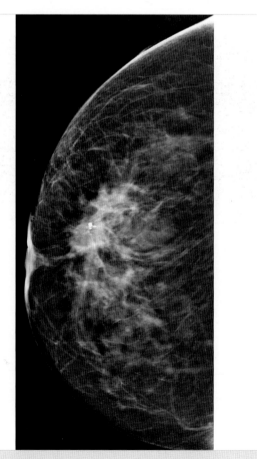

Fig. 82.12 Postbiopsy right craniocaudal (RCC) mammogram.

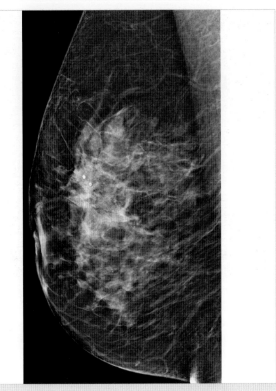

Fig. 82.13 Postbiopsy right mediolateral (RML) mammogram.

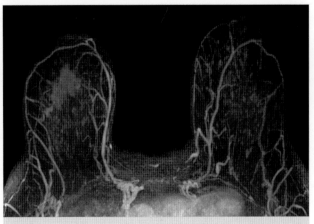

Fig. 82.14 Magnetic resonance (MR) maximum-intensity projection (MIP) image.

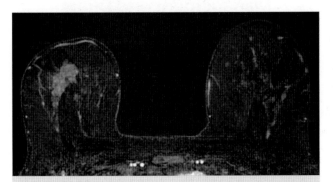

Fig. 82.15 Axial subtraction magnetic resonance (MR) image.

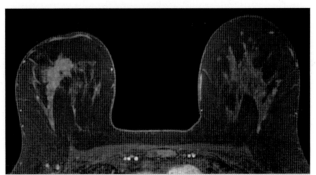

Fig. 82.16 Axial dynamic fat-saturation magnetic resonance (MR) image.

83 Palpable Breast Mass

Tanya W. Moseley

83.1 Presentation and Presenting Images

(▶ Fig. 83.1, ▶ Fig. 83.2, ▶ Fig. 83.3)

A 78-year-old male who felt a lump in his right breast while showering presents for diagnostic mammographic evaluation.

83.2 Key Images

(▶ Fig. 83.4, ▶ Fig. 83.5, ▶ Fig. 83.6, ▶ Fig. 83.7, ▶ Fig. 83.8)

83.2.1 Breast Tissue Density

There are scattered areas of fibroglandular density.

83.2.2 Imaging Findings

The imaging of the left breast is normal (*not shown*). The palpable finding in the right breast is denoted by the triangular marker (*arrow* in ▶ Fig. 83.4 and ▶ Fig. 83.5). The right breast demonstrates a high-density mass with indistinct margins and heterogeneous calcifications (*circle*) at the 7 o'clock position in the middle depth 2 cm from the nipple (▶ Fig. 83.4, ▶ Fig. 83.5, and ▶ Fig. 83.6). The right digital breast tomosynthesis (DBT) confirms with the mammographic findings and demonstrates that the mass has indistinct margins and corresponds to the palpable abnormality felt by the patient. The triangular marker localizes to the inferior aspect of the right breast (▶ Fig. 83.7 and ▶ Fig. 83.8).

83.3 Diagnostic Images

(▶ Fig. 83.9)

83.3.1 Imaging Findings

Sonography demonstrates a hypoechoic mass with angular and indistinct margins (▶ Fig. 83.9). It corresponds to the mass seen mammographically.

83.4 BI-RADS Classification and Action

Category 5: Highly suggestive of malignancy

83.5 Differential Diagnosis

1. ***Breast cancer***: Although rare, breast cancer does occur in men. This palpable mass is highly suspicious for malignancy.
2. *Gynecomastia*: Gynecomastia is usually eccentric to the nipple and retroareolar in location.
3. *Simple cyst*: The mass is hypoechoic and does not meet strict criteria for a cyst at ultrasound. Simple cysts are round or oval circumscribed masses with an imperceptible wall and posterior acoustic enhancement.

83.6 Essential Facts

- Gynecomastia is described as hyperplasia of the ductal and stromal elements of the male breast. It typically presents as a soft, mobile, painful mass.
- Male breast cancer is significantly less common than gynecomastia. It accounts for 1% of all breast cancers and 0.17% of all cancers in men.
- Male breast cancer typically presents as a hard, fixed, painless mass.
- Most male breast cancers are either in situ or invasive ductal carcinomas, because breast lobules are rare in males.

83.7 Management and Digital Breast Tomosynthesis Principles

- DBT can be performed on male breasts.
- As the parts of the breast tissue are viewed separately in slices with DBT, suspicious lesions may be quickly identified and accurately characterized.
- The conventional mammographic and DBT images can be acquired with one compression.
- The addition of DBT to conventional mammography significantly improves the diagnostic accuracy of conventional mammography.

83.8 Further Reading

[1] Appelbaum AH, Evans GFF, Levy KR, Amirkhan RH, Schumpert TD. Mammographic appearances of male breast disease. Radiographics. 1999; 19 (3):559–568

[2] Stavros AT, Rapp CL, Parker SH. Breast Ultrasound. Philadelphia, PA: Lippincott, Williams, & Wilkins; 2004.

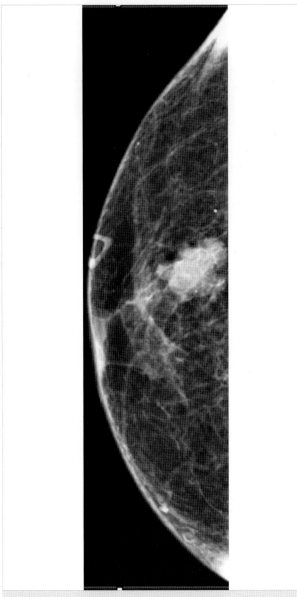

Fig. 83.1 Right craniocaudal (RCC) mammogram.

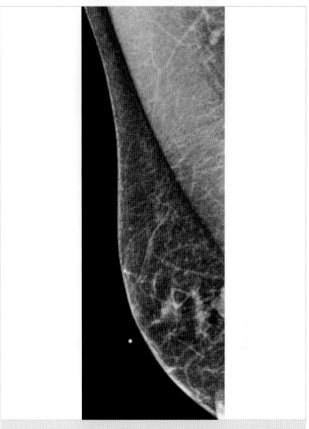

Fig. 83.2 Right mediolateral oblique (RMLO) mammogram.

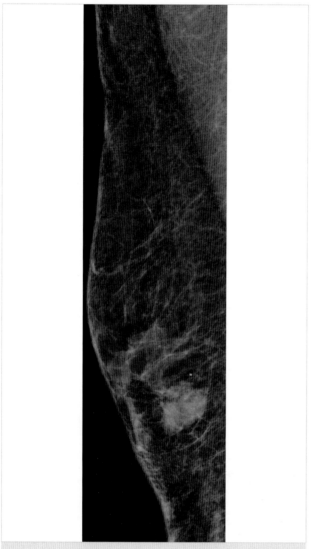

Fig. 83.3 Right lateromedial (RLM) mammogram.

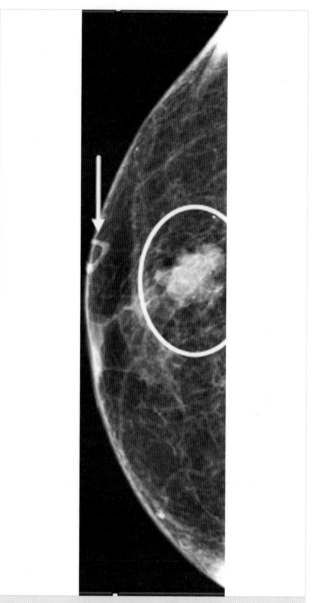

Fig. 83.4 Right craniocaudal (RCC) mammogram with label.

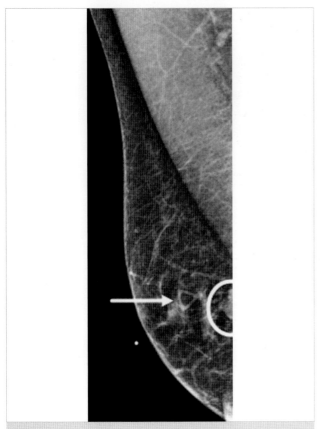

Fig. 83.5 Right mediolateral oblique (RMLO) mammogram with label.

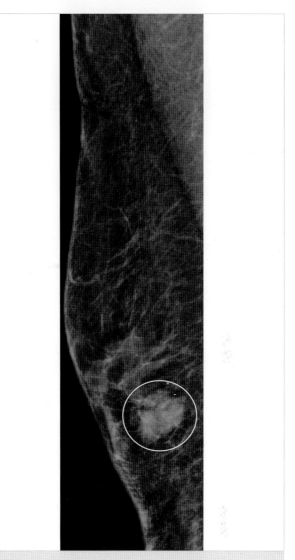

Fig. 83.6 Right lateromedial (RLM) mammogram with label.

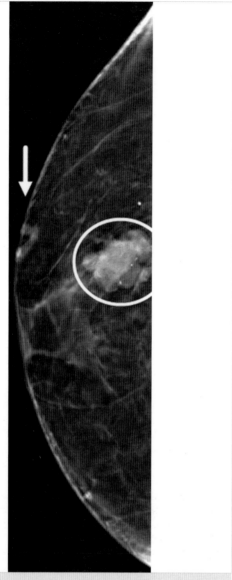

Fig. 83.7 Right craniocaudal digital breast tomosynthesis (RCC DBT), slice 15 of 48 with label.

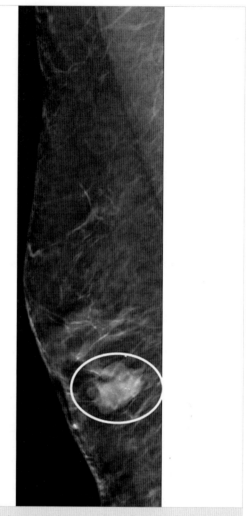

Fig. 83.8 Right lateromedial digital breast tomosynthesis (RLM DBT), slice 25 of 52 with label.

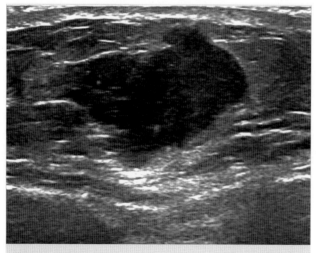

Fig. 83.9 Right breast ultrasound.

84 Palpable Mass on First Mammogram

Lonie R. Salkowski

84.1 Presentation and Presenting Images

(► Fig. 84.1, ► Fig. 84.2, ► Fig. 84.3, ► Fig. 84.4, ► Fig. 84.5, ► Fig. 84.6, ► Fig. 84.7, ► Fig. 84.8, ► Fig. 84.9)

A 39-year-old female presents for a second opinion of the palpable mass in her right breast. Prior to these evaluations, she has had no other mammograms. The palpable area was not marked.

84.1.1 Breast Tissue Density

The breasts are heterogeneously dense, which may obscure small masses.

84.1.2 Imaging Findings

The diagnostic imaging confirms the irregular mass with spiculated margins and grouped amorphous calcifications in the right breast at the 11 o'clock location, 3 cm from the nipple (► Fig. 84.1, ► Fig. 84.2, ► Fig. 84.3, ► Fig. 84.4, and ► Fig. 84.5). The calcifications appear to be confined to the mass and not located beyond the mass (► Fig. 84.8 and ► Fig. 84.9). This mass corresponds to the recently reported palpable finding (area of concern was not marked with a skin marker). The digital breast tomosynthesis (DBT) images better define the margins and determine that the mass is a portion of the dense tissue located in the upper outer quadrant (► Fig. 84.6 and ► Fig. 84.7). Although it is ill-defined mammographically, the mass measures approximately 3 × 3 cm. An ultrasound is recommended.

84.2 Key Images

(► Fig. 84.10, ► Fig. 84.11)

84.2.1 Imaging Findings

The ultrasound localizes the 2.4 × 2 × 2.4 cm irregular hypoechoic mass with angular and indistinct margins at the 11 o'clock location, 3 cm from the nipple (► Fig. 84.10 and ► Fig. 84.11). Within the mass, there are several echogenic microcalcifications.

84.3 BI-RADS Classification and Action

Category 5: Highly suggestive of malignancy

84.4 Differential Diagnosis

1. *Breast cancer*: The irregular shape with angular and indistinct margins and associated amorphous calcifications suggest that this mass is suspicious. On biopsy this mass was a grade 3 invasive ductal carcinoma (IDC).
2. *Fibroadenoma*: typically fibroadenomas are more circumscribed. A biopsy yielding a fibroadenoma result would be discordant.
3. Pseudoangiomatous stromal hyperplasia (*PASH*): PASH can have variable appearances including no mammographic findings, focal asymmetry, and circumscribed and partially circumscribed masses. PASH can often be palpable but rarely is it associated with calcifications and a mass with irregular margins such as this case demonstrates.

84.5 Essential Facts

- Although this lesion was not misinterpreted, it has factors that could easily lead to the reader missing the cancer.
- Steps that radiologists can take to increase their accuracy in mammographic interpretation are interpreting both screening and diagnostic mammograms, reviewing pertinent clinical data, adhering to proper positioning and technical requirements, and using ultrasound for palpable findings.
- When available, it is important to evaluate a mammogram with comparisons. Subtle changes, including developing asymmetries, can easily be missed.
- It is important to be alert for subtle signs of malignancy: areas of architectural distortion, small groups of amorphous calcifications, focal asymmetries, and relatively well-circumscribed masses.
- Only 39% of nonpalpable cancers demonstrate the classic signs of spiculated masses and linear calcifications.
- It is important to judge a lesion by it most malignant feature.

84.6 Management and Digital Breast Tomosynthesis Principles

- A synthesized mammogram is an image that is reconstructed from the images acquired during DBT.
- The synthesized mammogram differs from the conventional two-dimensional full-field digital mammogram (2D FFDM). It is meant to be read in conjunction with the DBT images and not as a standalone image.
- Early studies suggest that a synthesized 2D mammogram with DBT images is comparable to a conventional 2D FFDM with DBT images.

- The benefit of the synthesized 2D mammogram over FFDM is the dose reduction for the combination exam. No additional radiation is required for the synthesized mammogram.
- Computer-aided detection (CAD) can be applied to the synthesized mammogram.
- There is a learning curve to adjusting to the new look of the synthesized mammogram compared to the conventional FFDM.

84.7 Further Reading

[1] Majid AS, de Paredes ES, Doherty RD, Sharma NR, Salvador X. Missed breast carcinoma: pitfalls and pearls. Radiographics. 2003; 23(4):881–895

[2] Skaane P, Bandos AI, Eben EB, et al. Two-view digital breast tomosynthesis screening with synthetically reconstructed projection images: comparison with digital breast tomosynthesis with full-field digital mammographic images. Radiology. 2014; 271(3):655–663

[3] Zuley ML, Guo B, Catullo VJ, et al. Comparison of two-dimensional synthesized mammograms versus original digital mammograms alone and in combination with tomosynthesis images. Radiology. 2014; 271(3):664–671

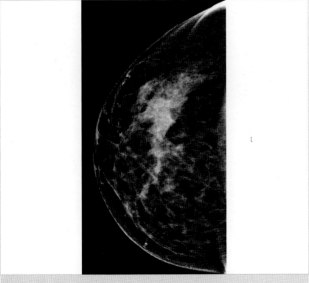

Fig. 84.1 Right craniocaudal (RCC) mammogram.

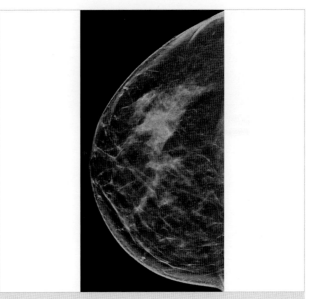

Fig. 84.2 Right craniocaudal (RCC) synthetic mammogram.

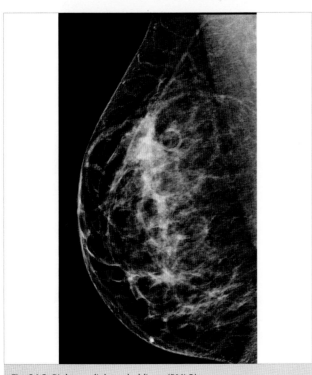

Fig. 84.3 Right mediolateral oblique (RMLO) mammogram.

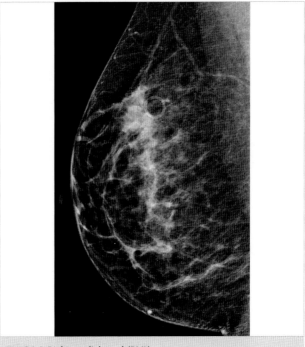

Fig. 84.4 Right mediolateral (RML) mammogram.

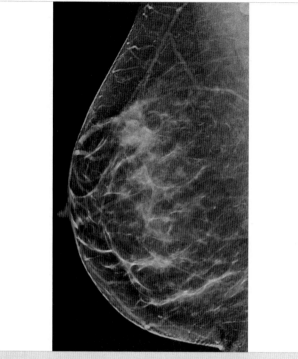

Fig. 84.5 Right mediolateral (RML) synthetic mammogram.

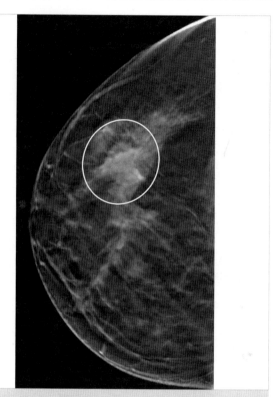

Fig. 84.6 Right craniocaudal digital breast tomosynthesis (RCC DBT), slice 42 of 74 labeled.

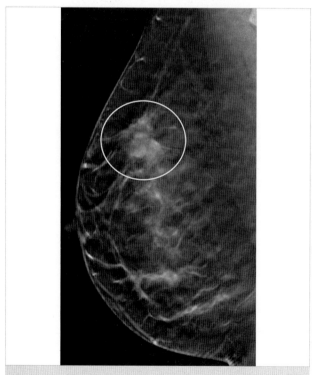

Fig. 84.7 Right mediolateral digital breast tomosynthesis (RML DBT), slice 31 of 72 labeled.

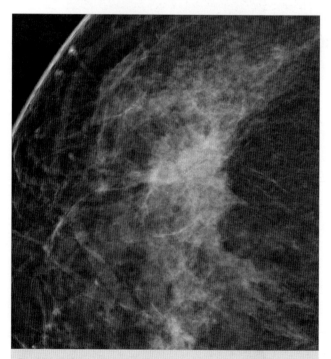

Fig. 84.8 Right craniocaudal (RCC) spot-magnification mammogram.

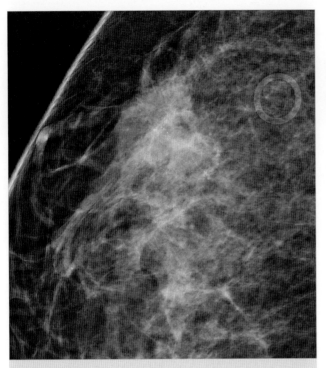

Fig. 84.9 Right mediolateral (RML) spot-magnification mammogram.

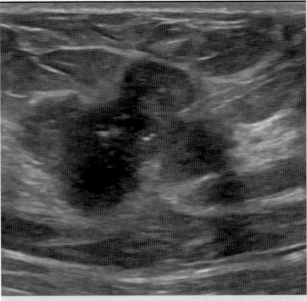

Fig. 84.10 Right breast ultrasound, transverse view.

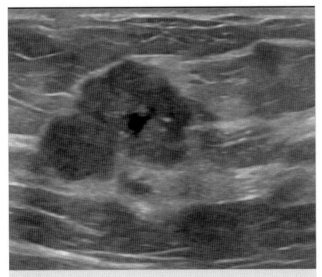

Fig. 84.11 Right breast ultrasound, longitudinal view.

85 Palpable Thickening

Lonie R. Salkowski

85.1 Presentation and Presenting Images

(▶ Fig. 85.1, ▶ Fig. 85.2, ▶ Fig. 85.3, ▶ Fig. 85.4, ▶ Fig. 85.5, ▶ Fig. 85.6, ▶ Fig. 85.7)

A 63-year-old female with a history of treated right breast cancer presents for evaluation of a palpable thickening in the left breast found 2 months ago. The area of concern is marked with a BB.

85.1.1 Breast Tissue Density

There are scattered areas of fibroglandular density.

85.1.2 Imaging Findings

The area of thickening marked with a BB is in the subareolar region. The conventional digital mammograms and the additional spot-compression mammograms do not reveal any focal finding (▶ Fig. 85.1, ▶ Fig. 85.2, ▶ Fig. 85.3, ▶ Fig. 85.6, and ▶ Fig. 85.7). The complexity of the subareolar region can easily obscure lesions. The digital breast tomosynthesis (DBT) images suggest an area of architectural distortion at the12 o'clock location in the subareolar region (▶ Fig. 85.4 and ▶ Fig. 85.5). An ultrasound was recommended for further evaluation.

85.2 Diagnostic Images

(▶ Fig. 85.8, ▶ Fig. 85.9, ▶ Fig. 85.10, ▶ Fig. 85.11, ▶ Fig. 85.12)

85.2.1 Imaging Findings

The targeted ultrasound of the thickening located at 12 o'clock reveals multiple irregular hypoechoic masses with angular margins with the epicenter 5 cm from the nipple (▶ Fig. 85.8 and ▶ Fig. 85.9). The masses span an area of 4 cm, larger than noted on DBT. The largest mass in this group measures 12 × 9 × 11 mm. Due to the suspicious nature of these masses and their extent, an axillary ultrasound was performed. In the axilla 13 cm from the nipple, there was an oval hypoechoic mass measuring 3.2 × 1.9 cm (▶ Fig. 85.10). Both areas were biopsied with ultrasound guidance. The ribbon clip is located in the area corresponding to where the patient noted thickening (▶ Fig. 85.11 and ▶ Fig. 85.12).

85.3 BI-RADS Classification and Action

Category 4C: High suspicion for malignancy

85.4 Differential Diagnosis

1. ***Invasive ductal cancer (IDC) with axillary metastases***: The mammographic and ultrasound presentation is not typical for cancer. The large area of involvement with the abnormal appearing axillary node raises suspicion and a biopsy is warranted. On biopsy, this lesion was a grade 3 IDC with axillary nodal metastases.
2. *Multiple abscesses with inflamed axillary lymph node*: Typically, for this diagnosis, there would be additional signs of skin thickening and edema within the parenchyma, which are not present.
3. *Papillomatosis*: This lesion typically presents as multiple small masses in a segmental distribution. It is not typical that they are accompanied by an enlarged and pathologic-appearing axillary lymph node.

85.5 Essential Facts

- This lesion was essentially mammographically occult. DBT suggested a small area of architectural distortion; however, this greatly underestimated the size of the lesion.
- In this case, the patient's clinical symptoms contributed most to detection of the lesion.
- Of breast cancers that are mammographically occult, 9 to 16% are detected only by palpation. Distinguishing between benign and malignant lesions on palpation alone is limited. Only 20% of surgical biopsies for palpable lesions detect malignancy.
- Patients with clinical symptoms and no overt signs on mammography that correlate to the symptoms warrant further evaluation with ultrasound.
- If mammogram and ultrasound are negative for a palpable mass, then the evaluation should be based on clinical symptoms. This may include close observation, patient reassurance, or a palpated-guided biopsy.

85.6 Management and Digital Breast Tomosynthesis Principles

- Some lesions will be occult on DBT, just as they can be occult on mammography.
- Most studies to date have compared DBT to FFDM. Larger studies are needed to determine the proportion of cancers detected by DBT that are mammographically occult, and what proportion of cancers are occult on DBT.
- Some cancers that have been reported occult on DBT can been seen on contrast-enhanced magnetic resonance (MR) imaging. Some of these lesions have been large. The reason why these lesions may not have been detected on DBT is the lack of, or missed, architectural distortion or the lack of distinct mass margins.

85.7 Further Reading

[1] Conant EF. Clinical implementation of digital breast tomosynthesis. Radiol Clin North Am. 2014; 52(3):499–518

[2] Georgian-Smith D, Taylor KJ, Madjar H, et al. Sonography of palpable breast cancer. J Clin Ultrasound. 2000; 28(5):211–216

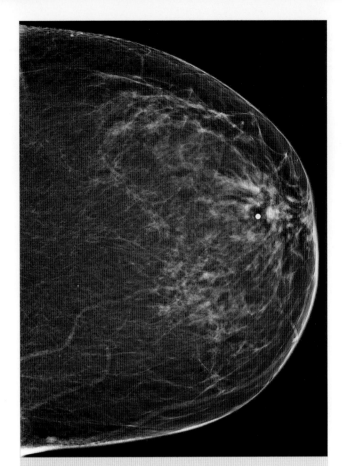

Fig. 85.1 Left craniocaudal (LCC) mammogram.

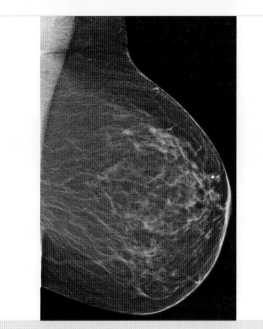

Fig. 85.2 Left mediolateral oblique (LMLO) mammogram.

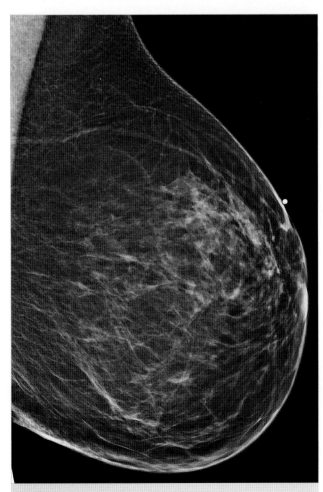

Fig. 85.3 Left mediolateral (LML) mammogram.

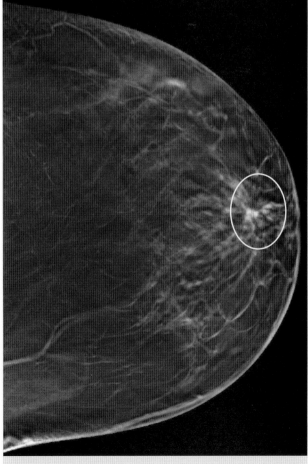

Fig. 85.4 Left craniocaudal digital breast tomosynthesis (LCC DBT), slice 53 of 82, with label.

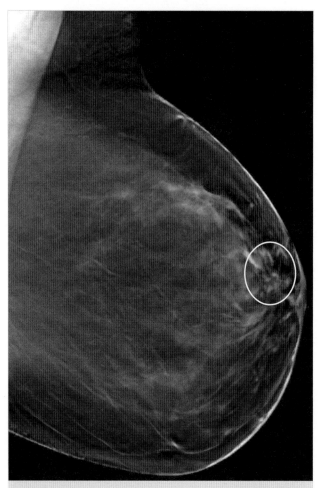

Fig. 85.5 Left mediolateral oblique digital breast tomosynthesis (LMLO DBT), slice 48 of 102, with label.

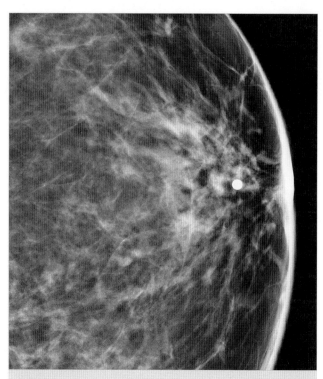

Fig. 85.6 Left craniocaudal (LCC) spot-compression mammogram.

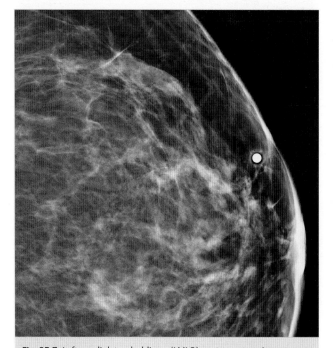

Fig. 85.7 Left mediolateral oblique (LMLO) spot-compression mammogram.

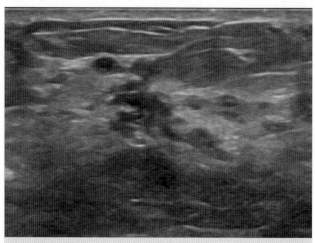

Fig. 85.8 Left breast ultrasound, transverse view.

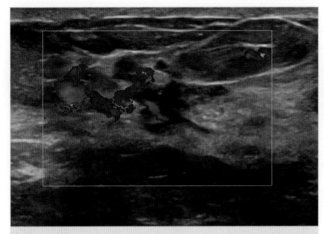

Fig. 85.9 Left breast Doppler ultrasound.

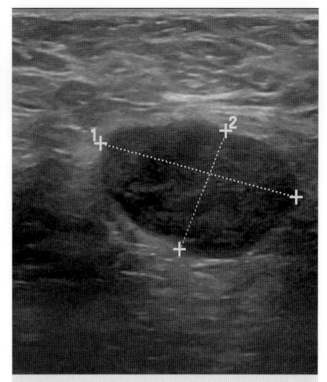

Fig. 85.10 Left breast ultrasound, left axilla at 13 cm from the nipple.

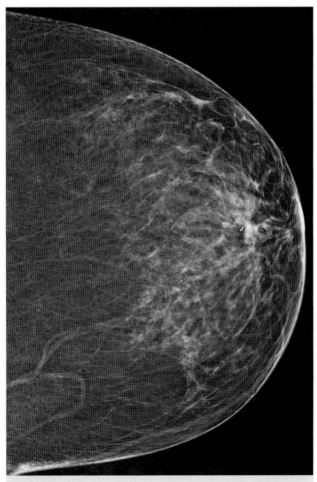

Fig. 85.11 Postbiopsy left craniocaudal (LCC) mammogram.

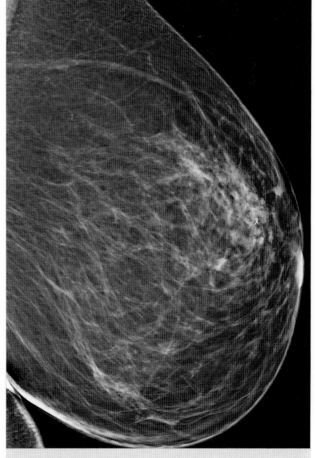

Fig. 85.12 Postbiopsy left mediolateral (LML) mammogram.

86 Right Breast Pain

Tanya W. Moseley

86.1 Presentation and Presenting Images

(▶ Fig. 86.1, ▶ Fig. 86.2, ▶ Fig. 86.3, ▶ Fig. 86.4, ▶ Fig. 86.5, ▶ Fig. 86.6, ▶ Fig. 86.7, ▶ Fig. 86.8, ▶ Fig. 86.9, ▶ Fig. 86.10, ▶ Fig. 86.11, ▶ Fig. 86.12)

A 56-year-old female presents for evaluation of generalized right breast pain. This is her baseline mammogram.

86.1.1 Breast Tissue Density

There are scattered areas of fibroglandular density.

86.1.2 Imaging Findings

There are no prior studies for comparison. The imaging of the left breast is normal (*not shown*). The right breast demonstrates oval masses (*circles*) at the 11 o'clock location in the anterior depth, 2 cm from the nipple, and at the 7 to 8 o'clock location in the middle depth, 5.5 cm from the nipple (▶ Fig. 86.7, ▶ Fig. 86.8, ▶ Fig. 86.9). Digital breast tomosynthesis shows the margins of both masses are well circumscribed (▶ Fig. 86.10, ▶ Fig. 86.11, and ▶ Fig. 86.12). No other masses are seen.

The patient is premenopausal and not at an increased risk to develop breast cancer (no family history or genetic predisposition). Ultrasound is recommended to further evaluate both masses.

86.2 Diagnostic Images

(▶ Fig. 86.13, ▶ Fig. 86.14)

86.2.1 Imaging Findings

Ultrasound was performed. The mass at the 11 o'clock position (3.3 cm from the nipple) was shown to be a well-circumscribed hypoechoic mass. The mass at the 7 o'clock position (5.8 cm from the nipple) was a well-circumscribed anechoic mass. The cyst is benign (7 o'clock mass); no further work-up is needed. The solid benign-appearing mass (11 o'clock mass) may be followed short-term with repeat sonography in 6 months.

86.3 BI-RADS Classification and Action

Category 3: Probably benign

86.4 Differential Diagnosis

1. **Benign and probably benign masses**: Both masses have benign sonographic findings. As this was a baseline exam, it was decided to follow the solid mass with benign features, but it could have been decided to biopsy instead. This decision should involve a discussion with the patient about the level of suspicion of malignancy and about her ability to follow an imaging finding for 2 years to assure it remains stable.
2. *Suspicious masses*: There are no suspicious sonographic findings associated with either mass.
3. *Summation artifacts*: Both masses persist on conventional mammography and DBT imaging, and again are confirmed on sonography.

86.5 Essential Facts

- Benign sonographic characteristics include the following: well-circumscribed margins, wider than tall orientation, less than three gentle lobulations, and the absence of any malignant characteristics.
- Malignant sonographic characteristics include the following: spiculated margins, taller than wider orientation, microlobulation, angular margins, and posterior acoustic shadowing.
- Conventional mammography plus DBT increases reader performance for identifying masses and architectural distortions over conventional mammography alone.
- DBT increases the detection of masses including invasive cancers in breasts of all parenchymal densities and reduces the recall rate while increasing the positive predictive value for both recalls and biopsies.

86.6 Management and Digital Breast Tomosynthesis Principles

- DBT is both a screening and diagnostic modality.
- DBT acquires several images of the breast at multiple angles. The individual images are reconstructed into a series of thin, high-resolution slices typically 1-mm thick, which can be viewed in the same manner as computed tomography (CT) or magnetic resonance (MR) images, as single slices or dynamically as a movie (cine).
- The ability to view images as a single slice or dynamically as a movie eliminates the effects of overlapping breast tissue and allows for better visualization and characterization of masses.
- Benign and malignant lesions may have similar appearances on mammography.
- Radiologists need to be careful not to dismiss all benign-appearing masses as benign.

86.7 Further Reading

[1] Rafferty EA, Park JM, Philpotts LE, et al. Assessing radiologist performance using combined digital mammography and breast tomosynthesis compared with digital mammography alone: results of a multicenter, multireader trial. Radiology. 2013; 266(1):104–113

[2] Rose SL, Tidwell AL, Bujnoch LJ, Kushwaha AC, Nordmann AS, Sexton R, Jr. Implementation of breast tomosynthesis in a routine screening practice: an observational study. AJR Am J Roentgenol. 2013; 200(6):1401–1408

[3] Stavros AT, Thickman D, Rapp CL, et al. Solid breast nodules: use of sonography to distinguish between benign and malignant lesions. Radiology. 1995;196(1):123-134

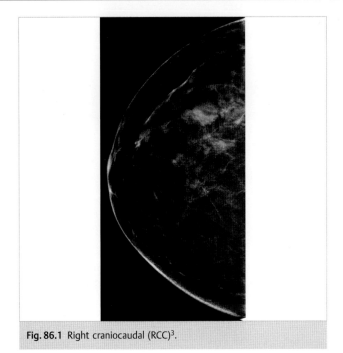

Fig. 86.1 Right craniocaudal (RCC)[3].

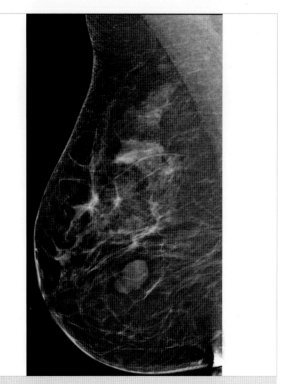

Fig. 86.2 Right mediolateral oblique (RMLO) mammogram.

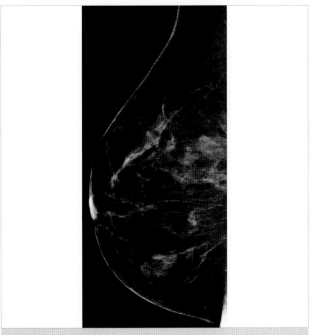

Fig. 86.3 Right lateromedial (RLM) mammogram.

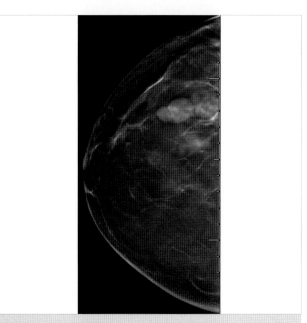

Fig. 86.4 Right craniocaudal digital breast tomosynthesis (RCC DBT), slice 17 of 79.

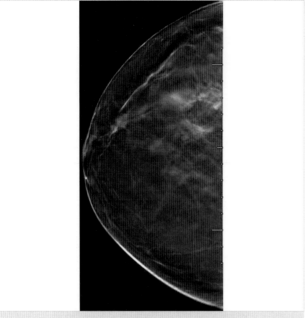

Fig. 86.5 Right craniocaudal digital breast tomosynthesis (RCC DBT), slice 35 of 79.

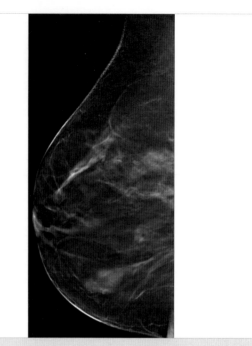

Fig. 86.6 Right lateromedial digital breast tomosynthesis (RLM DBT), slice 37 of 83.

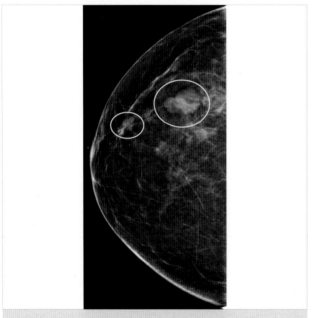

Fig. 86.7 Right craniocaudal (RCC) mammogram with label.

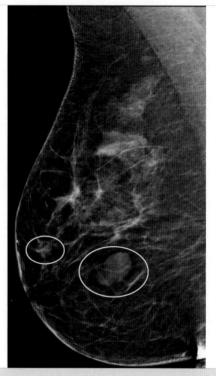

Fig. 86.8 Right mediolateral oblique (RMLO) mammogram with label.

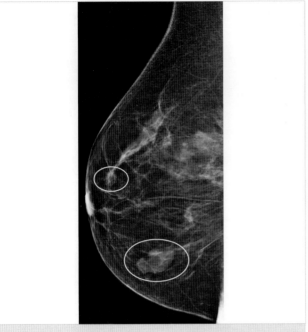

Fig. 86.9 Right lateromedial (RLM) mammogram with label.

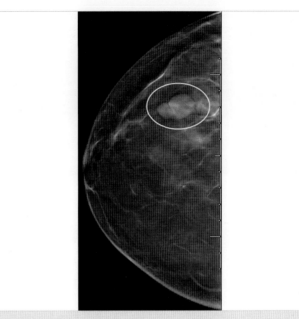

Fig. 86.10 Right craniocaudal digital breast tomosynthesis (RCC DBT), slice 17 of 79 with label.

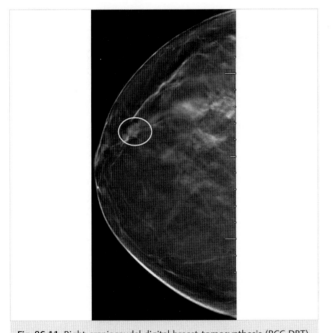

Fig. 86.11 Right craniocaudal digital breast tomosynthesis (RCC DBT), slice 35 of 79 with label.

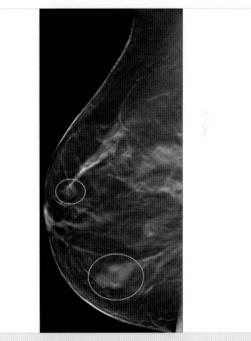

Fig. 86.12 Right lateromedial digital breast tomosynthesis (RLM DBT), slice 37 of 83 with label.

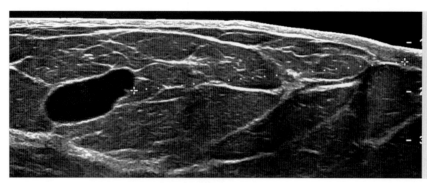

Fig. 86.13 Right breast ultrasound of 7 o'clock mass.

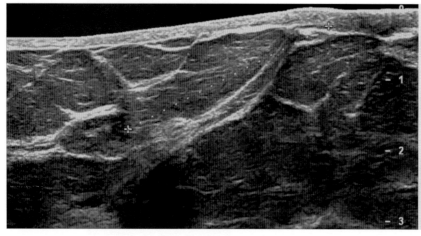

Fig. 86.14 Right breast ultrasound of 11 o'clock mass.

87 Breast Pain

Lonie R. Salkowski

87.1 Presentation and Presenting Images

(▸ Fig. 87.1, ▸ Fig. 87.2, ▸ Fig. 87.3, ▸ Fig. 87.4, ▸ Fig. 87.5, ▸ Fig. 87.6, ▸ Fig. 87.7, ▸ Fig. 87.8, ▸ Fig. 87.9, ▸ Fig. 87.10)

A 56-year-old female with a strong family history of breast cancer presents with left breast pain, marked with a BB.

87.1.1 Breast Tissue Density

The breasts are heterogeneously dense, which may obscure small masses.

87.1.2 Imaging Findings

The conventional digital and synthetic mammograms do not demonstrate a significant finding correlating to the area of pain noted by the patient (marked with a BB in ▸ Fig. 87.1, ▸ Fig. 87.2, ▸ Fig. 87.3, and ▸ Fig. 87.4). The digital breast tomosynthesis (DBT) images (▸ Fig. 87.5 and ▸ Fig. 87.6) reveal a 1.3-cm irregular mass with obscured and spiculated margins at the 2 o'clock location, slightly anterior and medial to the site marked as painful. This lesion is not readily apparent on the full-field digital mammograms (FFDM) or the synthetic mammograms. The additional spot-compression mammograms (▸ Fig. 87.7, ▸ Fig. 87.8, ▸ Fig. 87.9, and ▸ Fig. 87.10) of this region also demonstrate the mass that was seen on DBT due to the associated architectural distortion. An ultrasound is recommended for further characterization.

87.2 Diagnostic Images

(▸ Fig. 87.11, ▸ Fig. 87.12, ▸ Fig. 87.13, ▸ Fig. 87.14, ▸ Fig. 87.15)

87.2.1 Imaging Findings

The ultrasound of the mammographic mass that is near the area of pain reveals a 9 × 9 × 13 mm irregular hypoechoic mass with indistinct margins at the 2 o'clock location, 3 cm from the nipple. Adjacent to this mass is a similar smaller, 7 × 5 × 8 mm irregular hypoechoic mass with indistinct margins and posterior shadowing located at the 3 o'clock location, 2 cm from the nipple (▸ Fig. 87.11, ▸ Fig. 87.12, and ▸ Fig. 87.13). In retrospect, the second mass is not seen on the conventional digital mammogram, synthetic mammogram, or DBT. Both masses were biopsied. The coil marker clip was placed in the 2 o'clock mass, and the ribbon clip, in the 3 o'clock mass (▸ Fig. 87.14 and ▸ Fig. 87.15).

87.3 BI-RADS Classification and Action

Category 4C: High suspicion for malignancy

87.4 Differential Diagnosis

1. **Two cancers (invasive ductal carcinoma):** The patient's pain may have been a referred pain, but it did not directly relate to the masses. Her breast pain did bring her in for evaluation, and eventually for diagnosis of two adjacent cancers.
2. *Fat necrosis*: Fat necrosis can be symptomatic or asymptomatic. The patient has no history of trauma or surgical breast procedures. The imaging is too worrisome to dismiss the findings as fat necrosis. Biopsy of both lesions is warranted.
3. *Radial scars*: Radial scars are great mimickers of carcinoma. For this diagnosis to be concordant, the size of the imaging finding needs to match the size of the histopathologic finding. A smaller lesion would be discordant.

87.5 Essential Facts

- This case demonstrates two adjacent cancers; one is seen mammographically and the other is occult. Both are seen by ultrasound.
- Multifocal breast cancer is defined as multiple lesions (two or more) within 4 or 5 cm of each other.
- Multifocal breast cancer typically occurs within the same quadrant.
- Up to 27 to 34% of cancers are multifocal. Mammographically unifocal cancers were found to have additional foci at histopathologic aassessment.
- It is more common for invasive lobular carcinoma (ILC) to be multifocal than for invasive ductal carcinoma. (IDC).

87.6 Management and Digital Breast Tomosynthesis Principles

- Understanding the advantages and limitations of the breast imaging modalities allows one to optimize the use of these imaging modalities in detecting the majority of breast cancers. Ultrasound and magnetic resonance (MR) imaging can be useful adjunct tools in the detection of mammographically occult cancers.
- Early studies suggest that DBT was better at detecting architectural distortion when compared to FFDM. DBT detected those architectural distortions seen on FFDM and also those not detected on FFDM.

- Any new technology has a prevalence bias, that is, when first introduced, cancer detection rates are higher than observed in subsequent incident screening. This was observed when mammography and breast MRI were first introduced, and this may also now be happening with the introduction of DBT. Further studies are needed to determine the role that DBT will have in breast cancer detection.

87.7 Further Reading

[1] Berg WA, Gutierrez L, NessAiver MS, et al. Diagnostic accuracy of mammography, clinical examination, US, and MR imaging in preoperative assessment of breast cancer. Radiology. 2004; 233(3):830–849

[2] Partyka L, Lourenco AP, Mainiero MB. Detection of mammographically occult architectural distortion on digital breast tomosynthesis screening: initial clinical experience. AJR Am J Roentgenol. 2014; 203(1):216–222

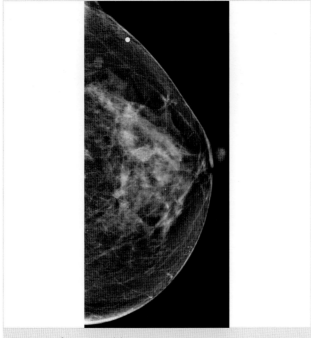

Fig. 87.1 Left craniocaudal (LCC) mammogram.

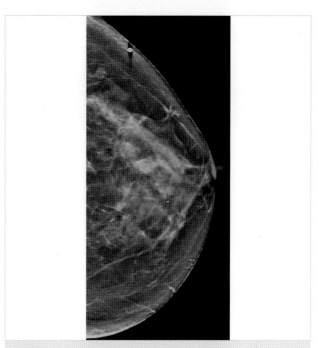

Fig. 87.2 Left craniocaudal (LCC) synthetic mammogram.

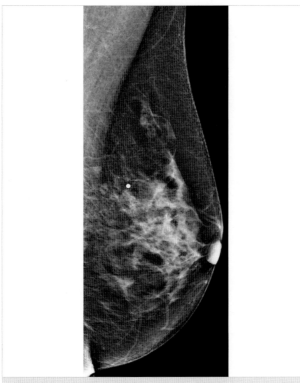

Fig. 87.3 Left mediolateral oblique (LMLO) mammogram.

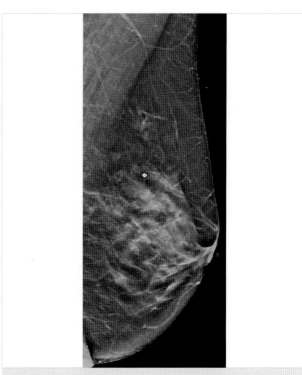

Fig. 87.4 Left mediolateral oblique LMLO synthetic mammogram.

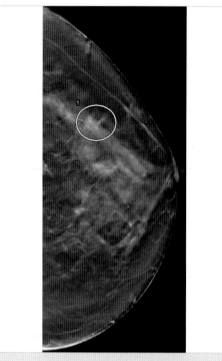

Fig. 87.5 Left craniocaudal digital breast tomosynthesis (LCC DBT), slice 32 of 61.

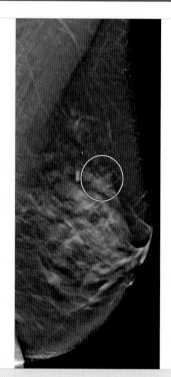

Fig. 87.6 Left mediolateral oblique digital breast tomosynthesis (LMLO DBT), slice 20 of 57.

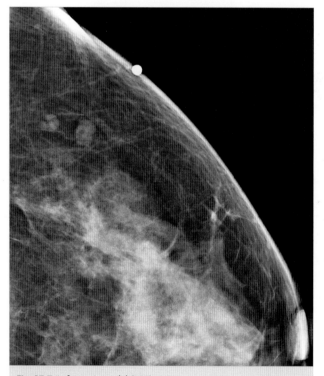

Fig. 87.7 Left craniocaudal (LCC) spot-compression mammogram.

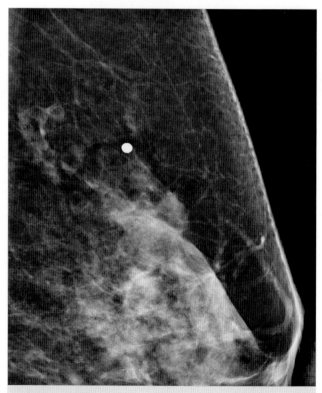

Fig. 87.8 Left mediolateral oblique (LMLO) spot-compression mammogram.

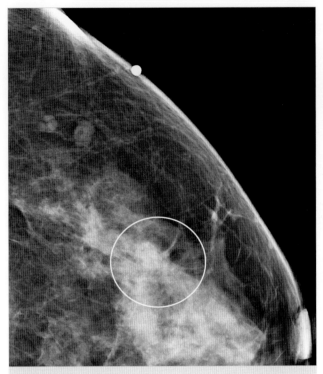

Fig. 87.9 Left craniocaudal (LCC) spot-compression mammogram with label.

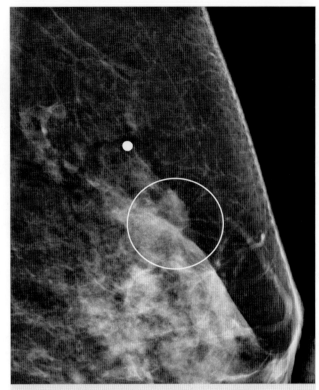

Fig. 87.10 Left mediolateral oblique (LMLO) spot-compression mammogram with label.

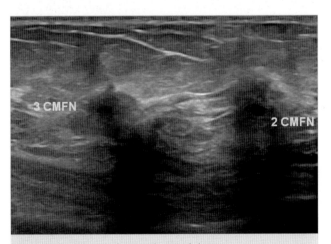

Fig. 87.11 Left breast ultrasound, antiradial view.

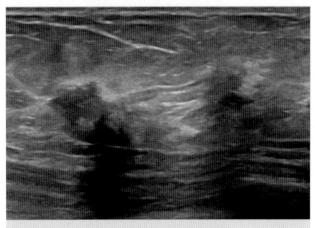

Fig. 87.12 Left breast ultrasound, longitudinal view.

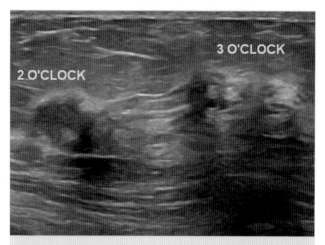

Fig. 87.13 Left breast ultrasound, longitudinal view with label.

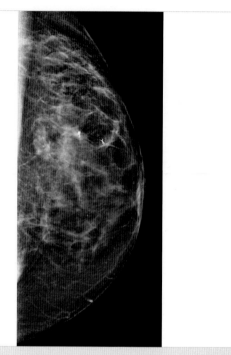

Fig. 87.14 Postbiopsy left craniocaudal (LCC) mammogram.

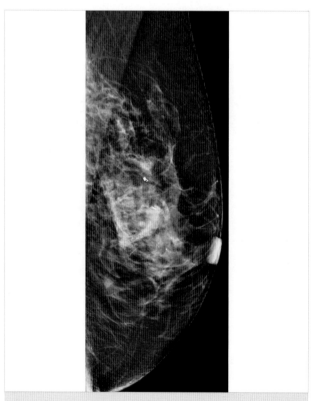

Fig. 87.15 Postbiopsy left mediolateral (LML) mammogram.

88 Palpable Axillary Mass

Tanya W. Moseley

88.1 Presentation and Presenting Images

(▶ Fig. 88.1, ▶ Fig. 88.2, ▶ Fig. 88.3, ▶ Fig. 88.4)

A 55-year-old female with a palpable abnormality in her right axilla presents for diagnostic mammography.

88.2 Key Images

(▶ Fig. 88.5, ▶ Fig. 88.6, ▶ Fig. 88.7, ▶ Fig. 88.8)

88.2.1 Breast Tissue Density

There are scattered areas of fibroglandular density.

88.2.2 Imaging Findings

The imaging of the left breast is normal and is shown for comparison (▶ Fig. 88.2 and ▶ Fig. 88.4). The palpable abnormality (triangular skin marker) in the right axilla corresponds with the abnormal lymph nodes (*circle* in ▶ Fig. 88.6 and ▶ Fig. 88.8). There is an area of architectural distortion (*arrows*) measuring 1.7 centimeters in the outer hemisphere of the right breast at the 9 to 10 o'clock location, 8 cm from the nipple (▶ Fig. 88.5 and ▶ Fig. 88.6). The digital breast tomosynthesis (DBT) movie confirms an area of architectural distortion in the right breast at the 9 o'clock location, 8 cm from the nipple (▶ Fig. 88.7 and ▶ Fig. 88.8).

88.3 Diagnostic Images

(▶ Fig. 88.9, ▶ Fig. 88.10)

88.3.1 Imaging Findings

Ultrasound shows an abnormal level I lymph node (▶ Fig. 88.9) that corresponds to the largest lymph node seen on the mammogram. The lymph node has lost its parallel orientation, reniform shape, and echogenic fatty hilum. This lymph node has an appearance suggestive of a metastatic lymph node.

Ultrasound of the breast shows a hypoechoic spiculated mass (*arrows* in ▶ Fig. 88.10) measuring approximately 2 cm maximally at the 9 o'clock location. This mass corresponds to the architectural distortion seen mammographically.

88.4 BI-RADS Classification and Action

Category 5: Highly suggestive of malignancy

88.5 Differential Diagnosis

1. *Invasive lobular carcinoma*: A discrete mass is less commonly seen with invasive lobular carcinoma compared with invasive ductal carcinoma; instead, there is a higher incidence of subtle mammographic signs, such as asymmetry or architectural distortion.
2. *Summation artifact*: The architectural distortion is noted and persists on both the conventional and DBT imaging.
3. *Radial scars*: Radial scars may present as an area of architectural distortion. However, the abnormal lymph node makes this diagnosis a less likely possibility.

88.6 Essential Facts

- Identifying invasive lobular carcinoma at screening mammography has been known to be a difficult task with false-negative rates ranging from 8 to 19%.
- The difficulty of detection is secondary to the spread of invasive lobular carcinoma through the breast parenchyma in a single file fashion and the tendency of the cells to grow circumferentially around ducts and lobules causing minimal interruption of the fundamental anatomical structures of the breast.
- Invasive lobular carcinoma presents more commonly as an asymmetry or an architectural distortion.
- Invasive lobular carcinoma is commonly less dense than or isodense to normal breast tissue.

88.7 Management and Digital Breast Tomosynthesis Principles

- DBT permits radiologists to scroll manually through the images or view the images as a movie and visualize the breast tissue in sections.
- These cross-sectional tomosynthesis images (slices) allow better visualization of lesions because of the elimination of breast tissue overlap and the reduction of the masking impact of tissue density.
- Architectural distortion is better seen and characterized on DBT than on conventional mammography.
- DBT identifies a subset of architectural distortions that are not identified on conventional mammography. Identification of these additional architectural distortions increases the cancer detection rate.

88.8 Further Reading

[1] Helvie MA, Paramagul C, Oberman HA, Adler DD. Invasive lobular carcinoma. Imaging features and clinical detection. Invest Radiol. 1993; 28(3):202–207

[2] Krecke KN, Gisvold JJ. Invasive lobular carcinoma of the breast: mammographic findings and extent of disease at diagnosis in 184 patients. AJR Am J Roentgenol. 1993; 161(5):957–960

[3] Partyka L, Lourenco AP, Mainiero MB. Detection of mammographically occult architectural distortion on digital breast tomosynthesis screening: initial clinical experience. AJR Am J Roentgenol. 2014; 203(1):216–222

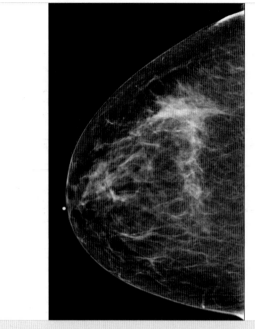

Fig. 88.1 Right craniocaudal (RCC) mammogram.

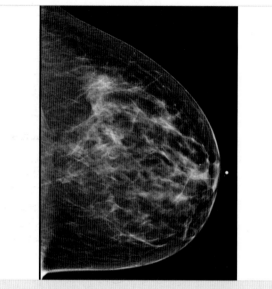

Fig. 88.2 Left craniocaudal (LCC) mammogram.

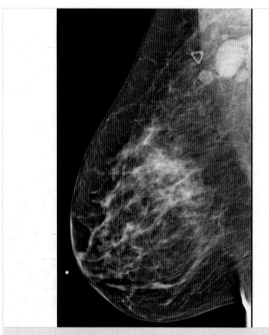

Fig. 88.3 Right mediolateral oblique (RMLO) mammogram.

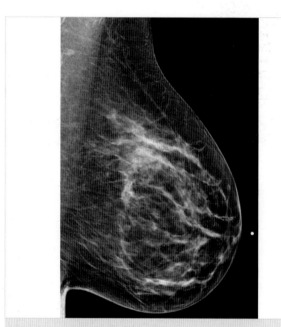

Fig. 88.4 Left mediolateral oblique (LMLO) mammogram.

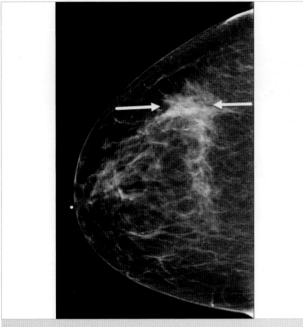

Fig. 88.5 Right craniocaudal (RCC) mammogram with label.

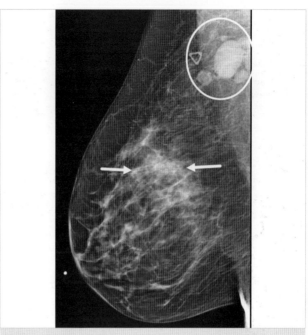

Fig. 88.6 Right mediolateral oblique (RMLO) mammogram with label.

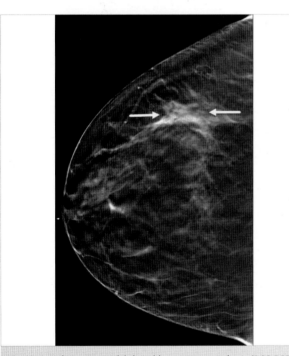

Fig. 88.7 Right craniocaudal digital breast tomosynthesis (RCC DBT), slice 25 of 74 with label.

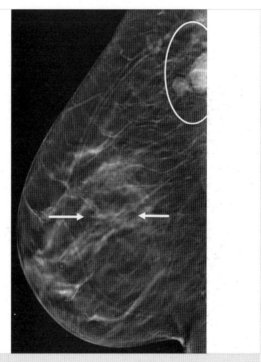

Fig. 88.8 Right mediolateral oblique digital breast tomosynthesis (RMLO DBT), slice 49 of 75 with label.

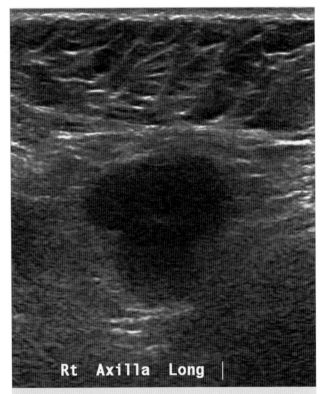

Fig. 88.9 Right breast ultrasound Axilla.

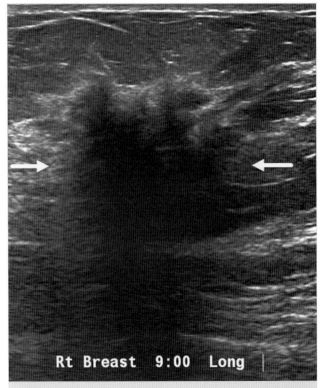

Fig. 88.10 Right breast ultrasound.

89 Spiculated Retroareolar Mass with Linear Calcifications

Tanya W. Moseley

89.1 Presentation and Presenting Images

(▶ Fig. 89.1, ▶ Fig. 89.2)

A 78-year-old female with chronic obstructive pulmonary disease (COPD) presents for a chest computed tomogram (CT). She has a history of bilateral reduction mammoplasties.

89.1.1 Imaging Findings

The chest CT shows bilateral pleural effusions (*arrows*) and left nipple-areolar skin thickening and distortion (*circle*) in the left retroareolar region (▶ Fig. 89.1 and ▶ Fig. 89.2). These findings prompted mammographic evaluation (▶ Fig. 89.3, ▶ Fig. 89.4 and ▶ Fig. 89.5).

89.2 Key Images

(▶ Fig. 89.3, ▶ Fig. 89.4, ▶ Fig. 89.5, ▶ Fig. 89.6, ▶ Fig. 89.7, ▶ Fig. 89.8, ▶ Fig. 89.9, ▶ Fig. 89.10, ▶ Fig. 89.11)

89.2.1 Breast Tissue Density

There are scattered areas of fibroglandular density.

89.2.2 Imaging Findings

The mammographic imaging of the left breast reveals a spiculated mass with associated linear heterogeneous calcifications (*oval*) in the retroareolar region. A radiopaque BB (*broken arrow*) marks the nipple in the lateromedial (LM) view (▶ Fig. 89.8). An abnormal lymph node (*solid arrow*) is seen in the low axilla on the mediolateral oblique (MLO) and LM views (▶ Fig. 89.7 and ▶ Fig. 89.8). Digital breast tomosynthesis (DBT) views help to delineate the linear orientation of the calcifications (▶ Fig. 89.9 and ▶ Fig. 89.10). The right breast (*not shown*) shows postreduction changes and no suspicious findings.

89.3 Diagnostic Images

(▶ Fig. 89.11 and ▶ Fig. 89.12)

89.3.1 Imaging Findings

These spot-magnification views of the retroareolar calcifications noted on the DBT reveal pleomorphic calcifications in a linear orientation (▶ Fig. 89.11 and ▶ Fig. 89.12). These are not in the skin.

89.4 BI-RADS Classification and Action

Category 5: Highly suggestive of malignancy

89.5 Differential Diagnosis

1. ***Breast cancer (in situ and invasive ductal carcinoma):*** A spiculated mass with pleomorphic calcifications and axillary adenopathy are all suspicious findings for malignancy.
2. *Post–reduction-mammoplasty changes*: The patient has had bilateral reduction mammoplasties, but the current imaging findings show the breasts as asymmetrical. While asymmetrical findings are possible, in this case the findings are suspicious for malignancy and warrant biopsy.
3. *Fibrocystic changes*: The morphology (pleomorphic) and orientation (linear) of the calcifications are inconsistent with fibrocystic changes.

89.6 Essential Facts

- The morphology (pleomorphic) and orientation (linear) of the calcifications are inconsistent with fibrocystic changes.
- Chest CT can identify incidental breast lesions. Moyle and colleagues (2010) found that 30% of the incidental breast lesions that were detected on CT in their study were unsuspected breast cancers, particularly the spiculated masses.
- Indeterminate and suspicious CT-identified breast lesions should be further evaluated with mammography.

89.7 Management and Digital Breast Tomosynthesis Principles

- Because DBT images present with reduced tissue overlap and structural noise, indeterminate and suspicious lesions are seen better, which leads to improved reader confidence.
- Two-view tomosynthesis imaging is required. Orthogonal reconstructions cannot be generated from DBT as from CT or magnetic resonance imaging (MRI). Elongated, planar, or nonspherical etiologies may be better seen in one view than another on DBT.
- Magnification cannot be performed with DBT. Thus, for optimal breast imaging, tomosynthesis systems must support both conventional mammography and DBT.
- Tomosynthesis-directed stereotactic biopsy may be used to biopsy calcifications, masses, and/or architectural distortions.

89.8 Further Reading

[1] Harish MG, Konda SD, MacMahon H, Newstead GM. Breast lesions incidentally detected with CT: what the general radiologist needs to know. Radiographics. 2007; 27 Suppl 1:S37–S51

[2] Moyle P, Sonoda L, Britton P, Sinnatamby R. Incidental breast lesions detected on CT: what is their significance? Br J Radiol. 2010; 83(987):233–240

[3] Muir TM, Tresham J, Fritschi L, Wylie E. Screening for breast cancer post reduction mammaplasty. Clin Radiol. 2010; 65(3):198–205

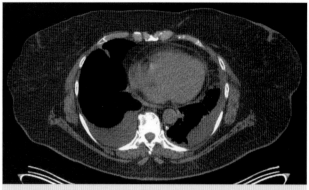

Fig. 89.1 Axial noncontrast computed tomogram (CT) of the chest.

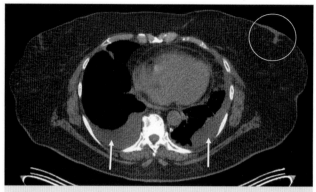

Fig. 89.2 Axial noncontrast computed tomogram (CT) of the chest with label.

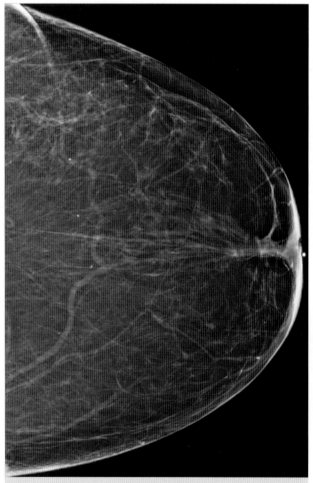

Fig. 89.3 Left craniocaudal (LCC) mammogram.

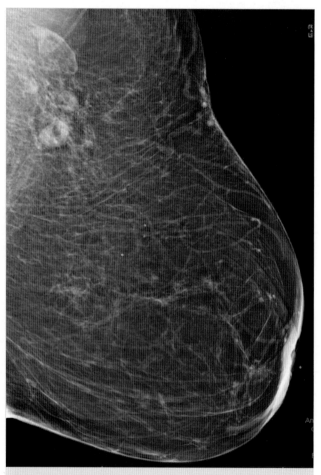

Fig. 89.4 Left mediolateral oblique (LMLO) mammogram.

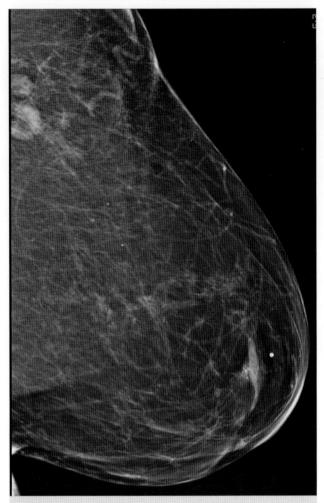

Fig. 89.5 Left lateromedial (LLM) mammogram.

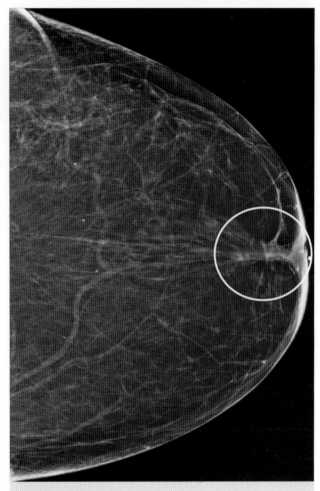

Fig. 89.6 Left craniocaudal (LCC) mammogram with label.

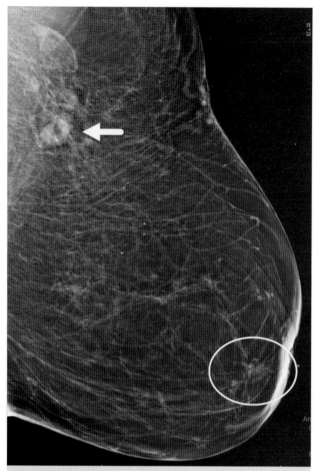

Fig. 89.7 Left mediolateral oblique (LMLO) mammogram with label.

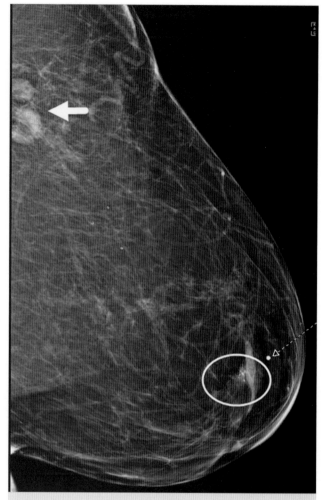

Fig. 89.8 Left lateromedial (LLM) mammogram with label.

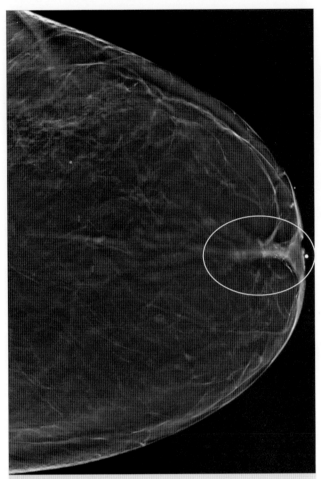

Fig. 89.9 Left craniocaudal digital breast tomosynthesis (LCC DBT), slice 22 of 71 with label.

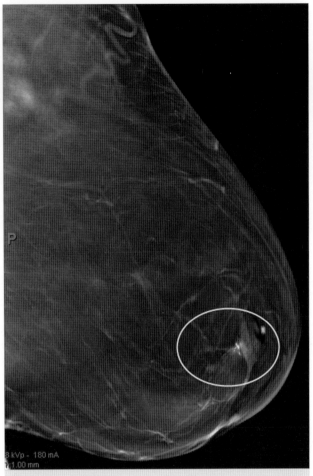

Fig. 89.10 Left lateromedial digital breast tomosynthesis (LLM DBT), slice 17 of 87 with label.

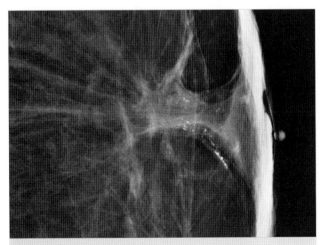

Fig. 89.11 Left craniocaudal (LCC) spot-magnification mammogram.

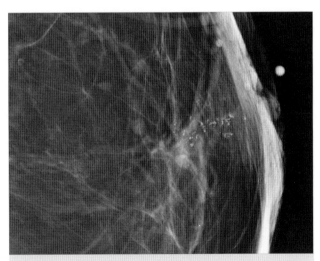

Fig. 89.12 Left lateromedial (LML) spot-magnification mammogram.

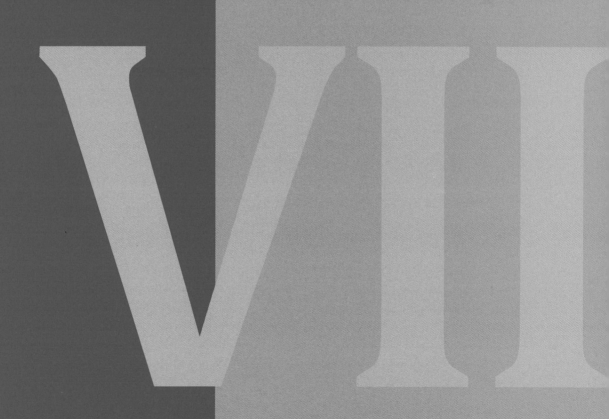

Part VII

Cases with Known Cancer Diagnosis Needing Additional Evaluation

90 Oval Mass Seen on Digital Breast Tomosynthesis

Tanya W. Moseley

90.1 Presentation and Presenting Images

(▶ Fig. 90.1, ▶ Fig. 90.2, ▶ Fig. 90.3, ▶ Fig. 90.4, ▶ Fig. 90.5)

A 52-year-old female with a left breast biopsy performed at an outside institution that was consistent with intraductal carcinoma (DCIS) and invasive ductal carcinoma presents for diagnostic mammography and evaluation.

90.2 Key Images

(▶ Fig. 90.6, ▶ Fig. 90.7, ▶ Fig. 90.8, ▶ Fig. 90.9, ▶ Fig. 90.10, ▶ Fig. 90.11, ▶ Fig. 90.12, ▶ Fig. 90.13, ▶ Fig. 90.14, ▶ Fig. 90.15)

90.2.1 Breast Tissue Density

There are scattered areas of fibroglandular density.

90.2.2 Imaging Findings

The imaging of the right breast is normal (*not shown*). The left breast demonstrates the known malignancy (*circle* in ▶ Fig. 90.6, ▶ Fig. 90.7, ▶ Fig. 90.8, ▶ Fig. 90.9, and ▶ Fig. 90.10) as an area of architectural distortion with associated pleomorphic calcifications and a postbiopsy clip located at the 2 to 3 o'clock location in the anterior depth, 3 cm from the nipple. The architectural distortion is confirmed on digital breast tomosynthesis (DBT) imaging (▶ Fig. 90.11 and ▶ Fig. 90.12). Note that the biopsy marker clip (*arrow* in ▶ Fig. 90.12) is at the superior margin of the architectural distortion. This is helpful to know when planning preoperative localization.

There is an 8-mm oval mass (*arrows* in ▶ Fig. 90.13 and ▶ Fig. 90.14) at 9 o'clock in the middle depth of the left breast, 4.5 cm from the nipple, on slice 28 of 67 of the craniocaudal (CC) tomosynthesis movie (▶ Fig. 90.13) and slice 29 of 77 of the lateromedial (LM) tomosynthesis movie (▶ Fig. 90.14). This finding is not seen on conventional mammography.

Sonography reveals an anechoic mass (▶ Fig. 90.15) with posterior acoustic enhancement that is the same size and distance from the nipple as the tomosynthesis finding.

90.3 BI-RADS Classification and Action

Category 2: Benign
  Category 6: Known biopsy-proven malignancy

90.4 Differential Diagnosis

1. **Cyst**: Cysts are often multiple, usually bilateral, and may be painful and fluctuate in size. They are most common in 30- to 50-year-old patients. Cysts can be found in the same breast that has a diagnosed cancer.

2. *Fibroadenoma*: Fibroadenomas are the most common benign masses in young women. They are multiple in 10 to 15% of patients. This is a reasonable benign diagnosis; however, it is not supported by the ultrasound findings.

3. *Invasive ductal carcinoma*: In this patient with a known malignancy, it is important to exclude multicentric and multifocal malignancy. The ultrasound reveals a cyst; thus, this is not a likely diagnosis.

90.5 Essential Facts

- It is important to identify true mass lesions and to dismiss pseudomasses or summation artifacts.
- The spiculated mass was easily identified on both conventional mammography and DBT imaging. In this case, it would have been difficult to identify the oval mass on conventional mammography. Before DBT, additional imaging including spot-compression views would have been necessary to confirm the finding.
- Determination that the mass is oval does not confirm benignity. Ultrasound was necessary to further characterize this mass as a cyst.
- If ultrasound had not identified this mass and biopsy was deemed necessary, tomosynthesis-directed stereotactic biopsy could have been performed.

90.6 Management and Digital Breast Tomosynthesis Principles

- The detection of lesions obscured by overlapping breast parenchyma is a limitation of conventional two-dimensional (2D) analog and digital mammography.
- Overlapping breast parenchyma may obscure cancers resulting in missed cancer diagnoses. Conversely, overlapping parenchyma or superimposed normal structures may create pseudomasses or summation artifacts, resulting in false-positive diagnoses and unnecessary biopsies.
- Spiculated masses are suspicious on conventional mammography and DBT imaging. The management of oval masses detected on tomosynthesis is less straightforward. Rafferty and colleagues (2013) found that some circumscribed cancers were misclassified as benign. Until there is a sufficient body of research or experiential knowledge regarding the management of these masses, additional imaging may need to be performed.

90.7 Further Reading

[1] Friedewald SM, Rafferty EA, Rose SL, et al. Breast cancer screening using tomosynthesis in combination with digital mammography. JAMA. 2014; 311 (24):2499–2507

[2] Rafferty EA, Park JM, Philpotts LE, et al. Assessing radiologist performance using combined digital mammography and breast tomosynthesis compared with digital mammography alone: results of a multicenter, multireader trial. Radiology. 2013; 266(1):104–113

[3] Rose SL, Tidwell AL, Bujnoch LJ, Kushwaha AC, Nordmann AS, Sexton R, Jr. Implementation of breast tomosynthesis in a routine screening practice: an observational study. AJR Am J Roentgenol. 2013; 200(6):1401–1408

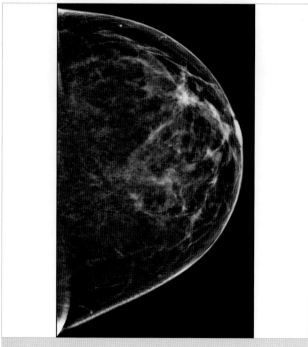

Fig. 90.1 Left craniocaudal (LCC) mammogram.

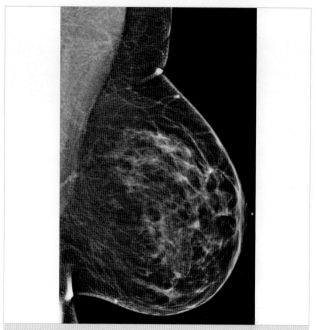

Fig. 90.2 Left mediolateral oblique (LMLO) mammogram.

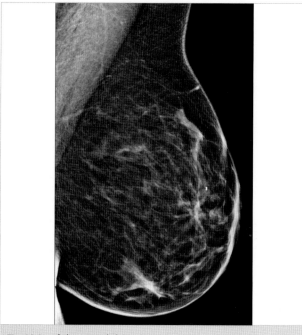

Fig. 90.3 Left lateromedial (LLM) mammogram.

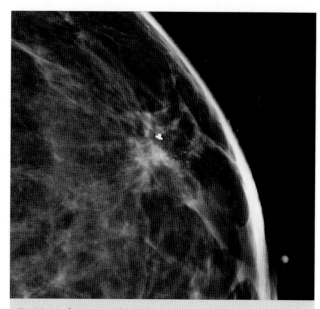

Fig. 90.4 Left craniocaudal (LCC) spot-magnification mammogram.

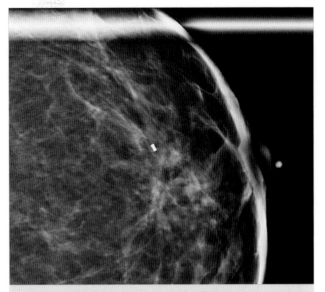

Fig. 90.5 Left lateromedial (LLM) spot-magnification mammogram.

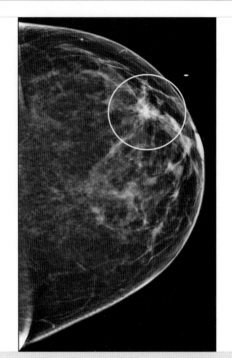

Fig. 90.6 Left craniocaudal (LCC) mammogram with label.

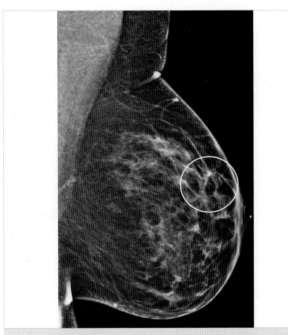

Fig. 90.7 Left mediolateral oblique (LMLO) mammogram with label.

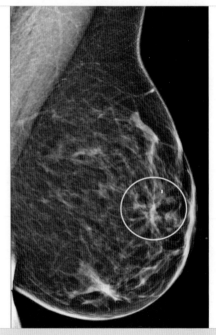

Fig. 90.8 Left lateromedial (LLM) mammogram with label.

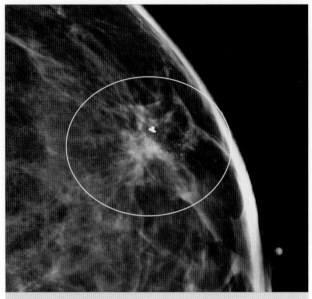

Fig. 90.9 Left craniocaudal (LCC) spot-magnification mammogram with label.

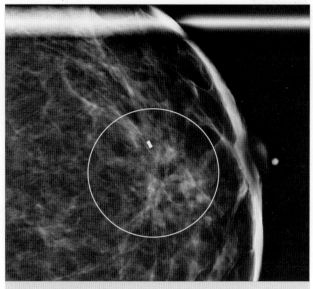

Fig. 90.10 Left lateromedial (LLM) spot-magnification mammogram with label.

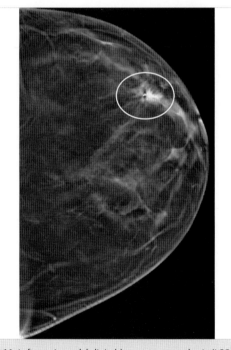

Fig. 90.11 Left craniocaudal digital breast tomosynthesis (LCC DBT), slice 46 of 67 with label.

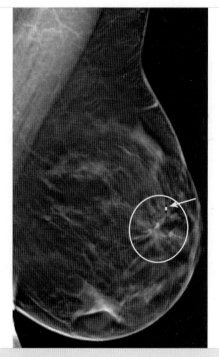

Fig. 90.12 Left lateromedial digital breast tomosynthesis (LLM DBT), slice 53 of 77 with label.

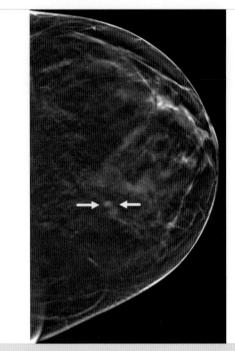

Fig. 90.13 Left craniocaudal digital breast tomosynthesis (LCC DBT), slice 28 of 67 with label.

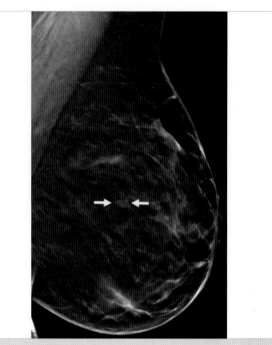

Fig. 90.14 Left lateromedial digital breast tomosynthesis (LLM DBT), slice 29 of 77 with label.

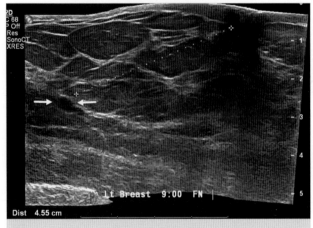

Fig. 90.15 Left breast ultrasound with label.

91 Retroareolar Extension

Tanya W. Moseley

91.1 Presentation and Presenting Images

(▶ Fig. 91.1, ▶ Fig. 91.2, ▶ Fig. 91.3, ▶ Fig. 91.4)

A 46-year-old female recently diagnosed with multifocal invasive ductal carcinoma of the right breast presents for a second opinion on treatment options.

91.2 Key Images

(▶ Fig. 91.5, ▶ Fig. 91.6, ▶ Fig. 91.7)

91.2.1 Breast Tissue Density

The breasts are heterogeneously dense, which may obscure small masses.

91.2.2 Imaging Findings

The imaging of the left breast is normal (*not shown*). The right breast demonstrates a 3-cm irregular mass at the 1 o'clock location, 7.5 cm from the nipple (*circle* in ▶ Fig. 91.5 and ▶ Fig. 91.6) with spiculated margins and an associated postbiopsy clip. In the retroareolar region there is a postbiopsy clip (*arrow*).

Tomosynthesis was only done in the craniocaudal (CC) projection and slices 1 to 38 of 82 suggest that the retroareolar findings extend to the base of the nipple; however, there is the suggestion of a fat plane behind the nipple on the mediolateral oblique (MLO) conventional mammogram (*broken arrow* in ▶ Fig. 91.6). This is difficult to assess on the digital breast tomosynthesis (DBT) imaging (▶ Fig. 91.7) because the nipple (marked with a BB) is not in profile.

91.3 Diagnostic Images

(▶ Fig. 91.8, ▶ Fig. 91.9, ▶ Fig. 91.10, ▶ Fig. 91.11)

91.3.1 Imaging Findings

Both masses seen on mammography are seen on sonography. On mammography there was the suggestion that the retroareolar mass extended to the base of the nipple. Sonography confirms that the retroareolar mass (*circle*) extends to the base of the nipple (*arrow*) (▶ Fig. 91.8 and ▶ Fig. 91.9).

Magnetic resonance imaging (MRI) demonstrates that the retroareolar mass (*circle*) extends to and involves the nipple (▶ Fig. 91.10 and ▶ Fig. 91.11).

91.4 BI-RADS Classification and Action

Category 6: Known biopsy-proven malignancy

91.5 Differential Diagnosis

1. ***Multifocal malignancy***: In this case, the diagnosis of multifocal malignancy is already known. The task for the radiologist with a known cancer diagnosis is to determine if there are additional foci of malignancy in the same or another quadrant of the breast. Determining multifocality versus multicentricity will help the patient and the surgeon decide the appropriate surgical options.
2. *Multiple radial scars*: Radial scars may present as spiculated lesions. The clinical history is not appropriate for this diagnosis.
3. *Multiple summation shadows*: The 1 o'clock mass persisted and was well seen, not compatible with a summation shadow. The retroareolar mass was better seen on the CC view suggestive of the possibility of a pseudomass; however, ultrasound and MRI confirm a true lesion.

91.6 Essential Facts

- Additional imaging is necessary when DBT findings are equivocal. Spot-compression tomosynthesis imaging was not performed but may have been helpful to evaluate the retroareolar region of the right breast.
- Multifocal or multicentric breast cancer is defined as the presence of two or more tumor foci within one quadrant of a breast or within different quadrants of a breast, respectively.
- Breast-conserving lumpectomy may be performed in patients with multifocal and multicentric breast cancer if the disease can be completely removed with good cosmesis.

91.7 Management and Digital Breast Tomosynthesis Principles

- The ability of DBT to eliminate the effects of overlapping breast tissue may result in an increase in the diagnosis of multifocal and multicentric malignancies.
- Although there is an 8-hour training program for radiologists prior to interpreting DBT images, confidence with using this new modality will be gained with continued usage.
- The suggestion of a fat plane on the MLO view in this case did not confer benignity.
- Radiologists must be cautious and not incorrectly conclude that the presence of fat within a mass is synonymous with benignity. The presence of fat suggests benignity with encapsulated or pseudoencapsulated masses. DBT is excellent in defining capsules and pseudocapsules.

91.8 Further Reading

[1] Freer PE, Wang JL, Rafferty EA. Digital breast tomosynthesis in the analysis of fat-containing lesions. Radiographics. 2014; 34(2):343–358
[2] Gentilini O, Botteri E, Rotmensz N, et al. Conservative surgery in patients with multifocal/multicentric breast cancer. Breast Cancer Res Treat. 2009; 113(3): 577–583

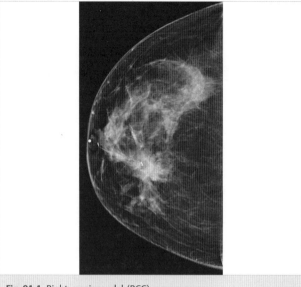

Fig. 91.1 Right craniocaudal (RCC) mammogram.

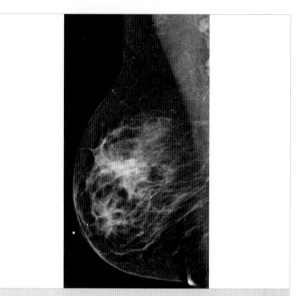

Fig. 91.2 Right mediolateral oblique (RMLO) mammogram.

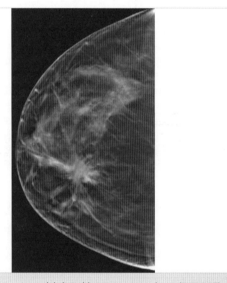

Fig. 91.3 Right craniocaudal digital breast tomosynthesis (RCC DBT), slice 44 of 82.

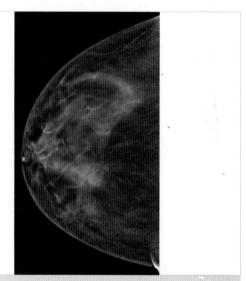

Fig. 91.4 Right craniocaudal digital breast tomosynthesis (RCC DBT), slice 4 of 82.

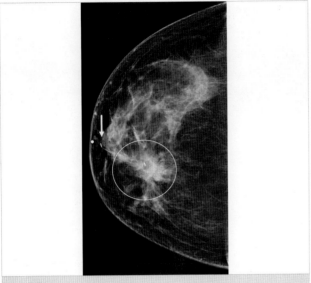

Fig. 91.5 Right craniocaudal (RCC) mammogram with label.

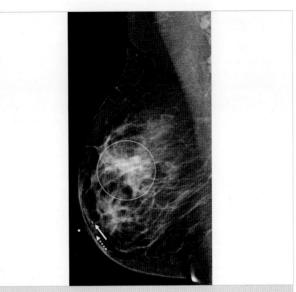

Fig. 91.6 Right mediolateral oblique (RMLO) mammogram with label.

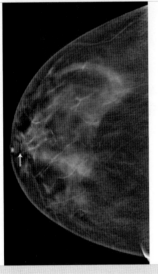

Fig. 91.7 Right craniocaudal digital breast tomosynthesis (RCC DBT), slice 4 of 82 with label.

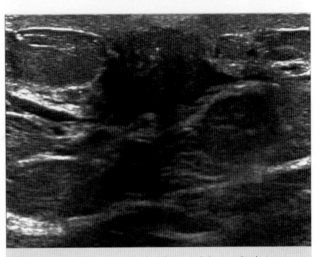

Fig. 91.8 Right breast retroareolar ultrasound, longitudinal view.

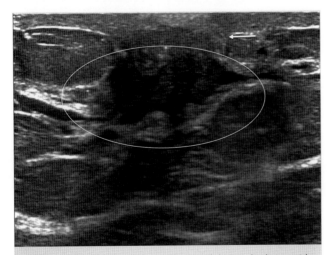

Fig. 91.9 Right breast retroareolar ultrasound, longitudinal view with label.

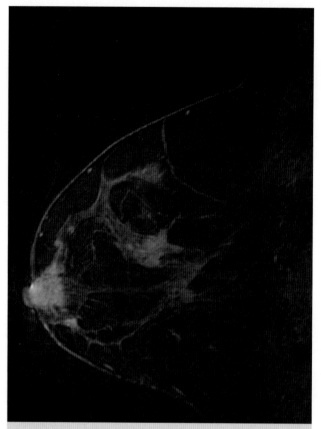

Fig. 91.10 Right breast sagittal subtraction magnetic resonance image (MRI).

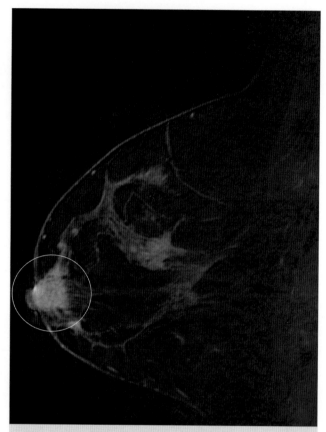

Fig. 91.11 Right breast sagittal subtraction magnetic resonance image (MRI) with label.

92 Regional Calcifications

Tanya W. Moseley

92.1 Presentation and Presenting Images

(▶ Fig. 92.1, ▶ Fig. 92.2, ▶ Fig. 92.3, ▶ Fig. 92.4, ▶ Fig. 92.5)

A 40-year-old female with a history of abnormal calcifications and a biopsy performed at an outside institution presents for diagnostic mammography and evaluation.

92.2 Key Images

(▶ Fig. 92.6, ▶ Fig. 92.7, ▶ Fig. 92.8, ▶ Fig. 92.9, ▶ Fig. 92.10)

92.2.1 Breast Tissue Density

The breasts are heterogeneously dense, which may obscure small masses.

92.2.2 Imaging Findings

The imaging of the right breast is normal (*not shown*). The left breast demonstrates heterogeneous, pleomorphic calcifications measuring 8 cm with a regional distribution (*wavy line* in ▶ Fig. 92.6, ▶ Fig. 92.7, ▶ Fig. 92.8, ▶ Fig. 92.9, and ▶ Fig. 92.10). There is an associated postbiopsy clip (*arrow*) in the upper outer region of the calcifications; however, it does not demonstrate the extent of the calcifications. The calcifications extend from the base of the nipple to the pectoralis muscle and superior to inferior across the posterior nipple line.

92.3 BI-RADS Classification and Action

Category 6: Known biopsy-proven malignancy

92.4 Differential Diagnosis

1. ***Ductal carcinoma in situ (DCIS)***: Pleomorphic calcifications in a linear or segmental distribution are a typical appearance for DCIS. Calcifications associated with benign disease are generally more rounded and uniform in density and size.
2. *Fat necrosis*: Occasionally fat necrosis may demonstrate pleomorphic calcifications with an appearance that can be difficult to differentiate from malignancy. This differential is less likely given there is no history of trauma or surgery.

3. *Pleomorphic lobular carcinoma in situ (LCIS)*: Pleomorphic LCIS may demonstrate imaging features that overlap with DCIS.

92.5 Essential Facts

- Given the regional distribution and the pleomorphic morphology of the calcifications, ultrasound is recommended to evaluate for a mass lesion. Although no mass lesions were seen with DBT, it does not detect all masses.
- When suspicious calcifications involve an area larger than 2 cm, it is helpful to biopsy near the ends of the calcifications, rather than just in a central group. This can provide the surgeon valuable information about the extent of disease and assist in making decisions about breast-conserving therapy or mastectomy options.
- Although the calcifications are seen on DBT, the morphology and distribution of the calcifications are better evaluated with magnification views performed with conventional mammography.
- DBT can perform spot-compression views, but not magnification views.

92.6 Management and Digital Breast Tomosynthesis Principles

- DBT is superior in the detection of masses and architectural distortions but is limited in the evaluation of the distribution and morphology of calcifications.
- Conventional two-dimensional (2D) mammography can more quickly detect calcifications and is better at evaluating the morphology and distribution of calcifications.
- Calcifications are less easily appreciated and evaluated with DBT because calcifications can traverse multiple tomosynthesis slices.
- One way to evaluate calcifications is to increase the width of the tomosynthesis movie slice.

92.7 Further Reading

[1] Spangler ML, Zuley ML, Sumkin JH, et al. Detection and classification of calcifications on digital breast tomosynthesis and 2D digital mammography: a comparison. AJR Am J Roentgenol. 2011; 196(2):320–324

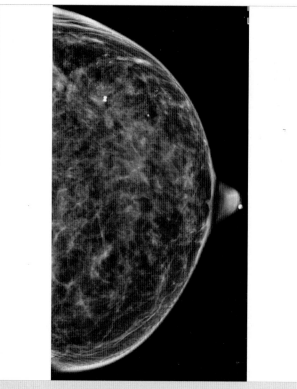

Fig. 92.1 Left craniocaudal (LCC) mammogram.

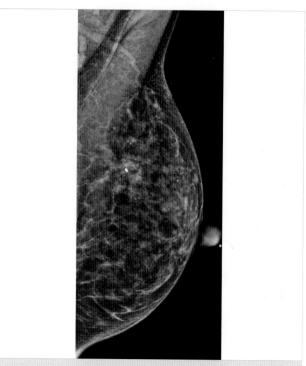

Fig. 92.2 Left mediolateral oblique (LMLO) mammogram.

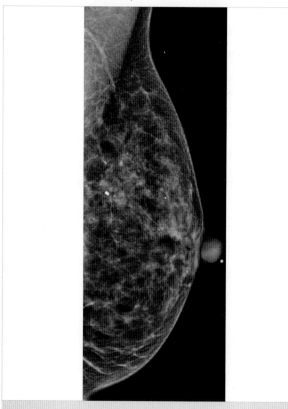

Fig. 92.3 Left lateromedial (LLM) mammogram.

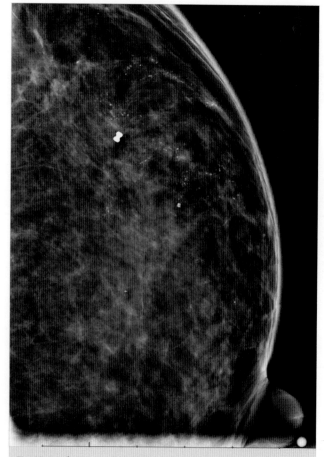

Fig. 92.4 Left craniocaudal (LCC) spot-magnification mammogram.

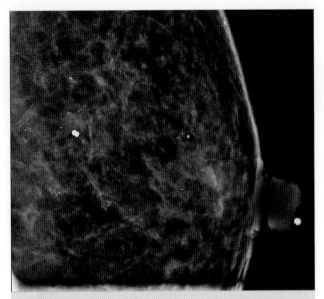

Fig. 92.5 Left lateromedial (LLM) spot-magnification mammogram.

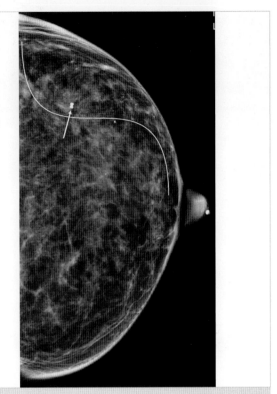

Fig. 92.6 Left craniocaudal (LCC) mammogram with label.

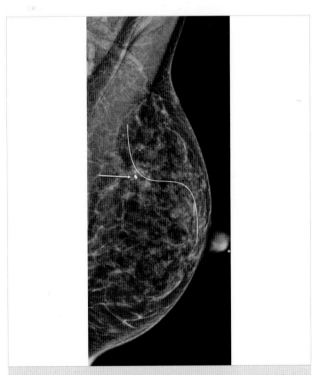

Fig. 92.7 Left mediolateral oblique (LMLO) mammogram with label.

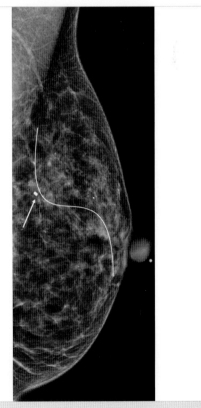

Fig. 92.8 Left lateromedial (LLM) mammogram with label.

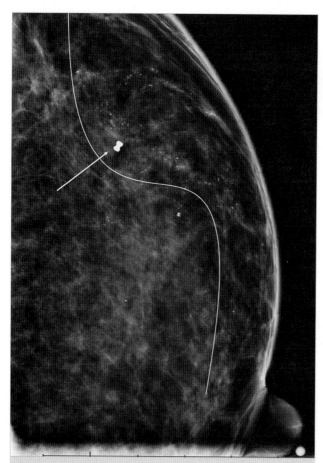

Fig. 92.9 Left craniocaudal (LCC) spot-magnification mammogram with label.

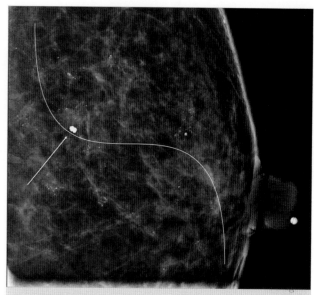

Fig. 92.10 Left lateromedial (LLM) spot-magnification mammogram with label.

93 Fine-Linear Branching Calcifications

Tanya W. Moseley

93.1 Presentation and Presenting Images

(▶ Fig. 93.1, ▶ Fig. 93.2, ▶ Fig. 93.3, ▶ Fig. 93.4, ▶ Fig. 93.5, ▶ Fig. 93.6, ▶ Fig. 93.7)

A 51 year-old-female with a recent left breast biopsy at an outside institution consistent with ductal carcinoma in situ and invasive ductal carcinoma presents for diagnostic mammography and evaluation.

93.2 Key Images

(▶ Fig. 93.8, ▶ Fig. 93.9, ▶ Fig. 93.10, ▶ Fig. 93.11, ▶ Fig. 93.12, ▶ Fig. 93.13, ▶ Fig. 93.14)

93.2.1 Breast Tissue Density

The breasts are heterogeneously dense, which may obscure small masses.

93.2.2 Imaging Findings

The imaging of the right breast is normal (*not shown*). The left breast demonstrates fine-linear branching calcifications, an associated tissue density, and a postbiopsy clip at the 3 o'clock location in the middle to posterior depth, 6 cm from the nipple. (*circle*) (▶ Fig. 93.1, ▶ Fig. 93.2, ▶ Fig. 93.3, ▶ Fig. 93.8, ▶ Fig. 93.9, ▶ Fig. 93.10). While tomosynthesis (▶ Fig. 93.4, ▶ Fig. 93.5, ▶ Fig. 93.11, ▶ Fig. 93.12) diminishes the effects of the tissue density which is consistent with a postbiopsy hematoma and allows the full extent of the calcifications to be seen, spot-magnification views (▶ Fig. 93.6, ▶ Fig. 93.7, ▶ Fig. 93.13, ▶ Fig. 93.14) are needed to evaluate the morphology of the calcifications.

93.3 BI-RADS Classification and Action

Category 5: Highly suggestive of malignancy (for new finding of fine-linear branching calcifications)
   Category 6: Known biopsy-proven malignancy

93.4 Differential Diagnosis

1. ***Ductal carcinoma in situ***: Fine-linear branching calcifications is a typical presentation of ductal carcinoma in situ. This morphology of calcifications warrants a BIRADS category 5.

2. ***Invasive ductal carcinoma***: Typically invasive carcinomas do not present as calcifications.

3. ***Ductal carcinoma in situ and invasive ductal carcinoma***: If the density was a mass lesion and not postbiopsy changes, this finding would be suspicious for ductal carcinoma in situ and invasive ductal carcinoma.

93.5 Essential Facts

- The postbiopsy changes obscure findings on the conventional two-dimensional (2D) mammography. This masking is eliminated with DBT.
- DBT allows the full extent of calcifications to be evaluated and measured, but it is unable to perform magnification views to characterize the calcifications. Characterization of the morphology of calcifications must be performed with 2D mammography.
- Having an accurate size measurement helps to adequately stage the malignancy and to develop an appropriate treatment plan.
- Although magnification views cannot be performed with DBT and calcifications may be on multiple slices, in this example, the calcifications were shown to be more extensive on tomosynthesis than seen on the conventional mammography.

93.6 Management and Digital Breast Tomosynthesis Principles

- Tomosynthesis systems must support both conventional mammography and tomosynthesis because magnification views cannot be performed with tomosynthesis.
- Spangler and colleagues (2011) found conventional mammography to be slightly more sensitive than DBT for the detection of calcifications, but, with improvements in processing algorithms and display, DBT could potentially improve.
- Kopans and colleagues (2011) found that calcifications can be demonstrated with the same or better clarity on DBT as on conventional mammography, which allows the same and perhaps improved analysis of calcifications.
- In this case DBT removed the postbiopsy changes that obscured the calcifications, allowing them to be visualized.

93.7 Further Reading

[1] Kopans D, Gavenonis S, Halpern E, Moore R. Calcifications in the breast and digital breast tomosynthesis. Breast J. 2011; 17(6):638–644

[2] Spangler ML, Zuley ML, Sumkin JH, et al. Detection and classification of calcifications on digital breast tomosynthesis and 2D digital mammography: a comparison. AJR Am J Roentgenol. 2011; 196(2):320–324

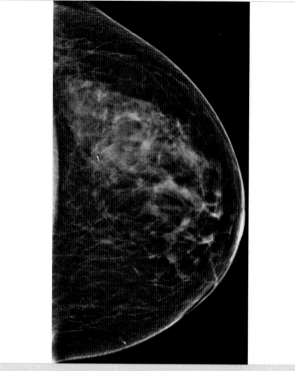

Fig. 93.1 Left cranciocaudal (LCC) mammogram.

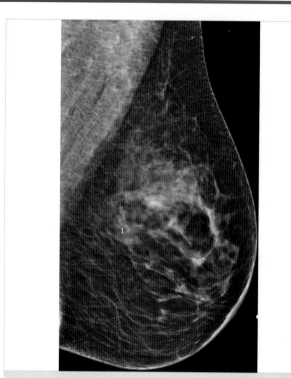

Fig. 93.2 Left mediolateral oblique (LMLO) mammogram.

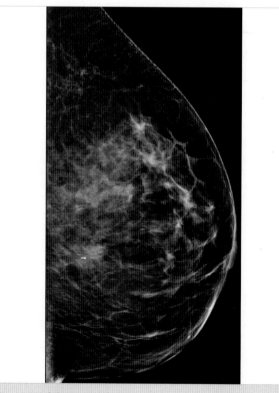

Fig. 93.3 Left lateromedial (LLM) mammogram.

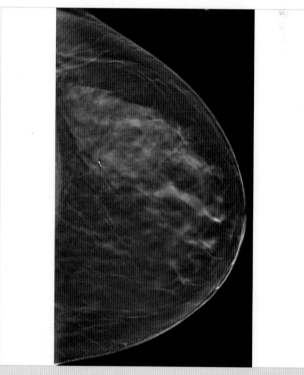

Fig. 93.4 Left digital breast tomosynthesis (LCC DBT), slice 26 of 83.

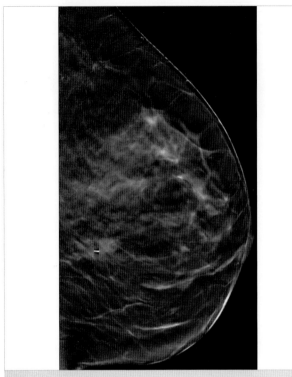

Fig. 93.5 Left digital breast tomosynthesis (LLM DBT), slice 36 of 70.

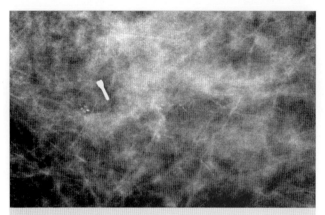

Fig. 93.6 Left cranciocaudal (LCC) spot-magnification mammogram.

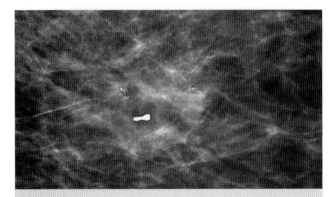

Fig. 93.7 Left lateromedial (LLM) spot-magnification mammogram.

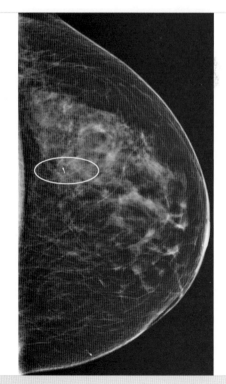

Fig. 93.8 Left cranciocaudal (LCC) mammogram with label.

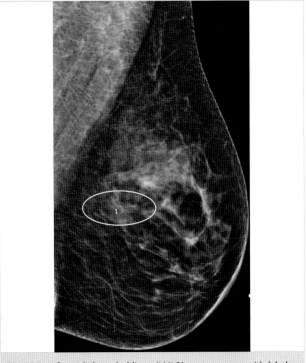

Fig. 93.9 Left mediolateral oblique (LMLO) mammogram with label.

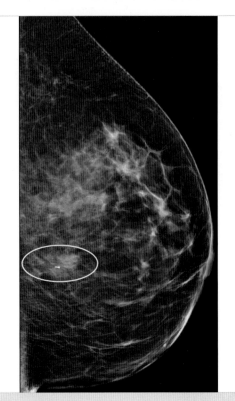

Fig. 93.10 Left lateromedial (LLM) mammogram with label.

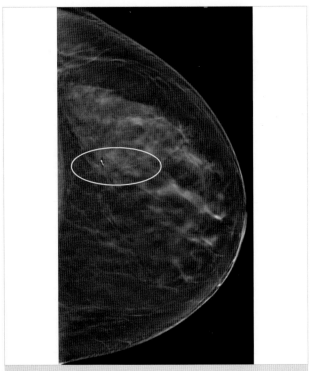

Fig. 93.11 Left cranciocaudal digital breast tomosynthesis (LCC DBT), slice 26 of 83 with label.

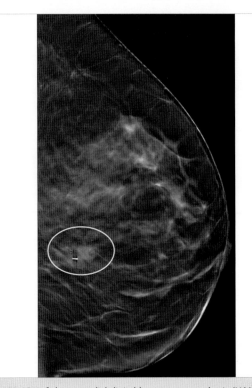

Fig. 93.12 Left lateromedial digital breast tomosynthesis (LLM DBT), slice 36 of 70 with label.

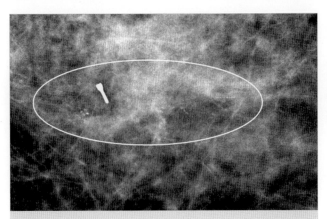

Fig. 93.13 Left cranciocaudal (LCC) mammogram, spot magnification with label.

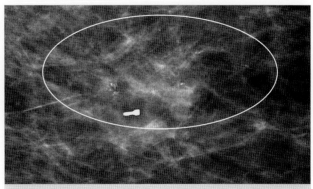

Fig. 93.14 Left lateromedial (LLM) mammogram, spot magnification with label.

94 Regional Calcifications

Tanya W. Moseley

94.1 Presentation and Presenting Images

(▶ Fig. 94.1, ▶ Fig. 94.2, ▶ Fig. 94.3, ▶ Fig. 94.4, ▶ Fig. 94.5, ▶ Fig. 94.6, ▶ Fig. 94.7, ▶ Fig. 94.8, ▶ Fig. 94.9)

A 69-year-old female recently diagnosed with high-grade ductal carcinoma in situ (DCIS) of the right breast presents for diagnostic mammography and evaluation.

94.2 Key Images

(▶ Fig. 94.10, ▶ Fig. 94.11, ▶ Fig. 94.12, ▶ Fig. 94.13, ▶ Fig. 94.14, ▶ Fig. 94.15, ▶ Fig. 94.16)

94.2.1 Breast Tissue Density

The breasts are heterogeneously dense, which may obscure small masses.

94.2.2 Imaging Findings

The imaging of the left breast is normal (*not shown*). The right breast demonstrates pleomorphic calcifications in a regional distribution with an associated postbiopsy clip and a high-density mass at the 10 to 11 o'clock location (*circle* in ▶ Fig. 94.10, ▶ Fig. 94.11, ▶ Fig. 94.12, ▶ Fig. 94.13, and ▶ Fig. 94.14). The high-density mass was not present on the prebiopsy mammogram (▶ Fig. 64.6 and ▶ Fig. 64.7) and is consistent with a postbiopsy hematoma. Digital breast tomosynthesis images clearly demonstrate the malignant calcifications, and the benign vascular calcifications are adjacent to the known malignancy (*broken arrow*; ▶ Fig. 94.15 and ▶ Fig. 94.16). The postbiopsy clip at the 8 o'clock location (*short solid arrow* in ▶ Fig. 94.10, ▶ Fig. 94.11, and ▶ Fig. 94.12) denotes the site of a prior benign biopsy. An abnormal lymph node (*long solid arrow* in ▶ Fig. 94.11) is noted in the right axilla.

94.3 BI-RADS Classification and Action

Category 6: Known biopsy-proven malignancy

94.4 Differential Diagnosis

1. *Ductal carcinoma in situ (DCIS) and postbiopsy hematoma*: DCIS may present as pleomorphic calcifications. The absence of the high-density mass on the prebiopsy mammogram makes this finding more consistent with a postbiopsy hematoma.
2. *Ductal carcinoma in situ and invasive ductal carcinoma*: Suspicious calcifications and a high-density mass are concerning for ductal carcinoma in situ and invasive ductal carcinoma.

The absence of the high-density mass on the prebiopsy mammogram makes this mass more consistent with a postbiopsy hematoma than a malignant mass. Even excluding the mass as malignant, the abnormal axillary lymph node makes this a likely possibility.

3. *Fat necrosis*: Although fat necrosis has many appearances, the presence of the abnormal lymph node makes this an unlikely possibility.

94.5 Essential Facts

- DBT is helpful in evaluating the distribution of both the suspicious calcifications and the benign vascular calcifications.
- Comparison of the two-dimensional (2D) mammography and DBT images helped resolve that the density associated with the calcifications was a postbiopsy change and not an associated mass lesion.
- Theoretically DCIS of the breast is considered a preinvasive and/or noninvasive lesion without potential for lymph node or distant metastases. Tan and colleagues (2007) found no risk factors that were predictive for sentinel lymph node biopsy; however, some authors believe that there is a subset of patients with DCIS who would benefit from sentinel lymph node biopsy.
- Axillary metastases at sentinel lymph node sampling are uncommon in patients with DCIS, but have been reported in up to 15% of patients.
- Most axillary metastases are likely due to occult invasive cancer in patients with high-grade or large volume DCIS. A small invasive cancer can go undetected at histopathologic diagnosis.

94.6 Management and Digital Breast Tomosynthesis Principles

- Axillary views may be performed with DBT; however, the likely yield using DBT to evaluate axillary lymph nodes is low.
- Although limited with respect to the inability to magnify calcifications, DBT can identify and localize calcifications.
- If this finding were visualized only on DBT and biopsy needed to be performed, you would want to target away from the vascular calcifications.

94.7 Further Reading

[1] Boler DE, Cabioglu N, Ince U, Esen G, Uras C. Sentinel lymph node biopsy in pure DCIS: is it necessary? ISRN Surg. 2012; 2012:394095

[2] Khakpour N, Zager JS, Yen T, et al. The role of ultrasound in the surgical management of patients diagnosed with ductal carcinoma in situ of the breast. Breast J. 2006; 12(3):212–215

[3] Tan JCC, McCready DR, Easson AM, Leong WL. Role of sentinel lymph node biopsy in ductal carcinoma-in-situ treated by mastectomy. Ann Surg Oncol. 2007; 14(2):638–645

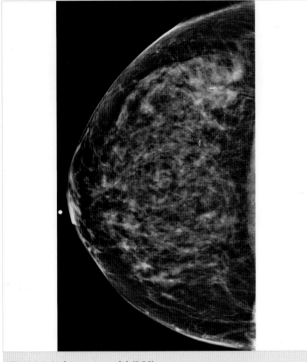

Fig. 94.1 Right craniocaudal (RCC) mammogram.

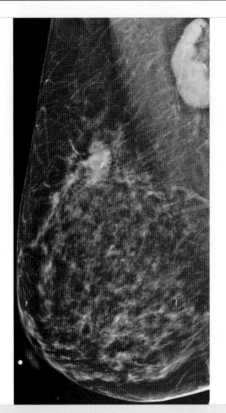

Fig. 94.2 Right mediolateral oblique (RMLO) mammogram.

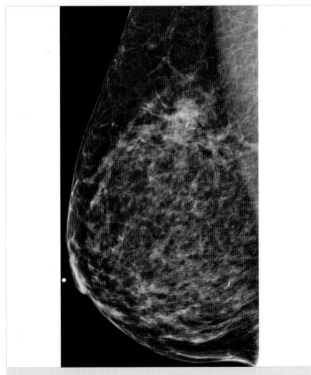

Fig. 94.3 Right lateromedial (RLM) mammogram.

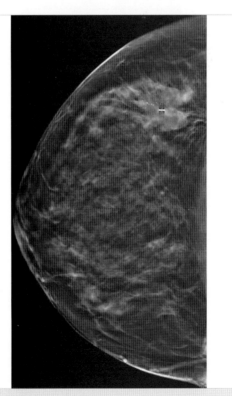

Fig. 94.4 Right craniocaudal digital breast tomosynthesis (RCC DBT), slice 36 of 73.

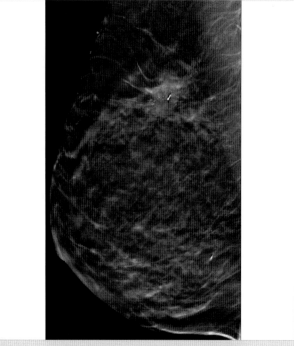

Fig. 94.5 Right digital breast tomosynthesis (RLM DBT), slice 43 of 70.

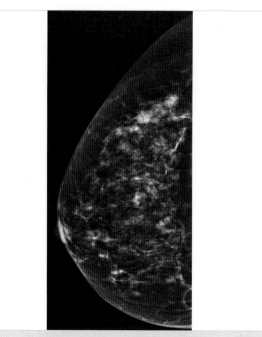

Fig. 94.6 Right craniocaudal (RCC) mammogram comparison.

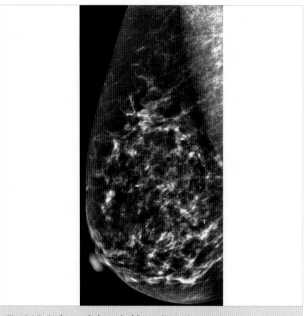

Fig. 94.7 Right mediolateral oblique (RMLO) mammogram comparison.

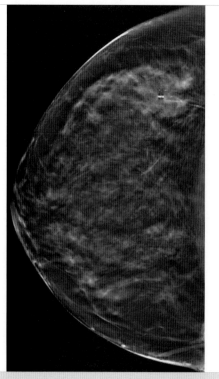

Fig. 94.8 Right craniocaudal digital breast tomosynthesis (RCC DBT), slice 32 of 73.

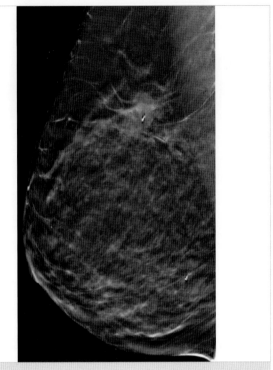

Fig. 94.9 Right lateromedial digital breast tomosynthesis (RLM DBT), slice 36 of 70.

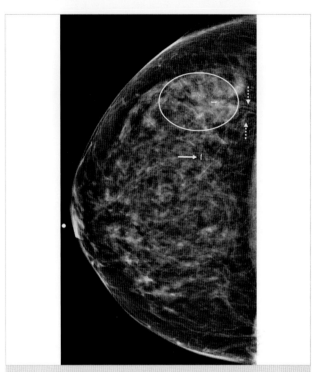

Fig. 94.10 Right craniocaudal (RCC) mammogram with label.

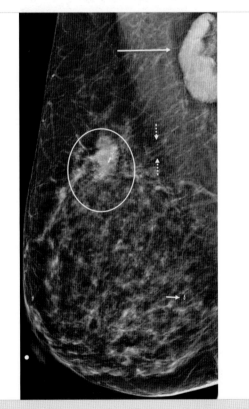

Fig. 94.11 Right mediolateral oblique (RMLO) mammogram with label.

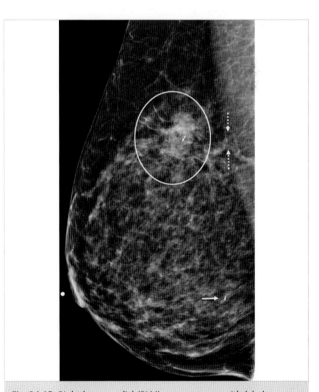

Fig. 94.12 Right lateromedial (RLM) mammogram with label.

453

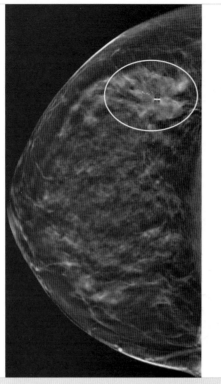

Fig. 94.13 Right craniocaudal digital breast tomosynthesis (RCC DBT), slice 36 of 73 with label.

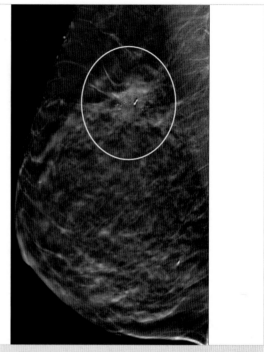

Fig. 94.14 Right lateromedial digital breast tomosynthesis (RLM DBT), slice 43 of 70 with label.

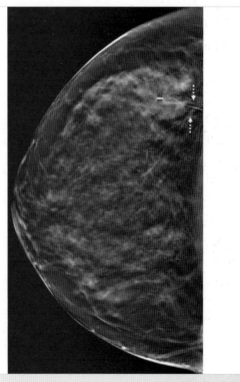

Fig. 94.15 Right craniocaudal digital breast tomosynthesis (RCC DBT), slice 32 of 73 with label.

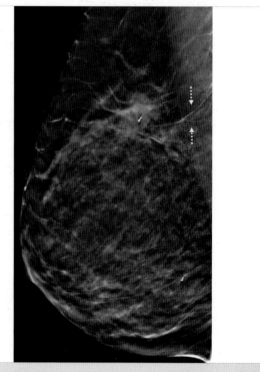

Fig. 94.16 Right lateromedial digital breast tomosynthesis (RLM DBT), slice 36 of 70 with label.

95 Cancer Occult to Imaging

Tanya W. Moseley

95.1 Presentation and Presenting Images

(▶ Fig. 95.1, ▶ Fig. 95.2, ▶ Fig. 95.3, ▶ Fig. 95.4, ▶ Fig. 95.5, ▶ Fig. 95.6, ▶ Fig. 95.7, ▶ Fig. 95.8, ▶ Fig. 95.9)

A 46-year-old female recently diagnosed with invasive ductal carcinoma (IDC) with lobular features of the right breast presents for diagnostic mammography and evaluation.

95.1.1 Breast Tissue Density

The breasts are extremely dense, which lowers the sensitivity of mammography.

95.1.2 Imaging Findings

The imaging of the left breast is normal (*not shown*). The right breast contains a ribbon clip (*broken arrow*) in the retroareolar location and a coil clip (*solid arrow*) at the 10 to 11 o'clock position (▶ Fig. 95.1, ▶ Fig. 95.2, ▶ Fig. 95.5, ▶ Fig. 95.6, ▶ Fig. 95.7, ▶ Fig. 95.8, and ▶ Fig. 95.9). The clips denote the sites of biopsy-proven malignancy; however, no discreet masses are seen on conventional mammography or on digital breast tomosynthesis (DBT) Additionally, there is no appreciable change since the comparison mammogram (▶ Fig. 95.3 and ▶ Fig. 95.4).

95.2 BI-RADS Classification and Action

Category 6: Known biopsy-proven malignancy

95.3 Differential Diagnosis

1. **Breast cancer (invasive ductal carcinoma with lobular features):** The lesions in this case were biopsied and clips placed at the site of each biopsy. Even with knowledge of the lesion location, the lesions remain occult mammographically and on DBT.
2. *Normal study*: Although the findings are not detected by mammography, this is not a normal study. This case represents cancers that remain undetected by conventional mammography or DBT.
3. *Summation artifacts*: Summation artifacts create mass lesions. DBT demonstrates that summation artifacts are the result of parenchymal overlap. This is not the case here.

95.4 Essential Facts

- The pathology for this patient's malignancy is invasive ductal carcinoma with lobular features. This likely accounts for its occult nature.
- Invasive lobular carcinoma has a single file tumor growth pattern that is often very difficult to detect on breast imaging.
- The ease of detection of cancers on mammography varies by tumor type. Invasive ductal carcinoma is easier to identify mammographically than invasive lobular carcinoma.
- Invasive lobular carcinomas which often present as subtle asymmetries and architectural distortions are better seen with DBT than with conventional mammography.

95.5 Management and Digital Breast Tomosynthesis Principles

- DBT detects and characterizes the majority of masses in women regardless of breast density.
- DBT reduces breast tissue overlap effectively revealing breast lesions that may have gone undetected.
- Not all masses are detected by DBT, as seen in this case.
- Most breast cancers are identified on both views; however, even with DBT imaging, some cancers are well seen on only one view. Therefore, in order to identify the majority of breast malignancies, the use of two views is recommended for diagnostic imaging with DBT.
- In a letter to the *Radiology* editor (2013), Dr. Daniel Kopans describes masses that will be undetected on both conventional and DBT imaging as masses that don't have edges outlined by fat, that don't distort the architecture of the breast, and that don't make calcifications.

95.6 Further Reading

[1] Baker JA, Lo JY. Breast tomosynthesis: state-of-the-art and review of the literature. Acad Radiol. 2011;18(10):1298–1310
[2] Kopans DB. Digital breast tomosynthesis: a better mammogram. Radiology. 2013;267(3):968–969

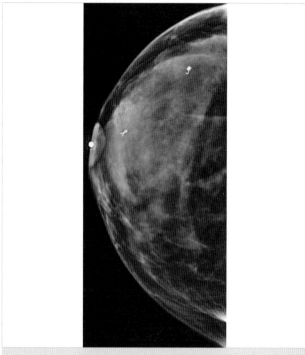

Fig. 95.1 Right craniocaudal (RCC) mammogram.

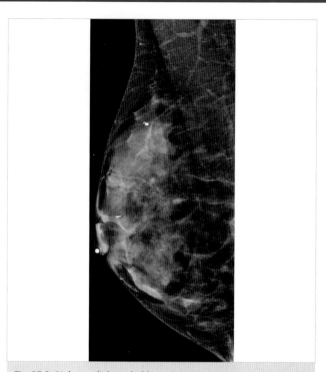

Fig. 95.2 Right mediolateral oblique (RMLO) mammogram.

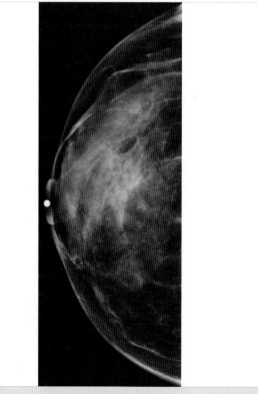

Fig. 95.3 Right craniocaudal (RCC) mammogram comparison.

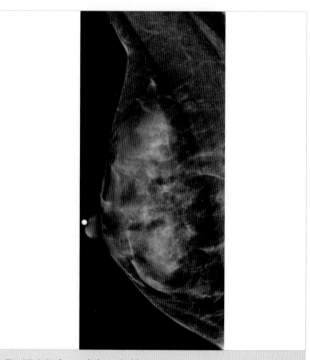

Fig. 95.4 Right mediolateral oblique RMLO mammogram comparison.

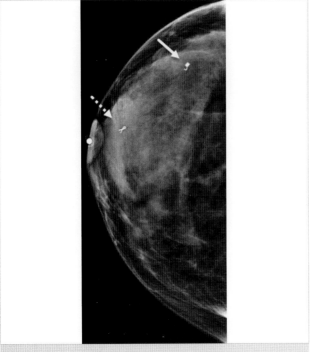

Fig. 95.5 Right craniocaudal (RCC) mammogram with label.

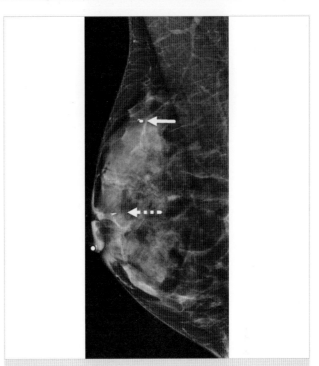

Fig. 95.6 Right mediolateral oblique (RMLO) mammogram with label.

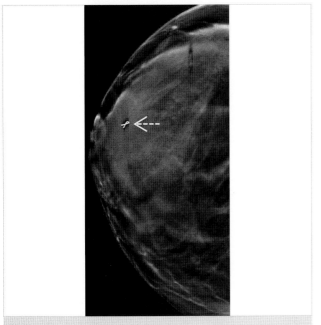

Fig. 95.7 Right craniocaudal digital breast tomosynthesis (RCC DBT), slice 17 of 47 with label.

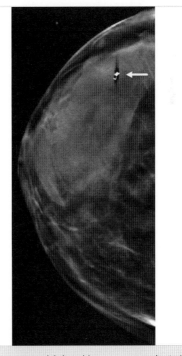

Fig. 95.8 Right craniocaudal digital breast tomosynthesis (RCC DBT), slice 37 of 47 with label.

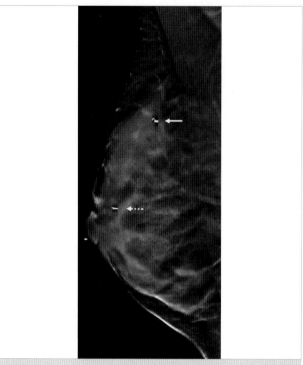

Fig. 95.9 Right lateromedial digital breast tomosynthesis (RLM DBT), slice 26 of 42 with label.

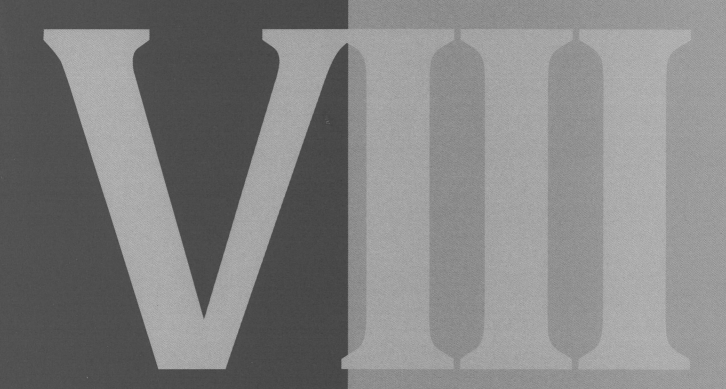

Part VIII

Intervention: Biopsy Using Tomosynthesis or Stereotactic Guidance

96 Introduction to Localization and Biopsy Using Tomosynthesis

Tanya W. Moseley

Digital breast tomosynthesis acquires several images of the breast at multiple angles. The individual images are reconstructed into a series of thin, high-resolution slices typically 1-mm thick, which can be viewed like computed tomography (CT) or magnetic resonance (MR) images as a single slice or stacked in dynamic cine mode. The ability to view images as a single slice or in dynamic mode eliminates the effects of overlapping breast tissue, which allows for better visualization and characterization of masses.

Conventional two-dimensional (2D) mammography plus digital breast tomosynthesis increases reader performance for identifying masses and architectural distortions over conventional mammography alone. DBT can find lesions not seen on conventional 2D mammography. The addition of DBT reduces callbacks for false-positive lesions and has a higher breast cancer detection rate than conventional mammography alone, specifically in the detection of small invasive, node-negative cancers. Although DBT is excellent at characterization of benign and malignant features, definitive diagnosis is proven by histopathologic analysis.

Many small architectural distortions detected by tomosynthesis may not be seen with sonography, thereby negating sonographic biopsy. Prone stereotactic vacuum-assisted biopsy of an architectural distortion is susceptible to targeting error because the imager may not be able to identify the architectural distortion on both stereo pair images. Also, the biopsy window for prone stereotactic biopsies is small, requiring a skilled technologist to properly position the finding within the biopsy window. Tomosynthesis-directed stereotactic biopsy uses the full detector for imaging and biopsy. Additionally, calcifications are often better biopsied with stereotactic biopsy than with ultrasound.

The three-dimensional (3D) capability of tomosynthesis allows lesions to be detected at the correct depth. Tomosynthesis-directed stereotactic biopsy has the advantage over prone stereotactic biopsy of calculating the distance from skin to lesion on the orthogonal images and thus facilitating the most efficacious approach for biopsy. Tomosynthesis-directed stereotactic seems better for low-contrast lesions such as uncalcified masses and architectural distortions. Tomosynthesis-directed biopsy can be performed quickly and safely without major complications. One limitation is that needle averse patients may have difficulty seeing the biopsy needle. One solution is an eye mask or using a prone stereotactic table.

The cases in this section can be found online at mediacenter.thieme.com.

96.1 Further Reading

[1] Alleva DQ, Smetherman DH, Farr GH, Jr, Cederbom GJ. Radial scar of the breast: radiologic-pathologic correlation in 22 cases. Radiographics. 1999; 19 (Spec No):S27–S35, discussion S36–S37

[2] Bernardi D, Caumo F, Macaskill P, et al. Effect of integrating 3D-mammography (digital breast tomosynthesis) with 2D-mammography on radiologists' true-positive and false-positive detection in a population breast screening trial. Eur J Cancer. 2014; 50(7):1232–1238

[3] Caumo F, Bernardi D, Ciatto S, et al. Incremental effect from integrating 3D-mammography (tomosynthesis) with 2D-mammography: Increased breast cancer detection evident for screening centres in a population-based trial. Breast. 2014; 23(1):76–80

[4] Ciatto S, Houssami N, Bernardi D, et al. Integration of 3D digital mammography with tomosynthesis for population breast-cancer screening (STORM): a prospective comparison study. Lancet Oncol. 2013; 14(7):583–589

[5] Freer PE, Niell B, Rafferty EA. Preoperative tomosynthesis-guided needle localization of mammographically and sonographically occult breast lesions. Radiology. 2015; 275(2):377–383

[6] Frouge C, Tristant H, Guinebretière JM, et al. Mammographic lesions suggestive of radial scars: microscopic findings in 40 cases. Radiology. 1995; 195(3):623–625

[7] Haas BM, Kalra V, Geisel J, Raghu M, Durand M, Philpotts LE. Comparison of tomosynthesis plus digital mammography and digital mammography alone for breast cancer screening. Radiology. 2013; 269(3):694–700

[8] Houssami N, Skaane P. Overview of the evidence on digital breast tomosynthesis in breast cancer detection. Breast. 2013; 22(2):101–108

[9] Lee E, Wylie E, Metcalf C. Ultrasound imaging features of radial scars of the breast. Australas Radiol. 2007; 51(3):240–245

[10] Schrading S, Distelmaier M, Dirrichs T, et al. Digital breast tomosynthesis-guided vacuum-assisted breast biopsy: initial experiences and comparison with prone stereotactic vacuum-assisted biopsy. Radiology. 2015; 274(3):654–662

[11] Shetty MK. Radial scars of the breast: sonographic findings. Ultrasound Q. 2002; 18(3):203–207

[12] Skaane P, Bandos AI, Gullien R, et al. Comparison of digital mammography alone and digital mammography plus tomosynthesis in a population-based screening program. Radiology. 2013; 267(1):47–56

[13] Skaane P, Bandos AI, Gullien R, et al. Prospective trial comparing full-field digital mammography (FFDM) versus combined FFDM and tomosynthesis in a population-based screening programme using independent double reading with arbitration. Eur Radiol. 2013; 23(8):2061–2071

[14] Spangler ML, Zuley ML, Sumkin JH, et al. Detection and classification of calcifications on digital breast tomosynthesis and 2D digital mammography: a comparison. AJR Am J Roentgenol. 2011; 196(2):320–324

[15] Svahn TM, Chakraborty DP, Ikeda D, et al. Breast tomosynthesis and digital mammography: a comparison of diagnostic accuracy. Br J Radiol. 2012; 85 (1019):e1074–e1082

[16] Waldherr C, Cerny P, Altermatt HJ, et al. Value of one-view breast tomosynthesis versus two-view mammography in diagnostic workup of women with clinical signs and symptoms and in women recalled from screening. AJR Am J Roentgenol. 2013; 200(1):226–231

Index

Note: Page numbers set **bold** or *italic* indicate headings or figures, respectively.